MEDICINE
IN
GREAT BRITAIN
FROM THE RESTORATION
TO THE
NINETEENTH CENTURY,
1660–1800

Recent Titles in
Bibliographies and Indexes in Medical Studies

Federal Information Sources in Health and Medicine: A Selected Annotated Bibliography
Mary Glen Chitty, compiler, with the assistance of Natalie Schatz

Viruses and Reproduction: A Bibliography
Ernest L. Abel, compiler

The History of Cancer: An Annotated Bibliography
James S. Olson, compiler

New Literature on Fetal Alcohol Exposure and Effects: A Bibliography, 1983-1988
Ernest L. Abel, compiler

Sociodemographic Factors in the Epidemiology of Multiple Sclerosis: An Annotated Bibliography
George W. Lowis, compiler

Prostitutes in Medical Literature: An Annotated Bibliography
Sachi Sri Kantha, compiler

Vital and Health Statistics Series: An Annotated Checklist and Index to the Publications of the "Rainbow Series"
Jim Walsh and A. James Bothmer, compilers

MEDICINE IN GREAT BRITAIN FROM THE RESTORATION TO THE NINETEENTH CENTURY, 1660–1800

An Annotated Bibliography

Compiled by
SAMUEL J. ROGAL

Bibliographies and Indexes in Medical Studies, Number 8

GREENWOOD PRESS
New York • Westport, Connecticut • London

Library of Congress Cataloging-in-Publication Data

Rogal, Samuel J.
    Medicine in Great Britain from the Restoration to the nineteenth century, 1660-1800 : an annotated bibliography / compiled by Samuel J. Rogal.
    p. cm.—(Bibliographies and indexes in medical studies, ISSN 0896-6591 ; no. 8)
    Includes indexes.
    ISBN 0-313-28115-7 (alk. paper)
    1. Medicine—Great Britain—History—Bibliography. I. Title. II. Series.
Z6661.G7R63 1992
[R486]
016.61'0941'09033—dc20   91-39004

British Library Cataloguing in Publication Data is available.

Copyright © 1992 by Samuel J. Rogal

All rights reserved. No portion of this book may be reproduced, by any process or technique, without the express written consent of the publisher.

Library of Congress Catalog Card Number: 91-39004
ISBN: 0-313-28115-7
ISSN: 0896-6591

First published in 1992

Greenwood Press, 88 Post Road West, Westport, CT 06881
An imprint of Greenwood Publishing Group, Inc.

Printed in the United States of America

The paper used in this book complies with the Permanent Paper Standard issued by the National Information Standards Organization (Z39.48-1984).

10 9 8 7 6 5 4 3 2 1

DEDICATION

As always, to Susan, Geoffrey, and James

"The Combatants to the Enterprize consent,
And the next day smil'd on the great Event."

Sir Samuel Garth, *The Dispensary*, 1699 (4:240-241)

Contents

	Preface	ix
I.	General Practice and Commentary upon Medicine	1
II.	Anatomy and Physiology	29
III.	Medicines, Cures, and Healing Agents	37
IV.	Waters	57
V.	General Surgery, Wounds, Dissection, Embalming, Rupture, Testicles	77
VI.	Plague/Epidemic, Fever, Scarlet Fever, Yellow Fever, Small Pox, Cow Pox, Inoculation, Venereal Diseases	91
VII.	Cold, Sore Throat, Croup, Catarrh, Whooping Cough, Asthma, Consumption, Respiration, Lungs, Scrofula, Dropsy, Influenza	123
VIII.	Gout, Rheumatism, Arthritis, Goiter, Back, Bones, Palsy	135
IX.	Distemper, Epilepsy, Apoplexy, Lock Jaw, Rabies, Swelling, Suppuration, Poison, Infection	145
X.	Stone, Urinary Diseases and Disorders, Liver, Jaundice	153
XI.	Stomach, Dysentery, Colic, Bowels	161
XII.	Cancer, Ulcers, Tumors	165
XIII.	Nutrition and Exercise, Scurvy, Indigestion, Spirits, Diabetes, Worms	169

XIV.	Heart, Spleen, Pulse, Blood, Bleeding, Sweating, Weakness	175
XV.	Muscles, Nerves	181
XVI.	Head, Hair, Skin	185
XVII.	Eyes, Ears	187
XVIII.	Teeth, Gums, Salivating	193
XIX.	Pregnancy, Birth, Midwifery, Infants and Children, Women	195
XX.	Seamen, Soldiers and Sailors, Farmers	209
XXI.	History, Biography, Hospitals, Institutions and Organizations, Dictionaries, Glossaries, General References	215
XXII.	Medical Conditions outside Britain	227
XXIII.	Professional Concerns	231
XXIV.	Some Contemporary Medical Periodicals	235
	Index of Subjects	237
	Index of Names	243

Preface

The sheer quantity of volumes relating to medicine and the state of general health published in England, Scotland, Ireland, and Wales between the Restoration and the end of the eighteenth century stands, perhaps, as the strongest evidence to support George Macaulay Trevelyan's observation that during the period from 1660 to 1800, "the medical profession was moving out of the dark ages of sciolism and traditional superstition into the light of science" (Illustrated English Social History [Harmondsworth: Penguin Books, Ltd., 1964], 3:91). Certainly, from the brightest side of the scientific light, that movement produced its share of prominent contributors: Sir Hans Sloane, John Hunter, Edward Jenner, Alexander Monro (both elder and younger), William Smellie, and William Hunter. They and other physicians, scientists, and humanitarians contributed significantly toward the improvement of medical knowledge; if not altogether perfect or accurate, they at least helped to persuade enlightened Britons of the late seventeenth century and the century following that life might become somewhat more comfortable for them than it had been during the generations of their ancestors. However, the disciplines of medicine, physic, and surgery did not belong entirely to a legion of significant and conscientious discoverers. Hundreds (thousands?) of lesser known and obscure practitioners of physic and medicine, a substantial number of theoretical non-practitioners, and an uncontrollable representation of unadulterated quacks seemed deeply intent upon promoting the general health and condition of humankind. Those individuals tested their ideas not only in homes and hospitals, but they set forth their theories and observations upon the pages of treatises, practical handbooks, and dictionaries; they focused upon problems ranging from midwifery to inoculation, from sea bathing to bleeding, from crude mercury to Peruvian bark; they generated attention and, most often, sparked heated and public controversy.

Therefore, as the title of this project indicates, the following list of over two thousand books and bound volumes has been compiled and annotated for the purpose of surveying the production and publication of medical tracts, treatises, narratives, guides, and references published in England, Ireland, Scotland, and Wales during one of the most significant periods in the overall history of science in the Western world. Although the list of entries that follows should be embraced as thorough and representative rather than be considered as complete, it does present legitimate variety and depth; thus, it will prove useful to historians of medicine and to scholars whose work transports them into the social and scientific niches of life on the British Isles during the Restoration and the eighteenth century. Further, the compiler has exercised care to insure that the checklist does include references to the principal practitioners and theorists of the period, as well as to identify the specific areas of their studies. To achieve those purposes described, no less than one hundred and ten distinct problems of prime concern to physicians and surgeons of the times have been categorized into twenty-four chapters; each entry within the main list includes the writer (when known), descriptive title, place and date of initial publication, and dates of the principal editions issued on or before 1800. The years of the writer's birth and death--as well as pertinent biographical, bibliographical, and historical information--have been included whenever such details have been proven accurate or made available through standard sources.

The principal sources consulted during the preparation for this checklist include the Dictionary of National Biography (Oxford: Oxford University Press, 1882-1900); The Biographia Britannica (London, 1734-1792); Robert Watt's Bibliotheca Britannica (London, 1824); Alexander Chalmers' Biographical Dictionary (1812-1817); Eminent Literary and Scientific Men of Great Britain (London, 1836); Samuel Austin Allibone's Critical Dictionary of English Literature and British and American Authors, 3 vols. (Philadelphia: J.B. Lippincott and Company, 1872-1877); Dr. Edward John Waring's Bibliotheca Therapeutica, 2 vols. (London: The New Sydenham Society, 1879); Medicine. Rare Books in the History of Medicine from the Collection of Warren Gerald Atwood, M.D., 2 parts (San Francisco: John Howell, Books, 1976); H.G. Bohn's A Catalogue of Books [The "Guinea Catalogue"] (London: Henry G. Bohn, 1841; rpt. 2 vols. New York: AMS Press, 1974); John Blake's A Short Title Catalogue of Eighteenth-Century Printed Books in the National Library of Medicine (Bethesda, Maryland: National Library of Medicine, 1979); Bernice Hamilton's "The Medical Professions in the Eighteenth Century," Economic History Review (4:1951).

Finally, additional biographical, bibliographical, and historical sources will be found within the specific entries to which they apply.

MEDICINE
IN
GREAT BRITAIN
FROM THE RESTORATION
TO THE
NINETEENTH CENTURY,
1660–1800

I

General Practice and Commentary upon Medicine

1. Adair, James Makittrick (1728-1802). <u>Commentaries on the Principles and Practices of Physick</u>. London, 1772. 605pp. A native of Inverness, Adair earned the M.D. from Edinburgh (1766); practiced at Antigua, Andover, Guildford, and Bath; wrote a volume of medical cautions for invalids residing at Bath (see #3 directly below).
2. _____. <u>Essays on Fashionable Diseases. . .by Benjamin Goosequill and Peter Paragraph</u>. London, 1790 (?). 260pp.
3. _____. <u>Medical Cautions</u>. Bath, 1786. 215pp.; 2nd ed., Bath, 1787. 543pp.
4. _____. <u>A Philosophical and Medical Sketch of the Natural History of the Human Body and Mind</u>. Bath, 1787. 318pp.
5. Aiken, John (1747-1822). <u>A Manual of Materia Medica</u>. Yarmouth, 1785. 194pp. Born at Kibworth, Harcourt, the brother of Anna Letitia Aiken Barbauld; studied with John Hunter prior to earning the M.D. at Leyden; his literary fame, however, rests with critical and biographical works co-authored with his sister.
6. Allen, John (1660?-1741). <u>Synopsis Medicinae: or, a Summary View of the Whole Practice of Physick</u>. 2 vols. London, 1719; four eds. through 1761. A practical treatise abstracted from the "best" physicians and practices of the past and the present.
7. Alston, Charles (1683-1760). <u>Lectures on the Materia Medica</u>. 2 vols. London, 1770. Educated at Glasgow, Alston studied medicine under Boerhaave at Leyden; later lectured in botany and materia medica at Edinburgh, as well as superintended the botanical gardens in the Scottish capital.
8. <u>Animadversions on the Constitution of Physick in this Kingdom. . .Interspersed with Reflections on. . .the College of Physicians</u>. London, 1768. 76pp.
9. Apperley, Thomas (1673?-1735). <u>Observations in Physick, Both Rational and Practical</u>. London, 1731. 300pp.
10. Arbuthnot, John (1667-1735). <u>An Essay concerning the Nature of Ailments</u>. London, 1731. 232pp.; Dublin, 1731. 108pp.; four London eds. through 1756. A native of Arbuthnot, near Montrose, the writer

studied at Aberdeen and earned the M.D. there; he went to London and became involved with the philosophers and the <u>literati</u> of that city, particularly Swift and Pope.

11. Archer, John (fl.1660-1684). <u>Every Man His Own Doctor</u>. London, 1671. The writer attempts to publicize his own remedies and nostrums; a second ed. in 1673.

12. Armstrong, John (1709-1779). <u>The Art of Preserving Health: A Poem</u>. London, 1744. 134pp.; eds. through 1795. Armstrong, who earned the M.D. from Edinburgh in 1732, maintained a fair reputation as a writer, of verse and travel literature; thus, this work exists as a didactic poem in four books and in blank verse.

13. _____. <u>An Essay for Abridging the Study of Physick</u>. London, 1735. 52pp.

14. _____. <u>Medical Essays</u>. London, 1773. 41pp.

15. Arnaud, Jasper. <u>An Alarm to All Persons Touching Their Health and Lives</u>. London, 1740. 24pp.

16. Aymes, John. <u>A Rich Storehouse for the Diseased</u>. London, 1760.

17. Baker, Sir George (1722-1809). <u>Opuscula Medica. Iterum Edita</u>. London, 1771. The writer served as physician in ordinary to Queen Charlotte and then to George III; he also held a term as president of the College of Physicians.

18. Balgrave, John. <u>Supplement to the English Physician, by Nicolas Culpeper</u>. London, 1666. Culpeper (1616-1664), described as a "student in physick and astrology" and as a "violent opponent" of the Royal College of Physicians, published his <u>English Physician</u> in 1652.

19. Ball, John (1704?-1779). <u>The Modern Practice of Physick</u>. 2 vols. London, 1760; three eds, through 1768.

20. Barker, John (1708-1749). <u>An Essay on the Agreement between Ancient and Modern Physicians</u>. London, 1747; 2nd ed., London, 1748; French eds. in 1749, 1767. The work draws comparisons among the practices of Hippocrates, Galen, Sydenham, and Boerhaave.

21. Barrow, John. <u>A New Essay on the Practice of Physick</u>. London, 1767.

22. Barwick, Peter (1619-1705). <u>Medicorum Animos Exagitant</u>. London, 1671. The writer a physician-in-ordinary to Charles II and a defender of William Harvey's theories upon the circulation of the blood.

23. Basse, John H. <u>Catechism of Health</u>. London, 1794.

24. Baynard, Edward (1641?--). <u>Health; a Poem. Shewing How To Keep and Preserve It. By Dabry Dawne</u>. London, 1719. 48pp.; nine (9) eds. through 1764. Born at Preston, Lancashire, the writer studied medicine (1671) at Leyden; became a fellow of the College of Physicians of London (1687); practiced medicine at Preston, Bath, and London.

25. Beale, Bartholomew (fl.1680-1706). <u>An Essay Attempting a More Certain and Satisfactory Discovery of the True Causes of All Diseases</u>. London, 1706. 240pp.

General Practice and Commentary upon Medicine

26. Beddoes, Thomas (1760-1808), ed. <u>Contributions to Physical and Medical Knowledge.</u> Bristol, 1799. 539 pp. Born at Shiffnall, Shropshire, Beddoes studied at Oxford; he eventually shifted the focus of his interests from chemistry, physiology, mineralogy, botany, and medicine to politics, education, and political economy.
27. _____. <u>A Lecture Introductory on the Constitution of the Human Body.</u> Bristol, 1797. 72pp.
28. Bellers, John (1654-1725). <u>An Essay toward the Improvement of Physick. In Twelve Proposals.</u> London, 1714. 58pp. The writer, a Quaker, not trained nor did he practice as a physician; a philanthropist and a close friend of Sir Hans Sloane.
29. Betts, John (d.1695). <u>Medicinae cum Philosophia Naturali Consensus.</u> London, 1692. The writer a Roman Catholic and a a physician in ordinary to Charles II.
30. Bickerton, George. <u>Accurate Disquisitions in Physick.</u> London, 1719. 223pp.
31. Bisset, Charles (1717-1791). <u>The Medical Constitution of Great Britain, to which is added Observations on the Weather and the Diseases which appeared during the period from 1st January 1758 to the Summer Solstice of 1760. Together with an Account of the Throat Distemper and Military Fever which were Epidemic in 1760.</u> London, 1760. Various translations into the German by J.G. Moeller, at Breslau, between 1779 and 1781. Although an M.D., Bisset served in the Royal Army and published widely on various subjects related to military fortifications.
32. Blackburne, Thomas (1749-1782). <u>De Medici Institutis.</u> Edinburgh, 1775. The writer educated at Cambridge and Edinburgh (M.D.).
33. Blagrave, Joseph (1610-1682). <u>Astrological Practice of Physick, Discovering the True Method of Curing All Kinds of Diseases by Such Herbs and Plants as Grow in Our Nation.</u> London, 1671. The writer maintains that astrology exists as a prerequisite for the practice of medicine.
34. Blair, Patrick (d.1728). <u>Miscellaneous Observations on the Practice of Physick, Anatomy, and Surgery, with Remarks on Botany.</u> Boston [Lincolnshire], 1718. A Scottish botanist, physician, and surgeon, Blair attracted attention by dissecting an elephant that had died at Dundee in 1706.
35. Blizard, Sir William (1743-1835). <u>Of the Expediency and Utility of Teaching the Several Branches of Physick and Surgery by Lectures at the London Hospital.</u> London, 1783. In conjunction with Dr. Robert Maclurin, Sir William established (1785) the first regular school of medical science in connection with the English Hospital; the institution became known as the London Medical School. Blizard, knighted in 1810 by George III, twice served as president of the Royal College of

Surgeons.
36. Bodley, James. _A Critical Essay upon the Works of Physicians_. London, 1741. A London physician, the writer held the M.D. degree.
37. Bradley, Richard (1688?-1732). _A Course of Lectures upon the Materia Medica_. London, 1730. 170pp. Bradley gained election as a felllow of the Royal Society (1720) and an appointment as professor of botany at Cambridge; a prolific writer, he concentrated his efforts upon botany and materia medica.
38. Brisbane, John (d.1776?). _Select Cases in the Practices of Medicine_. London, 1762-1772. 62pp. A Scottish physician, the writer served the Middlesex Hospital between 1758 and 1773.
39. Brocklesby, Richard (1722-1797). _Oeconomical and Medical Observations_. London, 1764. 320 pp. The writer studied at Edinburgh and Leyden (M.D. 1745); settled in London and became (1751) a licentiate of the College of Physicians; M.D. Cambridge in 1754, after which he gained election as a fellow to the College of Physicians; served in Germany with the army, then returned to London to practice medicine; associated with Edmund Burke and Samuel Johnson.
40. Brookes, Richard (fl.1721-1763). _The General Practice of Physick_. 2 vols. London, 1751; 6 eds. through 1771. A London M.D., Brookes wrote also on the distempers and sea fishing and published a geographical dictionary (1762; 18 eds, through 1827).
41. _____. _An Introduction to Physick and Surgery_. London, 1754. 556 pp.; 2nd ed., London, 1763. 390pp.
42. Brown, John (1735-1789). _Elements of Medicine; or, a Translation of the Elementa Medicinae Bruonis_. 2 vols. London, 1780; 2nd ed., London, 1795; Fairhaven, New Hampshire, 1797; Edinburgh, 1780; further eds. at Milan (1792), Hildburgshausen (1794), Philadelphia (ed. Dr. Benjamin Rush, 1790), Frankfurt-am-Main (1795, 1798), Copenhagen (3 eds.), and Paris. A native of Berwickshire, Brown lectured at Edinburgh. The Bruonian theory regarded living tissues as excitable and life itself as nonexistent, except as a result of the action of external stimuli upon an organized body. Brown tested those theories upon himself, with opium and alcohol, and died from the abuse of the agents prescribed. _The Elements_ appeared in both English and Latin editions.
43. _____. _Observations on the Principles of the Old System of Physick, Exhibiting a Compound of the New Doctrine_. Edinburgh, 1787. 141pp. The work an attack upon William Cullen's doctrine of spasms. See #79, this chapter, below.
44. Brown, Joseph (fl.1700-1721). _An Essay towards the Forming a True Idea of Fundamentals in Physick_. London, 1709. 167pp. The writer, reported to have been a dishonest fellow, never earned the M.D. degree, although he claimed the title of "Doctor."
45. _____. _The Modern Practice of Physick Vindicated_. 2 parts. London, 1703. 194pp.; further eds. in 1704,

General Practice and Commentary upon Medicine

1705. The work, dedicated (without permission) to the Duke of Leeds, represents a defense of the writer's own suspect remedies and medical theories.

46. Buchan, William (1729-1805). Domestic Medicine; or, a Treatise on the Prevention and Cure of Disease by Regimen and Simple Medicines. Edinburgh, 1769. 624pp.; 9 London eds. through 1786; first American ed. 1771; 12 American eds. through 1797. In all, Buchan's tract went through nineteen editions and 80,000 copies during his lifetime. A native of Ancrum, Scotland, the writer practiced medicine at Ackworth, Sheffield, Edinburgh, and London.

47. Burdon, Henry. The Fountain of Health. London, 1734.

48. Burnet, Sir Thomas (1632-1715). Thesaurus Medicinae Practicae. London, 1672; abridged by the writer 1703; further complete eds. at London (1673, 1685), Geneva (1697, 1698), Edinburgh (1703). A physician to Charles II and then Queen Anne, the writer received one of the original appointments (1681) to the Royal College of Physicians at Edinburgh.

49. Carr, Richard (1651-1706). Epostolae Medicinales. London, 1691; English ed., London, 1714. 168pp. This work contains eighteen popular epistles addressed to patients rather than to their physicians; ranges in substance from dietetics to coffee.

50. Chamberlain, John (d.1723). A Treasure of Health, from the Italian. London, 1786.

51. Chamberlen, Hugh the elder (1664-1728). A Few Queries relating to the Practice of Physick. London, 1694. Educated at Trinity College, Cambridge, the writer (his name also spelled "Chamberlain") invented an obstetric forceps that he later sold to William Smellie, who then went on to perfect both the instrument and the technique for its application.

52. _____. Manuale Medicum; or, a Small Treatise of Physick in General and of Vomits and Jesuit Powder in Particular. London, 1685.

53. Champney, Thomas. Medical and Chirurgical Reform Proposed. London, 1797. 126pp.

54. Charleton, Walter (1619-1707). Enquiries into Human Nature. London, 1680. One of the first elected fellows of the Royal Society (1662), Charleton had been, at age twenty-four, a physician to Charles I. His Enquiries constitute six lectures on human anatomy and physiology, delivered in the New Theatre of the Royal College of Physicians, Warwick Lane, London; that structure had been erected the previous year by Sir Joshua Cutler, and to him Charleton dedicated this volume.

55. Cheyne, George (1671-1743). The English Malady; or, a Treatise of Nervous Diseases of All Kinds. London, 1733; 5th ed., London, 1735; further eds. between 1733 (Dublin) and 1739. A native of Scotland, Cheyne studied medicine at Edinburgh under Archibald Pitcairn (1652-1713), the principal physician at the University and the one who introduced the mechanic principle into medical science. The novelist Samuel

Richardson served as Cheyne's London printer and became one of the more noted among his patients.

56. _____. Essay of Health and Long Life. London, 1724; seven London eds. through 1726; further eds. in 1740, 1754, 1823, 1827.

57. _____. Essay on Regimen. Together with Five Discourses, Medical, Moral, and Philosophical. London, 1740; 3rd ed., London, 1753.

58. _____. The Natural Method of Cureing [sic] the Diseases of the Body, and the Disorders of the Mind Depending on the Body. London, 1742; five London eds. through 1753.

59. Clark, William (1698-1790?). A Medical Dissertation concerning the Effects of the Passions on Human Bodies. London, 1752. 63pp.

60. Clarke, Richard (fl.1790-1800). Medical Strictures. London, 1799. A London M.D., the writer also set down plans for increasing the size of the Royal Navy.

61. Clerke, Sir William Henry (1751-1818). Thoughts upon the Means of Preserving the Health of the Poor. London, 1790. 27pp. A native of Lancashire and educated at Oxford, Clerke became rector of Bury in 1778; he concerned himself with the physical health of his parishioners, particularly in vaccinating the children of the poor and advising them on treatments for fever; he also demonstrated an interest in agriculture.

62. Clifton, Francis (d.1736). The State of Physick, Ancient and Modern. London, 1732. 192pp. Clifton earned the M.D. from Leyden in 1724, then practiced at London; he came into contact with Sir Hans Sloane, who promoted him for election as a fellow of the Royal Society (1727); served as physician to the Prince of Wales; left London for Jamaica, where he died.

63. _____. Tabular Observations Recommended as the Plainest and Surest Way of Practicing and Improving Physick. London, 1731. 31pp.

64. Clossy, Samuel (1724-1786). Observations on Some of the Diseases of the Parts of the Body. London, 1673. 195pp.

65. Cockburn, William (1669-1739). The Danger of Improving Physick. London, 1730. 39pp. A London M.D., the writer published various tacts on medicine between 1696 and 1732.

66. Colbatch, Sir John (1670-1729). Collection of Medical and Chirurgical Tracts. London, 1700, 1704. A native of Worcester and an apothecary there, Colbatch came under ridicule by Sir Samuel Garth in the physician-poet's mock epic, The Dispensary (1699).

67. _____. Dr. Colbatch's Legacy; or, the Family Physician. London, 1733. Published posthumously.

68. _____. The Generous Physician; or, Medicine Made Easy. London, 1733. 90pp. Another posthumously published piece.

69. Cole, Abdiah (1610-1670), and Nicholas Culpeper

(1616-1664). <u>The Rational Physician's Library, out of the best Authors and from our own Experience</u>. London, 1661. Rather than distinguishing himself as a physician (since he merely claimed such a title), Cole translated and/or published the works of legitimate medical practitioners. Culpeper, also a translator, functionaed principally as a religious and political hack writer.

70. Collignon, Charles (1725-1785. <u>Medicina Politica; or, Reflection on the Art of Physick as inseparably connected with the Prosperity of a State</u>. London, 1765. 43pp. Collignon, of French extraction, held the professorship of anatomy at Cambridge, served as a general physician to the town, and wrote upon the nature of moral reflections.

71. Coltheart, Patrick. <u>The Quacks Unmasked</u>. London, 1727. 28pp.

72. Connor, Bernard (1666-1698). <u>Evangelicum Medici</u>. London, 1697; Amsterdam, 1699. A native of County Kerry, Connor served as physician to King John Sobieski of Poland, after which he practiced medicine at London. He attempted to relate the miraculous cures of Christ and His apostles to "natural principles."

73. Cope, Henry. <u>Demonstratio Medico-Practica Prognosticum Hippocratis</u>. Dublin, 1736.

74. Cordwell, John. <u>A New System of Physick</u>. 3 vols. London, 1668-1670.

75. Cornaro, Luigi [Lewis] (1475-1566). <u>Sure and Certain Methods of Attaining a Long and Healthful Life. To Which are added, Rules for Health, and Directions for Life, by Joseph Addison</u>. 5th ed., London, 1737; another London ed. in 1779. This volume essentially a translation of Cornaro's <u>Discorsi della Vita Sobria</u> (Padua, 1588), written during the Venetian's eighty-third year and attesting to the advantages of temperance.

76. Cornwell, Bryan. <u>The Domestic Physician; or, Guardian of Health</u>. London, 1788. 650pp.

77. Cowper, Ashley (d.1788). <u>The Progress of Physick. By Timothy Scribble</u>. London, 1743. 20pp.; 2nd ed., London, 1750. 20pp.

78. Cruso, Johann (fl.1642-1701). <u>Medicamentorum Euporiston Thesaurus</u>. London, 1701. 140pp.; another London ed., in English (with annotations, glossary, and index). London, 1771. 260pp. The writer also produced a tract on measuring encampments for the army.

79. Cullen, William (1712-1790). <u>Clinical Lectures</u>. London, 1765; another London ed. in 1797. 538pp. One of the founders of the medical college at Glasgow (1744), Cullen held the chairs of chemistry and medicine at Glasgow and Edinburgh; he delivered clinical lectures in England; in 1757, he became the first physician to lecture in <u>English</u>, rather than in Latin.

80. _____. <u>First Lines of the Practice of Physick</u>. 4 vols. Edinburgh, 1776-1783; another ed. 1796. The work

81. ____. Lectures on the Materia Medica. London, 1771, 1773; 2 vol. ed., London, 1789.
82. ____. Synopsis Nosologiae Methodicae in usum Studiosorum. Edinburgh, 1769. The writer divides diseases into fevers, neuroses, cachexias, and local disorders; he differentiates, also, thirty-four varieties of rheumatism. The work established Cullen's reputation, although an English edition did not come forth until 1800.
83. Curteis, Thomas. Essays on the Preservation and Recovery of Health. London, 1704. 234pp.
84. Dalton, Robert. Every Man His Own Physician; or, the Present Practice of Physick. London, 1780.
85. Dawne, Derby. Health: A Poem. London, 1724. An M.D., the "poet" practiced medicine at London.
86. Degravere, John. Thesaurus Remediorum. London, 1662.
87. Dennis, Thomas. The Way of Curing Diseases. London, 1668.
88. Dewell, Thomas. The Philosophy of Physick; or, Phlogistic System. Marlborough, 1784. The writer held the M.D. degree.
89. Dickinson, Edmund (1624-1707). Physica Vetus et Vera; sive, Tractatus de Naturali Veritate Hexaemeri Mosaici. London, 1702. 340pp.; further eds. at Rotterdam (1703) and Leoburg (1705). The writer served as physician to Charles II and James II.
90. Dixon, Roger (fl.1660-1665). Consultum Sanitatus: A Directory to Health. London, 1663. The writer also dispensed advice to and about the poor.
91. Dominicet, Robert (fl.1780-1790). Medical Anecdotes of the Last Thirty Years, Illustrated with Medical Truths. London, 1781. The writer held the M.D. degree.
92. Dray, Thomas. Observations of Chronic Diseases. London, 1772.
93. Duncan, Andrew (1744-1828). Medical Cases. Edinburgh, 1778. 370pp.; four eds. through 1790. Educated at St. Andrew's and Edinburgh (M.D. St. Andrew's, 1769), Duncan served on five occasions (beginning 1764) as president of the Royal Medical Society; traveled to China as a surgeon for the East India Company; licentiate of the Edinburgh College of Physicians (1770), lecturer at Edinburgh (1774-1776), and professor of physiology (1790) there; founded a public dispensary and lunatic asylum at Edinburgh, as well as a number of major medical journals.
94. Edwards, George (1752-1823). Diseases of the Human Body. London, 1791. The Edinburgh-born writer practiced medicine in London and Durham and published at least forty-two books between 1779 and 1819.
95. Elements of the Practice of Physick, for the use of those Students who attend the Lectures and read on this Subject at Guy's Hospital. 2 parts. London, 1798.

General Practice and Commentary upon Medicine

96. Elliott, Sir John (1736-1786). *The Medical Pocket Book*. London, 1781. 138pp.; 13 eds. through 1800. An M.D. who practiced at London, Elliott's collected works in medicine, physiology, and natural philosophy first reached publication in 1780.
97. *The Ensign of Peace. Shewing How the Health, both of Body and Mind, may be Preserved*. London, 1775. 215pp.
98. Este, Rev. Charles (1753-1829). *Tracts on Medical Subjects*. London, 1776. 39pp. The writer abandoned the stage for the study of medicine before eventually entering the Church.
99. *An Explanation of the Terms of Art in the Several Branches of Medicine*. London, 1769. 356pp.
100. Falconer, William (1744-1824). *A Dissertation on the Influence of the Passions upon Disorders of the Body*. London, 1788. 105pp.; three eds. through 1796. A native of Chester and an M.D., Falconer published on medicine, natural history, antiquity, and theology; according to Edward Thurlow, the Lord Chancellor, Falconer "knew every thing, and knew it better than any one else" (Allibone 1:577).
101. *The Family Guide to Health; or, a General Practice of Physick in a Familiar Way*. London, 1767. 331pp.
101a. *The Family Physician, containing some of the most approved Receipts and Opinions of Sydenham, Tissot . . . [et al]*. Manchester, 1798. 191pp.
102. Farr, Samuel (1741-1795). *Elements of Medical Jurisprudence*. London, 1788. 144pp. The writer a native of Taunton, Somerset; his *Elements* gained notice as the first English work on medical jurisprudence, although William Hunter had published an essay in 1783 on the signs of murder in bastard children. Essentially, this tract exists as a translation from Fascelius, with a number of Farr's own comments and observations.
103. _____. *A Philosophical Inquiry into the Nature, Origin, and Extent of Animal Motion, Deduced from Principles of Reason and Analogy*. London, 1771. 399pp.
104. Fisher, Joseph. *The Practice of Medicine Made Easy*. London, 1785. An M.D., the writer published several scientific tracts in the *Transactions* of the Royal Irish Academy.
105. Flowerden, Joseph. *A Compendium of Physick and Surgery*. London, 1769. 492pp.
106. Floyer, Sir John (1649-1734). *Medicina Gerocomica, or the Galenic Art of Preserving Old Men's Healths*. London, 1724. 135pp. Floyer a native of Hinters, Staffordshire, and educated at Oxford; he had formed an association with Michael Johnson, the Lichfield printer and the father of Samuel Johnson. He suggested (1712) the boy, then two and one-half years old, be touched by Queen Anne to rid him of his infant malady (scrofula). A proponent of cold baths, Floyer also became the first English physician to rely upon the "pulse watch" (see #107 below).

107. _____. The Physician's Pulse Watch. 2 vols.
London:
Printed for Michael Johnson at Lichfield, 1707,
1710. Outlines the physician's theory of counting
the number of a patient's pulse beats to the
minute.
108. _____. Touchstone of Medicine. 2 vols. Printed for
Michael Johnson at Lichfield, 1678-1690.
109. Fordyce, George (1736-1802). Elements of the Practice
of Physick. 2 parts. London, 1767-1770.; six eds.
through 1791. A native of Aberdeen. Fordyce took
his M.D. degree at Edinburgh, studied anatomy at
Leyden in 1758, and then settled in London to
practice and to lecture. The Elements served as a
textbook for his lectures.
110. Forster, William. A Treatise on the Causes and Cures
of Diseases. Leeds, 1745. 236pp.
111. Fothergill, Anthony (1732?-1813). Preservative Plan
or Hints for the Preservation of Persons Exposed to
those Accidents which suddenly suspend or
extinguish Vital Action. London, 1798. 43pp. Born
in Yorkshire, the writer studied medicine at
Edinburgh (M.D. 1763) and practiced at Northampton;
appointed (1774) physician to the Northampton
Infirmary and as a licentiate of the College of
Physicians; moved to London in 1780, then to Bath
in 1784, Philadelphia (1803), and back to London
(1812); interested in chemical analyses as well as
medicine.
112. Fothergill, John (1712-1780). Rules for the
Preservation of Health. London, 1762. 137pp. Born
at Carr End, Yorkshire, and a member of the Society
of Friends, the writer traveled on the Continent
before settling to practice at London; at its
height, his income reached £7,000 per year, and
upon his death his estate was valued at £80,000;
he endowed a seminary for young Quakers at
Ackworth (near Leeds), assisted Sydney Parkinson in
the writing of his Journal of a Voyage to the South
Seas in the Endeavour, Commanded by Captain Cook
(1773), and printed (at his own expense of £2000)
Anthony Purver's translation of the Bible from the
Hebrew and Greek (1764).
113. The Fountain of Knowledge; or, British Legacy. . .to
which is added Every One Their Own Physician.
London, 1760 (?). 130pp.
114. Fowler, Thomas (1736-1801). Dissertatio Medica.
Edinburgh, 1778. Fowler, born at York, practiced
at Stafford and York; in 1786, he introduced his
arsenic solution as a general remedy.
115. Freind, John (1675-1728). Opera Omnia, Nempe
Comentarii Novem de Febribus: De Pergantibus in
Secunda Variolarum Conflentum Febre Epistola:
Prealectiones Chymicae: Emmenologia. [bound with]
Historia Medicinae a Geleni Tempore usque as
Initium Saeculi Decimi Sexti. London, 1725-1726.
Freind achieved a reputation both as a classical
scholar and as a physician; he delivered the

Ashmolean lectures on chemistry in 1704, the Harveian Oration in 1720; his official duties included physician the English military and to Queen Caroline. Political involvements resulted in his imprisonment in the Tower, and he gained his release only through the efforts of Dr. Richard Mead.

116. ____. Opera Omnia Medica, ed. Dr. John Wigan. London, 1733; Paris, 1735; Leyden, 1734; 3 vols. London, 1750. A collection of Freind's medical tracts in Latin, in addition to a Latin version (by Wigan) of his History of Physick.

117. Freke, John (1688-1756). An Essay on the Art of Healing. London, 1748. 272pp. Born at London, Freke served as a surgeon's apprentice; he achieved election as assistant surgeon to St. Bartholomew's Hospital, London (1726), where he became the first curator of the hospital museum; rose to become one of the principal surgeons of London and developed intense interests in music and painting; elected a fellow of the Royal Society in 1729.

118. The Fundamental Laws of Physick. London, 1711. 29pp.

119. Garnett, Thomas (1766-1802). A Lecture on the Preservation of Health. Liverpool, 1797. 72pp.; 2nd ed., London, 1800. 115pp. In addition to his medical tracts, Garnett published (1800) a narrative of a tour through the Scottish Highlands and the western islands of Scotland.

120. Gataker, Thomas (d.1769). Essays on Medical Subjects. London, 1764. 284pp. The writer practiced surgery at London; his medical tracts appeared between 1749 and 1764.

121. Geach, Francis (1724-1798). Medical and Chirurgical Observations. London, 1766. 79pp. Geach practiced at Plymouth and published his medical tracts between 1766 and 1781.

122. Goddard, Jonathan (1617?-1675). Discourses concerning Physick. London, 1688; further eds. in 1670, 1678. Physician, chemist, botanist, and a promoter of the Royal Society, Goddard worked extensively with the telescope, developed a nostrum known as "Goddard drops," and dealt in antiquarian books. His Discourse directs itself against apothecaries and maintains that physicians should compound their own prescriptions.

123. Godfrey, Robert. A Treatise on Physick. London, 1673; another ed. in 1674.

124. Gordon, George Alexander. The Compleat English Physician; or, an Universal Library of Family Medicines. London, 1778. 80pp.; further eds. in 1779, 1780. The writer held the M.D. degree.

125. Graeme, William (fl.1725-1735). An Essay on the Method of Acquiring Knowledge in Physick. London, 1729. 60pp. The writer held the M.D. degree.

126. Graham, James (1745-1794). A Short Inquiry into the Present State of Medical Practice. London, 1726. 22pp. Born at Edinburgh, Graham studied medicine at the University there, but neither earned nor

received the M.D. degree; he practiced at Pontefract, traveled to America (1771-1774), returned to England, and settled at Bristol; known for his "quack" cures, particularly that of "earth bathing," and for his religious fervor that bordered upon lunacy.

127. Gregory, James (1753-1821). Conspectus Medicinae Theoreticas in usum Academicum. 2 vols. Edinburgh, 1780-1782. A native of Aberdeen, the writer served as professor of the practice of medicine at the University of Edinburgh; the Conspectus proved valuable because of its emphasis upon therapeutics.

128. ____. Dissertatio Medica: De Morbis Coeli Mutatione Mendendis. Edinburgh, 1774.

129. Gregory, John (1724-1773). Elements in the Practice of Physick. Edinburgh, 1772; 2nd ed., Edinburgh, 1774. A native of Aberdeen, Gregory studied medicine at Edinburgh, Leyden, and Paris; he served as professor of philosophy at King's College, Aberdeen; as professor of physic at the same college (1756-1766); and as professor of physic at the University of Edinburgh (1766-1773).

130. ____. Observations on the Duties, Offices, and Qualifications of a Physician, and of the Method of Prosecuting Enquiries in Philosophy. Edinburgh, 1770; further eds. at Edinburgh in 1772, 1805.

131. Grieve, James (d.1773). A. Cornelius Celsus. Of Medicine, in Eight Books. London, 1756; three eds. to 1837. A layman, Celsus wrote philosophical and medical exercises for his own education, as well as for other laymen; he selected his materials from a variety of sources. Grieve received appointments as physician to St. Thomas's Hospital, London, and to Charterhouse School.

132. Grosvenor, Benjamin (1676-1758). Health. An Essay on Its Nature, Value, Uncertainty, Preservation, and Best Improvement. London, 1716. 242pp.; 2nd ed., London, 1748. Although not a medical practitioner, but an Independent clergyman residing in London, Grosvenor did publish general tracts upon the subject of health.

133. Hall, Charles (1745?-1825?). Medical Family Instructor, with an Appendix on Canine Madness. Shrewsbury, 1785. Essentially an economist, Hall did study medicine and earned the M.D. degree from Leyden in 1765.

134. Hamey, Baldwin the younger (1600-1676). Dissertatio Epistolaris de Juramento Medicorum. London, 1693. The writer held degrees in medicine both from Leyden (1626) and Oxford (1629); he practiced at London until 1665. The Dissertatio did not see publication until this 1693 version, edited by Adam Littleton (1627-1694), rector of Chelsea and a prebendary of Westminster.

135. Hanselins, Johann Georg. Medicina Brevis. London, 1714.

136. Harris, John. The Divine Physician: Prescribing Rules for the cure of Diseases, as well as of the Body

General Practice and Commentary upon Medicine 13

and the Soul. London, 1676.
137. Harris, Walter (1647-1732). Dissertationes Medicae et Chirurgicae Habitae in Amphitheatro Colegii Regalis Medicorum Londinensium. London, 1725. Harris, of Gloucester, a protege of and follower of Sydenham, served as a physician-in-ordinary to Charles II and to William III; he advanced the notion that discharges from unwashed ears came about simply as a part of the overall scheme of nature. The Dissertationes comprise his Lumleian lectures.
138. Harvey, Gideon the elder (1640?-1700?). The Art of Curing Diseases by Expectation: With Remarks on a Supposed Great Case of Apoplectick Fits. London, 1689; a Latin ed. in 1694. The work comprises a collection of random criticisms of contemporary medical practice, in addition to a treatise on herbal medicine. Harvey, born in Holland, served as a physician to Charles II.
139. Harvey, James (fl.1700-1720). Praesagium Medicum; or, the Prognostic Signs of Acute Diseases. London, 1706. 216pp.; second ed. in 1713 and 1720.
140. Hill, Sir John (1716-1775). The Family Practice of Physick; or, a Plain. . .Method of Curing Diseases with the Plants of Our Own Country. London, 1769. Originally an apothecary, Hill settled in London (from Peterborough), where he published volumes on medicine, botany, natural philosophy, natural history, drama, and prose fiction. He engaged in controversy with the Royal Society, Charles Churchill, and David Garrick; in a letter to Dr. John Hawkesworth (? January 1759), Garrick penned the following concerning Dr. Hill:
> For Physick & Farces, his Equal there scarce is,
> His Farces are Physick, his Physick a Farce is.
> (The Letters of David Garrick, ed. D.M. Little and G.K. Kahrl [London: Oxford University Press, 1963] 1:299)

At least seventy-six volumes of Hill's work reached publication between 1740 and 1777.
141. Hillary, William (d.1763). An Inquiry into the Means of Improving Medical Knowledge. London, 1761. 461pp. An M.D., Hillary published medical tracts between 1735 and 1761.
142. Hodges, Nathaniel (1629-1688). Vindiciae Medicinae et Medicorum: An Apology for the Profession and Professors of Physick. London, 1666. Hodges achieved recognition for his professional services rendered during the London plague of 1664-1665. The Vindiciae has been described as a pedantic attack upon medical quackery.
143. Home, Francis (1719-1813). Clinical Experiments, Histories, and Dissertations. Edinburgh, 1780. 458pp.; 3rd ed., London, 1783. Professor of materia medica at the University of Edinburgh, Home experimented with inoculations for measles (1759) and described false membrane in diptheretic croup

(1765).
144. ____. *Medical Facts and Experiments*. Edinburgh and London, 1759. 288pp.
145. ____. *Principia Medicina*. Edinburgh, 1758; further eds. in 1770 (3rd) and 1783.
146. Hook, Andrew. *An Essay on Physick; or, an Attempt To Review the Practice of the Antients*. London, 1734. 89pp.; 2nd ed., London, 1736.
147. Hooper, Joseph (fl.1780-1790). *A Discourse on the Best Means of Improving the Science of Medicine*. London, 1788. 39pp.
148. Hunter, William (1718-1783). *Medical Commentaries . . .interspersed with Remarks on the Structure, Functions, and Diseases of the Human Body*. 2 parts. London, 1762-1764. After spending five years at the University of Glasgow studying for the ministry, Hunter turned his attention to medicine (1737), came to London in 1741, and began the study of anatomy at St. George's Hospital; from 1748, he confined his practice to midwifery; he then became physician to Queen Charlotte (1764), gained election to the Royal Society (1767), and received appointment as professor of anatomy to the Royal Academy (1768).
149. *The Ill State of Physick in Great Britain*. London, 1727. 71pp.
150. Jackson, Joseph (fl.1690-1700). *Enchiridion Theoretico-Medicum*. London, 1695.
151. James, Lewis. *Letters Relating to the College of Physicians*. London, 1688.
152. Johnson, James (fl.1775-1795). *Medical Guide*. London, 1792.
153. Johnstone, John (1768-1836). *Medical Jurisprudence*. London, 1800. A native of Annan, Scotland, the writer practiced medicine first at Kidderminster, and then at Worcester.
154. Jones, John. *Medical, Philosophical, and Vulgar Errors of Various Kinds Refuted*. London, 1797.
155. Jones, Robert (fl.1780-1790). *An Inquiry into the State of Medicine*. Edinburgh, 1781. 376pp. The writer held the M.D. degree.
156. Kirkpatrick, James (d.1743; ed. and trans.). *Tissot's Advice to the People in General with regard to their Health; with a Table of Remedies, translated, with Notes*. Dublin, 1766. Simon Andrew Tissot (1728-1797), an eminent Swiss physician, studied at Montpellier and practiced at Lausanne; he achieved a reputation for his treatments of the small pox and for his medical lectures at Pavia. This edition first published almost a quarter-century following Kirkpatrick's death.
157. Kite, Charles (1768-1811). *Essays and Observations, Physiological and Medical, on the Submersion of Animals and on the Resin of the Acoroides Resnifera, or Yellow Resin of Botany Bay* [together with] *Selected Histories of Diseases* [and] *Meteorological Tables*. London, 1795. 434pp. Kite, a member of the Corporation of Surgeons, London,

practiced medicine at Gravesend.
158. The Lamentable State of Physick in England. London, 1769. 22pp.
159. Langrish, Browne (d.1759). The Modern Theory and Practice of Physick. London, 1735. 371pp.; 2nd ed., London, 1738; 3rd ed., London, 1764. The writer, a member of the Royal Society, practiced medicine at Winchester; in this volume he discusses his clinical research and describes experiments in the analysis of excretia and the examination of the blood.
160. Lettsom, John Coakley (1744-1815). Hints Designed To Promote Beneficence, Temperance, and Medical Science. 3 vols. London, 1799-1802. Originally, from Little Vandyke, Virgin Islands, Lettsome became one of the original founders of the Medical Society of London, where he established the Lettsomian Lecture Foundation. He wrote essays on air, bread, tea, alcoholism, and drug addiction (see his History under Section XXI, #1889, below); in addition, he maintained social and professional relationships with Benjamin Franklin.
161. Lewis, William (1714-1781). Experimental History of Materia Medica. London, 1741; further eds. in 1768, 1784 (3rd), 1791 (4th, 2 vols.); German ed. in 1771. Lewis, born at Kingston, Surrey, practiced medicine at London and at Kingston-upon-Thames.
162. Litton, Edmond. Philosophical Conjectures on Aereal Influences the Probable Origin of Diseases. London, 1747. 57pp.; 2nd ed., London, 1750. 57pp.
163. Lobb, Theophilus (1678-1763). A Compendium of the Practice of Physick, in Twenty-Four Lectures. With a Letter shewing what is the proper Preparation of Persons for Inoculation. London, 1747. Son of the Rev. Stephen Lobb, an Independent minister, the writer also pursued a religious calling before turning his attention to the practice of medicine.
164. _____. The Practice of Physick in General, as delivered in a Course of Lectures on the Theory of Diseases, and the Proper Method of Treating Them. 2 vols. London, 1771. The work published posthumously from Lobb's own manuscripts.
165. The London Practice Physick. London, 1769. 327pp.; six eds. through 1797.
166. Lynch, Barnard (fl.1745-1755). A Guide to Health through the Various Stages of Life. London, 1744. 480pp.; another ed. in 1754.
167. MacBride, David (1726-1778). A Methodical Introduction to the Theory and Practice of Physick. London, 1772. 660pp.; 2nd ed., enlarged (2 vols.), Dublin, 1776. The writer, born at Ballymoney, County Antrim, and a recipient of the M.D. from Glasgow in 1764, practiced chemistry as well as medicine; he achieved success after 1764, his professional income rising beyond £1700 in 1777. The Methodical Introduction came from his lectures, a Latin version of which appeared at Utrecht in

1774.
168. Manning, Henry (fl.1771-1780). Modern Improvements in the Practice of Physick. London, 1780. 440pp. The writer held the M.D. degree.
169. Manningham, Sir Richard (1690-1759). The Use and Abuse of Physick. London, 1753. 38pp.; 2nd ed., London, 1754. Born at Eversley, Hampshire, and educated (LL.B. and M.D.) at Cambridge, the writer practiced midwifery at London and established himself at the head of his profession; a licentiate of the College of Physicians and knighted (1721) by George I; represented in Laurence Sterne's Tristram Shandy.
170. Marrett, Christopher (fl.1665-1670). Frauds of Apothecaries. London, 1667; another ed. in 1670. The writer held the M.D. degree.
171. Marryat, Thomas (1730-1792). The New Practice of Physick Founded on Irrefragable Principles. Dublin, 1764. 364pp. Born at London and educated for the Presbyterian ministry, Marryat entered Edinburgh as a student of physic and graduated M.D. in 1761; he studied at medical schools on the Continent, visited America, and returned to Britain to practice at Antrim, Ireland (1766-1774), Shrewsbury (1774-1785), and Bristol; he administered to the poorer classes and lectured on therapeutics.
172. Marten, John. Gonosdogium Novum; or, A New System of All the Secret Infirmities and Diseases. London, 1709. 150pp.
173. Martin, Charles. OEconomy of the Human Body. London, 1759. The writer held the M.D. degree.
174. Martine, George the younger (1702-1741). Essays and Observations, Medical and Philosophical. London, 1740. A Scot, Martine borrowed heavily from Sanctorius, Boerhaave, Haller, and De Haven in his attempts to treat scientifically the employment of instruments of precision in diagnosis. The Essays collect six pieces; two of them--"Essays and Observations on the Construction and Graduation of Thermometers" and "An Essay towards a Natural and Experimental History of the Various Degrees of Heat in Bodies"--came forth together as a second edition (Edinburgh, 1772, and again in 1792).
175. Mason, Simon (fl.1745-1756). Practical Observations in Physick. Birmingham, 1757. 265pp. The writer produced tracts on a variety of health related subjects, from tea to fevers and ague.
176. Mead, Richard (1673-1754). The Art of Getting in Practice in Physick. London, 1722. A native of Stepney, Mead studied medicine at Utrecht, Pitcairn, and Leyden, eventually taking his degree in philosophy and medicine at the University of Padua (1695); he began to practice medicine at Stepney in 1696, then associated himself with St. Thomas's Hospital and Crutched Friars (1703) before receiving the M.D. from Oxford in 1707. After receiving appointment as fellow of the College of

Physicians in 1716, he became a physician-in-ordinary to George II (1727); he even found time to treat the poet Alexander Pope. Both a bibliophile and a scholar, Mead published on the prevention of the plague and on inoculation; he established the wide practice of the latter in Britain.

177. ____. De Imperio Solis et Luna in Corpore Humano et Morbis inde Oriundus. London, 1704. An "iatromechanical" treatise upon the influence of the sun and the moon on the human body.

178. ____. Medica Sacra, sive de Morbis insignioribus qui in Biblis memorantur, Commentarius. London, 1749; Amsterdam, 1749; an English ed. (trans. Dr. Thomas Stark), London, 1755. The writer focuses his attention upon the diseases mentioned in Scriptures, contending that demonical possessions (to include lunacy and epilepsy) should be considered as diseases.

179. ____. Monota et Praecepta Medica. London, 1751. This work constitutes a summary of the London physician's practical medical experiences.

180. ____. The Medical Works of Dr. Richard Mead. 3 vols. London, 1762.; 2nd ed., Edinburgh, 1765.

181. Meadow, Thomas. A New Method of Reducing All Distortions of the Human Body. London, 1760.

182. Medical Essays and Observations Revised and Published by a Society in Edinburgh. 5 vols. Edinburgh, 1733-1744; four eds, through 1752.

183. The Medical Museum; or, A Repository of Cases, Experiments, Researches, and Discoveries. 3 vols. London, 1763-1764; 2nd ed., 4 vols., London, 1781.

184. Medical Observations and Inquiries. By a Society of Physicians in London. 6 vols. London, 1757-1784.

185. Mihlis, Samuel (fl.1745-1753). Medical Essays and Observations. 2 vols. London, 1745. The writer held the M.D. degree and practiced medicine in London.

186. Millar, John (1733-1805). Observations on the Management of the Prevailing Diseases in Great Britain. London, 1779. 320pp. A native of Scotland and an M.D. from Edinburgh, the writer began his medical practice at Kelso; appointed (1774) physician to the Westminster General Dispensary, London, after which he became an active promoter of the Medical Society of London; concentrated his practice on women and children, but found the time to write on a variety of medical and professional concerns.

187. The Modern Family Physician; or, The Art of Healing Made Easy. London, 1775. 279pp.

188. Morgan, Thomas (d.1743). The Mechanical Practice of Physick. London, 1731, 1735. 362pp. The writer, a Welsh Deist, took up the study of medicine after his dismissal from the ministry because of his "unorthodox" views; he identified himself as an "M.D." on the title pages of his books, but there exists no evidence of his medical education or practice.

189. ____. Philosophical Principles of Medicine. London, 1725. 440pp; further eds, 1728, 1730.
190. Morland, John. A Rational Account of the Causes of Chronic Diseases. London, 1742; 2nd ed., London, 1744.
191. Mortimore, Cromwell (d.1752). An Address to the Publick: Containing Narratives of the Effects of Certain Chemical Remedies. London, 1745. 104pp. The writer practiced medicine at London and became the object of several satirists' literary and artistic attacks. He served as a secretary of the Royal Society and as an editor and contributor to its Philosophical Transactions.
192. Moss, William (fl.1782-1799). A Medical Survey of Liverpool. Liverpool, 1784. The writer also published a guide toward the management of children.
193. Nevett, Thomas (fl.1697-1704). The Rational OEconomy of Human Bodies. London, 1704. The writer held the M.D. degree.
194. Newman, Jeremiah Whitaker (1759-1839). Medical Essays. London, 1787. Newman practiced surgery at Ringwood, Hampshire, then moved to Dover; in addition to his medical practice and works on medicine, he pursued studies in literary criticism, biography, poetry, and prose fiction.
195. Nisbet, William (1759-1822). The Clinical Guide: or, A Concise View of. . .Diseases; to which is subjoined, A Practical Pharmacopoeia. Edinburgh, 1793. 180pp.; three eds. through 1799. An Edinburgh physician and medical writer, Nisbet settled in London at the beginning of the nineteenth century; he gained election as a fellow of the Royal College of Surgeons, wrote on various diseases, and composed guides for surgeons and physicians.
196. O'Connell, Maurice. Morborum Acutorum et Chronicorum Quorundam, Observationes Medicinales Experimentales. Dublin, 1746. 416pp.
197. Of the Improvement of Medicine in London, on the Basis of Public Good. London, 1775. 56pp.
198. Okes, Thomas (1730-1797). Duae Dissertationes in Publicis Scholis Cantabrigiae Habitae. Canterbury, 1770. The writer practiced surgery at Cambridge; in his spare time, he fathered twenty children.
199. Parkinson, James (1755-1824). Medical Admonitions to Families. 2 vols. London, 1799; five eds. through 1809. A pupil of John Hunter, then a surgeon and apothecary at Hoxton, Parkinson will no doubt be remembered for his unique and classical description of paralysis agitans ("Parkinson's disease," 1817) and by his being the first to report, in English, a case of appendicitis (1812).
200. Paxton, Peter (d.1711). Directory Physico-Medical, Composed for the Use and Benefit of all such as designed to Study and Practice the Art of Physick, wherein Proper Method and Rules are prescrib'd for the better Understanding of that Art, and

Catalogues of Such Authors exhibited as are necessary to be consulted by all young Students. London, 1701; another ed. in 1707. The writer attended Pembroke College, Cambridge, before he moved on to London to practice medicine.

201. ____. An Essay concerning the Body of Man, wherein its Changes or Diseases are consider'd and the Operations of Medicine Observed. London, 1701. 392pp. The work attempts to trace the origins of all diseases to the fluids of the body.

202. ____. Specimen Physico-Medicum, de Corpore Humano, ejus Morbis. Or, An Essay concerning the Knowledge and Cure of Most Diseases afflicting Human Bodies. London, 1711. 364pp.

203. Pearson, Richard (1765-1836). A Practical Synopsis of the Materia Alimentaria and Materia Medica. 2 vols. London, 1797-1807. A native of Birmingham and M.D. from Edinburgh (1786), the writer developed an interest in clinical experimentation with electricity; after a tour of Europe, he settled at Birmingham, where he became (1792) physician to the General Hospital; he moved to London in 1701, then on to Reading, Sutton Coldfield, and back to Birmingham.

204. Percival, Thomas (1740-1804). Essays Medical and Experimental, to which are added Select Histories of Disease. 3 vols. London, 1767-1778. A native of Warrington, Lancashire, Percival received his education at Edinburgh, London, and Leyden (M.D.); in 1767, he settled at Manchester, where he developed a reputation as a philanthropist, scientist, and physician; he engaged in the investigation of epidemic diseases; the Essays proved popular and gained acceptance among the practitioners of the day.

205. Perry, Charles (1698-1780). A Treatise on Diseases in General incident to the Human Body, to which is subjoined a System of Practice. 2 vols. London, 1741. Perry, a native of Norwich, traveled extensively after having graduated M.D. from Cambridge (1727); between 1739 and 1742, he toured Western and Eastern Europe, after which he settled in London to practice physic; there he wrote on subjects related to medicine and travel.

206. Pitt, Robert (1653-1713). The Antidote; or, The Preservative of Health and Life and the Restorative of Physic; to its Sincerity and Perfection. London, 1704. 192pp. Pitt's medical tracts appeared regularly between 1694 and 1705.

207. The Present State of Physick and Surgery in London. London, 1701. 30pp.

208. Price, Philip Parry (fl.1790-1800). A Treatise on the Diagnosis and Prognosis of Diseases. 2 parts. London, 1791. An M.D., the writer wrote and practiced at London.

209. Prosser, Thomas (fl. 1769-1790). The Oeconomy of Quackery Considered. London, 1777. Prosser also published tracts on subjects ranging from bronchial

fever to fevers of horses.
210. Quincy, John (d.1722). *The English Dispensatory*. London, 1721; twelve eds. through 1749. The work contains a complete account of the materia medica and of therapeutics; a number of prescriptions recorded therein gained considerable and lengthy popularity; Quincy--a Dissenter, a Whig, and a friend of Dr. Richard Mead--practiced medicine and operated an apothecary shop in London.
211. ____. *An Examination of Dr. Woodward's State of Physick and Diseases*. London, 1719. The work constitutes a serious attack upon John Woodward (1665-1728) and his *The State of Physic and Diseases; with an Inquiry into the Late Increase of them, but more particularly of the Small Pox* (London, 1818; Latin ed., Tiguri, 1720; German ed., Zurich, 1722). See #1020 below.
212. ____. *Medicina Statica Britannica; or, a Translation of the Aphorisms of Sanctorius*. London, 1712; further eds. in 1720, 1723, 1728, 1737. Sanctorio Sanctorius (1561-1636), who in 1611 became professor of theoretical medicine at Padua, invented the clinical thermometer, a pulsimeter, and a hygrometer; he achieved wide recognition for his investigations into the fluctuations in body weight under different conditions and resulting from "insensible perspiration."
213. ____. *Syllabus to a Course of Pharmacy*. London, 1722. The last of Quincy's works published during his lifetime.
214. Quinton, John (fl.1707-1734). *Practical Observations in Physick and Mineral Waters*. London, 1711. An M.D. who practiced at London, Quinton published tracts on surgery and waters.
215. ____. *Practical Observations in Physick and Surgery*. London, 1707; another London ed. in 1711.
216. Rattray, Sylvester (fl.1650-1666). *Prognosis Medica ad usum Praxeos facili Methodo Digesta*. Glasgow, 1666. The writer, a native of Angus, held degrees in theology and medicine.
217. Riverius, Lazarus. *The Secrets of Lazarus Riverius. Newly Translated by E.P.* London, 1685. One "Eugenius Philander" published, in 1673, *A Quaere concerning Drinking Bath-Water Resolved*, but that hardly qualifies him as the translator of Riverius. Edward Pratt stands as another possibility. See #625 and #628 below.
218. Roberdes, John. *The Practice of Physick*. London, 1698.
219. Robinson, Lewis. *Every Patient His Own Doctor; or, The Sick Man's Triumph over Death and the Grave*. London, 1778. 56pp. The writer held the M.D. degree.
220. Robinson, Nicholas (1697?-1775). *A Discourse on the Nature and Cause of Sudden Deaths*. London, 1729; further eds. in 1732, 1735. Robinson, a native of Wales and a physician of Christ Hospital, London, delivered lectures on medicine in his own house; in

this <u>Discourse</u>, he maintained that certain cases of apoplexy ought not to be treated by bleeding; he also describes, from his own observations, the appearance of the cerebrum after opium poisoning.

221. ____. <u>A New Theory of Physick and Diseases, Founded on the Principles of Newtonian Philosophy</u>. London, 1724. The writer proclaimed the lack of a true, fallible authority in medicine.

222. Rowley, William (1742-1806). <u>The Rational and Improved Practice of Physick of William Rowley</u>. 4 vols. London, 1793; also a two-volume ed. in Latin. A native of London, M.D. from St. Andrews, and a surgeon in the Royal Navy (1760-1763), Rowley became a physician at the St. Marylebone Infirmary, London; he described himself as a "man midwife."

223. ____. <u>Schola Medicinae Universalis Nova</u>. 2 vols. London, 1793. Rowley subsequently published a single-volume English translation of this work, which consists of a compendium of various subjects related to medicine.

224. Russell, Alexander (1715?-1768). <u>Tentamen Medicum et Medicastorum Audacitate</u>. Edinburgh, 1739. Edinburgh, 1739. Born at Edinburgh, Russell served (1750-1754) as physician to the English factory at Aleppo, Syria (then a part of the Turkish Ottoman Empire), and later in the same capacity at St. Thomas's Hospital, London (1758 until his death); Samuel Johnson reviewed Russell's <u>Natural History of Aleppo</u> (1756) in <u>The Literary Magazine</u> (1756, 1:2, 80-86).

225. Russell, William (fl.1674-1696). <u>Physical Treatise on Medicine</u>. London, 1684. The writer also published tracts on the legitimacy of Quakerism and on psalm-singing.

226. Rutty, John (1698-1775). <u>Materia Medica Antiqua et Nova Expurgata et Illustrata</u>. London, 1777. A native of Dublin who embraced the Quakerism of his parents, Rutty practiced medicine in that city from 1724 until his death; he entertained John Wesley whenever the Methodist leader came to Dublin and either required medical assistance or friendly conversation; thus, on Thursday, 6 April 1775, only three weeks prior to the physician's death, Wesley "visited that venerable man, Dr. Rutty, tottering over the grave; but still clear in his understanding, full of faith and love, and patiently waiting till his change should come" (<u>Journal</u>, ed. Nehemiah Curnock [London: Charles H. Kelly, 1909-1916] 6:58-59); the <u>Materia Medica</u> became a standard reference work.

227. Salmon, William (1644-1713). <u>The Family Dictionary</u>. London, 1696. A general work on "domestic medicine" by the London practitioner; although not a licensed or even "legitimate" medical person,

228. ____. <u>Practical Physick</u>. London, 1692. Salmon included in this volume the philosophic works of Hermes, Trismegistus, Kalid, Geber, Artephius, Nicholas Flammel, Roger Bacon, and George Ripley.

229. _____. *Synopsis Medicinae, or, a Compendium of Astrological, Galenical, and Chymical Physick*. 3 books. London: Richard Jones at the Golden Lion in Little Britain, 1671; 2nd ed., 1681; reissue in 1685; 4th ed., 1689. The work contains a quantity of lauditory verses by astrologers and second-rate philosophers.

230. Samson, William (fl.1770-1780). *Rational Physick; or, the Art of Healing. . .To which is added a Family Dispensary*. London, 1765. In 1768, Samson published a poem, *The Conciliade*, on the subject of disputes among physicians.

231. Saunders, Richard (1613-1687?). *The Astrological Judgment and the Practice of Physick, deduced from the Position of the Heavens at the Decumbiture of a Sick Person*. London, 1677. The work stands as a systematic explication of astrological therapeutics based largely upon examination of the urine and sputa by horoscopical methods; Saunders, born in Warwickshire, practiced astrology and compiled almanacs.

232. Saunders, William (1743-1817). *Elements of the Practice of Physick*. London, 1790. 136pp. The writer, an M.D. and senior physician to Guy's Hospital, London, published medical tracts on various subjects between 1765 and 1811.

233. Sermon, William (1629?-1679). *A Friend to the Sick, or the Honest English Man's Preservative. . .with a Particular Discourse of the Dropsie, Scurvie, and Yellow Jaundice*. London, 1673. The writer served as a physician to the Royal Army and practiced at Bristol before graduating M.D. from Cambridge (1670); he then moved to London, established a considerable practice, and gained appointment as a physician-in-ordinary to Charles II.

234. Shaw, Peter (1694-1763). *New Practice of Physick, on the Model of Dr. Sydenham*. 2 vols. London, 1726; further eds. in 1728, 1733, 1738; 7th ed., London, 1753. Shaw, a native of Lichfield, practiced medicine without a degree, but nonetheless served as a physician-in-ordinary to George II; he wrote largely on medicine and chemistry, in addition to editing works by Sir Francis Bacon and James Boyle.

235. Shebbeare, John (1709-1788). *The Practice of Physick, founded on Principles in Physiology and Pathology hitherto unapplied in Physical Enquiries*. 2 vols. London, 1755. A native of Bideford, Devonshire, Shebbeare resided in London and emerged as a political writer for the Tories; a number of his contemporaries appeared all too ready to proclaim that of his thirty-five published books, thirty had been forgotten; Samuel Johnson thought him "respectable," but (in the next century) Thomas Babington Macaulay, the historian and biographer, judged him (from a greater distance, perhaps) a "wretched scribbler."

236. Sibly, Ebenezer (1751-1800). *A Key to the Physic and to the Occult Sciences*. London, 1794. 395pp. The

writer studied surgery at London and eventually (1792) obtained the M.D. degree from King's College, Aberdeen; he resided at Ipswich, practicing medicine and studying astrology.

237. Sims, James (1741-1820). A Discourse on the Best Methods of Prosecuting Medical Enquiries. London, 1774; 2nd ed., 1774; French ed., Avignon, 1778; Italian ed., Venice, 1786. Born in County Down, Sims earned the M.D. degree from Leyden (1764); he practiced at Tyrone before coming to London; there he served as a physician to the General Dispensary in Aldersgate Street and to the Surrey Dispensary; he became the first chairman and vice president of the Philanthropic Society, and for twenty-two years presided over the Medical Society of London.

238. Simson, Thomas (1696-1764). De Erroribus circa Materiam Medicam. Edinburgh, 1726. Simson held the first professorship of medicine at St. Andrew's, Scotland, a chair established in 1721 by James Brydges, Duke of Chandos; he gained election as an honorary fellow of the Royal College of Physicians at Edinburgh.

239. ____. De Re Medici. Dissertationes Quatuor. Edinburgh, 1726. This piece focuses upon a variety of medical subjects, including the humors and secretions.

240. Smellie, William the younger (1740-1795). Thesaurus Medicus, seive Disputationum in Academia Edinensi adrem Medicum Pertinentium. 4 vols. Edinburgh, 1778-1785. Although never a physician in the academic or even legal sense, Smellie, a printer's apprentice who managed to acquire a superior education, developed a thorough knowledge of physic; his reputation arose from his associations with and contributions to the Encyclopaedia Britannica, The Scots Magazine, and The Edinburgh Magazine; he should not be confused with the elder William Smellie (see #1768 below), known for his work in anatomy and midwifery.

241. Smith, Brabazon. The Physician's Portable Library; or, Compendium of Modern Practice of Physick. London, 1800. 256pp. The writer, an M.D., practiced at London.

242. Smith, Hugh (1736?-1789). The Family Physician. London, 1750; five eds, through 1770. Graduated M.D. from Leyden in 1755, the writer practiced medicine at Hatton Garden, London; he published at least five separate works on various aspects of medical practice.

243. Smith, Hugh (d.1790). Formulae Medicamentorum; or, a Compendium of the Modern Practice of Physick. London, 1768. 159pp.; four eds, through 1781.

244. Smith, Timothy. Health and Long Life: Translated from L. Lessius and L. Cornaro. London, 1743. At age forty (c.1515), finding his health considerably impaired by intemperance, Luigi Cornaro (1475-1566) adopted strict rules both for meat and drink that served to prolong his life; at age eighty-three, he

published his <u>Discorsi della Vita Sobria</u> (1558); another English ed. of this work appeared in 1779.
245. Smith, William (fl.1755-1780). <u>Nature Studied with a View to Preserve and Restore Health</u>. London, 1774. 210pp. A practitioner of physic, Smith found time to write narratives of his travels to Guinea, a history of England, and tracts upon government and the prison systems.
246. ____. <u>A New and General System of Physick</u>. London, 1769. 581pp.
247. ____. <u>A Sure Guide to Sickness and Health</u>. London, 1776. 356pp.
248. Smythson, Hugh. <u>The Compleat Family Physician</u>. London, 1781. 1024pp.
249. Spens, Thomas, (fl.1792-1811). <u>Medical and Surgical Observations, from the German of Richter</u>. Edinburgh, 1794. August Gottlieb Richter (1742-1812) became one of the leading German surgeons of the eighteenth century; an M.D., Spens wrote and practiced medicine at Edinburgh.
250. Spilsbury, Francis B. <u>The Friendly Physician</u>. London, 1773. 51pp.
251. Sprackling, Robert. <u>Medela Ignorantiae; or, An Answer to Medela Medicinae</u>. London, 1665.
252. Sprengell, Sir Conrad (fl. 1708-1727). <u>The Aphorisms of Hippocrates and the Sentences of Celsus</u>. London, 1708; another ed. in 1735. The writer held the M.D. degree.
253. Squirrel, Robert (fl.1795-1806). <u>Maxims on Health</u>. London, 1798. The writer claimed the M.D. degree.
254. Stack, Richard William. <u>Some Medical Cases of Bath</u>. Bath, 1784. 118pp. An M.D., the writer practiced medicine at Bath.
255. Stanger, Christopher (1754-1834). <u>A Justification of the Right of every well-educated Physician of fair Character and mature Age, residing within the Jurisdiction of the College of Physicians of London to be admitted a Fellow if competent</u>. London, 1798. In this pamphlet, written after the denial of his own application for admission, the author demonstrates that Lord Chief Justice Mansfield had determined, in 1767, that the College had to admit all qualified licentiates of whatever university, not restrict admission to graduates of Oxford or Cambridge; Stanger, an M.D. graduate of Edinburgh, studied further in Europe and became associated with the London Foundling Hospital.
256. Stephenson, David (fl. 1744-1765). <u>Medicine Made To Agree with the Institution of Nature; or, A New Mechanical Practice of Physick</u>. London, 1744. 85pp. Stephenson also published (1746) a popular guide for the "gentleman" gardener.
257. Stewart, Alexander. <u>Medicial Discipline</u>. London, 1743.
258. Strother, Edward (1675-1737). <u>An Essay on Sickness and Health</u>. London, 1725. An M.D. from Utrecht, the writer practiced medicine at London; he authored at least ten medical tracts, as well as

several translations of works on physic.
259. Sutherland, Alexander (fl.1755-1765). <u>An Attempt To Revive Ancient Medical Dictrines</u>. 2 vols. London, 1763. The writer held the M.D. degree and practiced at London.
260. Tanner, John (fl.1670-1685). <u>The Hidden Treasure of the Art of Physick fully Discovered: in Four Books</u>. London, 1672.
261. Temple, Richard (d.1826). <u>The Practice of Physick</u>. London, 1792. 452pp.; 2nd ed., London, 1798. The writer held the M.D. degree.
262. Theobald, John (d.1760). <u>Every Man His Own Physician</u>. London, 1764. 48pp. Originally published in French at Paris, 1753; ten English eds. through 1770. A London M.D., the writer also published translations of works by Voltaire.
263. Thomas, Robert (1753-1835). <u>Medical Advice to the Inhabitants of Warm Climates</u>. London, 1790. 342pp. The writer practiced surgery on the island of Nevis, British West Indies, then settled at Salisbury.
264. Thomson, George (fl.1648-1679). <u>The Direct Method of Curing Chymically</u>. London, 1675. A Latin translation of this volume by one Gottfried Hennicken appeared at Frankfurt-am-Main in 1686, with a preface by Thomson dated 1684; an M.D. from Leyden (1648), Thomson resided for the greater part of his life at London, publishing a number of controversial tracts on diseases, plagues, and general physic; he incurred considerable and opposition when he challenged contemporary medical fads (such as bleeding).
265. Toulmin, George Hoggart (fl.1780-1810). <u>The Instruments of Medicine</u>. London, 1789. In addition to his tracts on medicine, the writer, an M.D., also published pieces on the "eternity" of the world and the universe.
266. Townsend, Joseph (1739-1816). <u>Elements of the Therapeutics; or, A Guide to Health</u>. 2 vols. London, 1799. Born at London, Townsend studied medicine at Edinburgh; he allied himself with the Calvinist Methodists; after traveling throughout Europe, he studied mineralogy in Cornwall and eventually became rector of Pewsey, Wiltshire; his published works focus upon religion, mineralogy, geology, and medicine.
267. Turner, Robert (fl.1654-1665). <u>The British Physician: or, The Nature and Vertues of English Plants</u>. London, 1664; a new ed. in 1687. The work reflects the writer's interest in the medicinal benefits from herbs, but it also contains "curious" incidental information; primarily an astrologer and a botanist, Turner graduated B.A. from Christ's College, Cambridge, in 1640.
268. Tweedie, James. <u>Hints on Temperance and Exercise</u>. London, 1799. 56pp.
269. Wallis, George (1740-1802). <u>The Art of Preventing Diseases and Restoring Health</u>. London, 1793; 2nd

ed., London, 1796; another ed. in 1798; German ed., Berlin, 1800. Wallis, born at York, lectured at that city on the theory and practice of physic, and he practiced medicine there; in addition to his medical tracts, he wrote comic drama and poetic satire.
270. Walwyn, William. Physick for Families. London, 1681. See, also, #272 below.
271. Webster, Charles (1740?-1795). Medicinae Praxeos Systema, ex Academiae Edinburgenae Disputationibus Inauguralibus Praecipue Depromptum, et Secundum Naturae Ordinem Digestum. 3 vols. Edinburgh, 1780-1871. In 1760, Webster went to Edinburgh from his native Dundee to practice physic; however, he became a minister of the nonjurors' Scottish Episcopal Church in Carrubber's Close, Edinburgh, then of St. Peter's Chapel, Roxburgh Place (which he built); James Boswell reports listening to Webster preach (4 April 1779) and partaking of claret and Welsh rabbit at his home (19 April 1779; see Joseph W. Reed and Frederick A. Pottle [eds.], Boswell, Laird of Auchinleck. 1778-1782 [New York: McGraw-Hill, 1977], pp. 65, 93).
272. Welwin, William. Physick for Families. London, 1696; another ed. in 1715. Allibone (3:2568, 2644) lists this title both under "William Welwin" and "William Walwyn" (see #270 above); undoubtedly, Physick for Families (eds. of 1681, 1696, 1715) belongs to a single writer.
273. Wesley, John (1703-1791). Advices with Respect to Health. Extracted from a Late Author. Bristol, 1769. The work represents the Methodist leader's edition of Avis au Peuple sur la Sante (1760), by Simon-Andre Tissot (1728-1797), a Swiss physician; the tract ran through ten editions in less than six years.
274. _____. Primitive Physick: or, an Easy and Natural Method of Curing Most Diseases. London, 1747. The work constitutes Wesley's attempt to dispense popular, remedies based upon commonly accepted cures of the day, to his Methodist followers throughout the British Isles; essentially, he sought to protect people from those greedy and incompetent medical practitioners whom he, himself, distrusted; one of the more popular volumes published in England during the eighteenth century, Primitive Physick had gone through twenty editions by the time of its writer's death on 2 March 1791.
275. Willis, Francis. Synopsis Physicae. London, 1690.
276. Willis, Thomas (1621-1675). Dr. Willis's Practice of Physick, being the Whole Works of that Renowned Physician: Translated by Samuel Pordage. London, 1681-1684; the original ed., in Latin, had appeared at Geneva and Lyon in 1676 (2 vols.) and again in Geneva in 1680 (2 vols). Son of a Wiltshire farmer, graduate of Christ's Church College, Oxford, Willis rose to become Sedleian professor of natural philosophy at Oxford (1660); in 1666, he

moved to London, where he emerged as the leading English exponent of the chemiatric theory, advancing the notion of diseases existing actually of disturbances of fermentation in the body, and thus had to be treated as such; supposedly, Willis, as an extremely devout individual, caused services to be performed at St. Martin's Lane Church early each morning so that he might worship before beginning on his daily rounds; further, he left 20 per year for the maintenance of those early services, as well as donated all of his Sunday fees for charitable purposes; he also served as a physician-in-ordinary to Charles II. Pordage, the translator (fl.1660-1680), stands as a less than minor poet and playwright of the Restoration; he once left a draft of his tragedy, Herod and Mariamne, with Lord Rochester, whose patronage he hoped to gain; Rochester responded with "Poet, whoe'er thou art,/God damn thee; Go hang thyself, and burn thy Mariamne" (see David M. Veith [ed.], The Complete Poems of John Wilmot, Earl of Rochester [New Haven and London: Yale University Press, 1968], pp. 161, 219).

277. _____. The London Practice of Physick: or, The Whole Practical Part of Physick Contained in the Works of Dr. Willis, Faithfully Made English and Printed Together for the Publick Good. London, 1685. Translator or editor unidentified; the volume contains a biographical sketch of Willis, parts one and two of his Pharmaceutice Rationalis (1674, 1675), and tracts on convulsive diseases, scurvy, brain disease, the nervous system, and fevers.

278. Wilson, Andrew (1718-1792). Short Remarks upon Autumnal Disorders of the Bowels. Newcastle-upon-Tyne, 1765; London, 1776. Wilson, whose father (Gabriel Wilson) served a Presbyterian church in Maxton, Scotland, earned the M.D. from Edinburgh and practiced medicine at Newcastle and then at London; at the latter city, he received appointment as physician to the London Medical Asylum; he also published, anonymously, several philosophical tracts.

279. Winter, George (fl.1790-1800). Dissertations on Different Diseases. London, 1799. The writer held the M.D. degree and also wrote a history of "animal magnetism."

280. Wintringham, Clifton the elder (1689-1748). A Treatise of Endemic Diseases. York, 1718. General Wintringham practiced medicine at York, received an appointment at the York County Hospital, and died in that city; his father, the Rev. William Wintringham, once attempted to weigh an individual spermatazoon; his son, Clifton Wintringham the younger (1710-1794), became physician-general to the British Army and a physician to George III.

281. Wirgman, George. Medical, Chirurgical, and Anatomical Observations, from the German of L. Heister. London, 1755. Lorenz Heister (1683-1758), one of

the leading German surgeons of the eighteenth century, performed the first post-mortem section of appendicitis (1711), introduced the term "tracheotomy" (1718), and published (1718) a work on surgery best remembered because of its detailed and particularly instructive illustrations.

282. Withers, Thomas (fl.1770-1795). <u>Observations on the Abuse of Medicine</u>. London, 1775. The writer, an M.D., practiced at Edinburgh and London.
283. _____. <u>Treatise on Medical Education</u>. London, 1794.
284. Woodman, Philip. <u>Medicus Novissimus; or, the Modern Physician</u>. London, 1712.
285. Yarwood, John. <u>Physick Refined</u>. London, 1683.
286. Young, James (fl.1679-1713). <u>Medicaster Medicatus</u>. London, 1685. Young practiced surgery at Plymouth and published tracts on head wounds, general surgery, and anatomy.
287. Y-Worth, William. <u>Chymicus Rationalis: or, the Fundamental Grounds of the Chemical Art, Rationally Stated and Demonstrated</u>. London, 1692. As an alchemical treatise, this tract focuses upon medically applicable chemical mixtures; the writer dedicated the work to William Boyle.

II

Anatomy and Physiology

288. Aitken, John (d.1790). <u>Principles of Anatomy and Physiology</u>. 2 vols. London, 1786. The writer studied medicine at Edinburgh, where he also lectured on surgery; he practiced physic, anatomy, midwifery, and surgery; recognition came as the result of his introducing an alternate mode of locking the midwifery forceps and from inventing a pair of forceps for dividing and diminishing the stone in the bladder when the object became too large to remove by lithotomy (surgical incision of the urinary bladder).

289. Albinus, Bernhard Siegfried (1697-1770). <u>Tables of the Skeleton and Muscles of the Human Body</u>. London, 1749. 92pp.; Edinburgh, 1777-1778. This tract represents the first edition in English of the <u>Tables</u>, originally published in Latin at Leyden in 1747; Andrew Bell (1726-1809), the foremost engraver then at Edinburgh, re-engraved the original plates; Albinus, a superior eighteenth-century anatomical illustrator, established a new standard of excellence in anatomical drawing; he also held the chairs of anatomy and surgery (1728) and medicine (1745) at Leyden.

290. Alexander, Benjamin (d.1768). <u>Morgagni's Seats and Causes of Diseases Investigated by Anatomy</u>. London, 1769. In 1761, at the age of seventy-nine, Giovanni Battista Morgagni (1682-1771) published his <u>Seats and Causes</u> (in Italian), which became the true foundation for modern pathological anatomy; for the first time, the records of post-mortem findings had been correlated with clinical records on a large scale; Morgagni spent his entire medical career as a professor at Padua; Alexander, the translator, held the M.D. degree.

291. <u>Anatomical Dialogues: or, A Breviary of Anatomy</u>. London, 1778; four eds. through 1796.

292. <u>An Anatomical Essay, in Two Discourses: I. Pointing at</u>

Many Things Curious. . .in the Structure of the Viscera. . . II. An Anatomical Explication, of the first six verses of the twelfth chapter of Ecclesiastes. Edinburgh, 1702. 196pp. These tracts attributed to Robert Elliott (1669-1714).
293. Anatomical Lectures; or, The Anatomy of the Human Bones, Nerves, and Lacteal Sac and Duct. London, 1775. 172pp.
294. Anatomy Epitomized and Illustrated; containing, I. A Concise and Plain Description of All Parts of the Human Body. . . II. A Large and Choice Collection of Sculptures. London, 1737. 182pp.
295. Bailie, Matthew (1761-1823). The Morbid Anatomy of Some of the Most Important Parts of the Human Body. London, 1793; Appendix. London, 1798; 2nd ed., London, 1797. A native of Shots, Lanarkshire, Scotland, Baillie studied at Balliol College, Oxford, and pursued medicine under the guidance of his uncle, William Hunter; in 1810, he received appointment as a physician to George III; his Morbid Anatomy stands as the first attempt, in English, to treat pathology as a subject in and for itself, as the writer described the morbid appearances of each human organ in systematic succession; Baillie's sister, Joanna (1762-1851), a close friend of Sir Walter Scott, gained a fair reputation as a poet and dramatist.
296. Baker, Robert. Cursus Osteologicus. London, 1697.
297. Bell, John (1763-1820). Engravings To Illustrate the Structure of the Bones, Muscles, and Joints. London, 1790; further eds. between 1794 and 1805. Bell, a celebrated Edinburgh anatomist and a brother of the noted artist Sir Charles Bell (1774-1842), proved more than competent as an illustrator in his own right; on more than one occasion, he provided illustrations for his own medical books.
298. ____. A System of the Anatomy of the Human Body. 4 vols. Edinburgh, 1793-1804.
299. Bibliotheca Anatomica, Medica, Chirurgica. . . containing a Description of the Several Parts of the Body. 3 vols. London, 1711-1714.
300. Charleton, Walter (1619-1707). Three Anatomy Lectures: (1) The Motion of the Blood through the Veins and Arteries; (2) The Organic Structure of the Heart; (3) The Efficient Cause of the Heart's Pulsation. London, 1683. In these lectures, Charleton clearly refuted the false belief that William Harvey had "borrowed" his theory of the circulation of the blood from Paul of Venice. See, also, #54, above.
301. Cheselden, William (1688-1752). The Anatomy of the Human Body. London, 1713; further eds. in 1722, 1726 (3rd, illustrated), 1730, 1741 (6th), 1778 (11th). Cheselden, a native of Somebry, Leceister-shire, became a surgeon at St. Thomas's Hospital, London (1718); ten years later (1728), he introduced a new operation for artificial pupil by way of a single iridotomy with a needle; the

Anatomy and Physiology

physician also found time to patronize boxing, establish a reputation as a competent draftsman, and prepare plans for Old Putney Bridge, London, and the Surgeon's Hall in the Old Bailey; he also gained a reputation for his speed in the operating theatre; prior to all of that, he had been a student of William Cowper (1666-1709).

302. ____. Osteographia, or Anatomy of the Bones; with Plates the Size of Life. London, 1728; another ed. in 1733; Gerard Van der Gucht supplied the illustrations for this volume.

303. ____. Syllabus of a Course of Lectures on Anatomy. London, 1771.

304. Collignon, Charles (1725-1785). Compendium Anatomico Medicum. London, 1756. See, also, #70, above.

305. ____. An Enquiry into the Structure the Human Body. Cambridge, 1764. 67pp.; 2nd ed., Cambridge, 1764. 67pp.

306. ____. Tyrocinium Anatomicum; or, An Introduction to Anatomy. Cambridge, 1763. 37pp.

307. Cook, John (fl.1730-1770). The New Theory of Generation, according to the Best and Latest Discoveries in Anatomy. 2 vols. London, 1762.

308. Cowper, William (1666-1709). The Anatomy of Human Bodies: Illustrated with 114 Copper-Plates. Oxford, 1698. A surgeon and anatomist, and originally from Hampshire, Cowper actually plagiarized 105 of the plates in this volume from a similar work on anatomy (1685) by the German Godfrey Bidloo; the latter attacked Cowper in his Gulielmus Cowper, Criminis Literati Citatus (Leyden, 1700); however, the text of The Anatomy and nine of its plates can be traced directly to Cowper; see, also, #301 above.

309. Cruikshank, William (1745-1800). Anatomy of the Absorbing Vessels of the Human Body. Edinburgh, 1786; 2nd ed., 1790. A native of Edinburgh who eventually became William Hunter's assistant and partner, Cruikshank developed a large private practice; on occasion, he would convert his private office into a public dispensary for the poor.

310. Dionis, Pierre (1643-1718). The Anatomy of Human Bodies Improv'd. London, 1703. This proves to have been the first English edition of the French text of 1690; Dionis, a Paris anatomist, became one of the earliest practitioners to offer (1673) courses on operative surgery on the cadaver; his published works on surgery and anatomy remained standard for well over fifty years; in fact there exists evidence of an edition of his tracts in Chinese.

311. Douglas, George (fl.1735-1763). A Treatise on Anatomy. Edinburgh, 1763. An M.D., the writer practiced physic in Edinburgh and London.

312. Douglas, James (1675-1742). Bibliographiae Anatomicae Specimen. London, 1715. 226pp. The writer, an M.D., gained the attention of the Gottingen physician Albrecht von Haller, who recommended him

highly.
313. ____. A Description of the Peritonaeum. London, 1730. 47pp.
314. ____. Nine Anatomical Figures. London, 1748. Published posthumously; the volume contains only the nine plates.
315. Douglas, John (d.1743). A Syllabus of what is to be perform'd in a Course of Anatomy, Chirurgical Operations, and Bandages. London, 1719. 48pp. An M.D., the writer served as a surgeon to the Westminster Infirmary, London.
316. Drake, James (1667-1707). Anthropologia Nova; or, a New System of Anatomy. 2 vols. London, 1707; 2nd ed., 1717; other eds. London, 1727-1728 and 1750. Drake devoted as much of his time to political attacks upon the government as he did to the practice of and writing about medicine.
317. Duncan, Andrew (1744-1828). Heads of Lectures on Pathological Physiology. Edinburgh, 1796. 87pp. See, also, #93, above.
318. ____. Heads of Lectures on Pathology. Edinburgh, 1782. 43pp. This volume a variation on #317, above.
319. Falconer, Magnus (1754-1778). Synopses of a Course of Lectures on Anatomy and Surgery. London, 1777; another ed. in 1779. The writer also produced (1776) a tract upon blood.
320. Free, John. Stadia Physiologica duo; or, Two Stages of Physiology. London, 1762. 267pp.
321. Fyfe, Andrew (1754-1824). A Compendium of the Anatomy of the Human Body. 3 vols. Edinburgh, 1800. Although a standard text in the London medical schools throughout the first quarter of the nineteenth century, Fyfe's Anatomy did not capture the favor of the entire British medical profession.
322. ____. A System of Anatomy and Physiology. 2 vols. London, 1787; four eds. through 1795.
323. Gibson, Thomas (1647-1722). The Anatomy of Humane Bodies Epitomized. London, 1682; further eds. in 1684, 1688, 1697, 1703, 1716 (7th ed.). The writer held the M.D.degree.
324. Glisson, Francis (1597-1677). Anatomia Hepatis. London, 1654. A native of Rampisham, Dorsetshire, Glisson received his degree from Cambridge, served as Regius Professor of Cambridge and as President of the Royal College of Physicians; although the Anatomia predates the guidelines for this bibliographical study by some six years, it needs to be considered: it contained the first accurate description of the capsule of the liver investing the portal vein (known as "Glisson's capsule") and its blood supply.
325. ____. Opera Medica Anatomica. 3 vols. London, 1691.
326. ____. De Ventriculo et Intestinis. London, 1677. The work focuses upon the concept of irritability as a specific property of all human tissues.
327. Harwood, Sir Busick (1745?-1814). A Synopsis of a Course of Lectures on Anatomy and Physiology.

Anatomy and Physiology 33

Cambridge, 1792. 94pp.; a third ed. at London, 1797. Born at Newmarket and apprenticed to an apothecary, Harwood qualified as a surgeon and gained an an appointment to a medical position in India; in 1790 he earned the M.D. from Cambridge; he conducted experiments in bleeding and transfusion, which resulted in his appointment as professor of anatomy at Cambridge.

328. ____. *A System of Comparative Anatomy and Physiology*. Cambridge, 1796. 72pp. The work includes fifteen engravings.

329. Haworth, Samuel (fl.1680-1685). *The Anatomy of Man's Soul and Body*. London, 1680. An M.D., the writer also published tracts on consumption and the value of mineral waters.

330. Hooper, Robert (1773-1835). *The Anatomist's Vade Macum*. London, 1797. 159pp.; three eds. through 1800. An M.D., the writer achieved recognition for his tracts on plants, physiology, morbid anatomy, and surgery; he also published (1798) a useful medical dictionary.

331. ____. *Observations on the Structure of the Intestinal Worms of the Human Body*. London, 1799. 64pp.

332. Hunter, William (1718-1783). *Anatomia Humani Uteri Gravidi Tabulus Illustrata*. Birmingham, 1774; English ed., Birmingham, 1774 (*The Anatomy of the Human Gravid Uterus Exhibited in Figures*). Hunter spent thirty years in the production of this volume; it represents a landmark in printing, anatomical drawing, fine engraving, and obstetrics; see, also, #148, above.

333. ____. *Two Introductory Lectures. . .delivered to his last Course of Anatomical Lectures, at His Theatre in Windmill Street. . .to which are added Some Papers Relating to Dr. Hunter's Intended Plan for Establishing a Museum in London*. London, 1784. The lectures, published posthumously, focus upon Leonardo's position as an anatomist; included, also, is a number of disparaging remarks about the work of William Harvey.

334. Huxham, John (1694-1768). *Anatomy*. London, 1756. A native of Halberton, Devonshire, and the son of a butcher, Huxham studied medicine under Hermann Boerhaave at Leyden and then practiced at Plymouth; his principal contributions to the medical profession may be found in the area of fevers (see, also, #860, #933, below).

335. Innes, John (1739-1777). *Eight Anatomical Tables*. Edinburgh, 1776. 52pp.; 2nd ed., Edinburgh, 1779. The writer held the position as a dissector at the University of Edinburgh.

336. Ireton, John. *Microcosmus: Anatomy of the Bodies of Men and Women*. London, 1670. This work essentially a translation of a tract by a Dr. Spaher.

337. Keill, James (1673-1719). *The Anatomy of the Human Body*. Edinburgh, 1698; eleven eds. through 1742. A native of Edinburgh, Keill practiced physic in

that city; between 1706 and 1719, he published essays on medicine in the Transactions of the Philosophical Society of Edinburgh.

338. Lower, Richard (1631-1691). Tractatus de Corde. Item de Mortu et Colore Sanguinis et Chyli in eum Transitu. London, 1669; another ed., Amsterdam, 1669. A native of Cornwall, Lower became a successful practitioner and physiologist; he gained recognition as the first physician to perform direct transfusion of the blood from one animal to another (February 1665) and the first, in England, to transfuse blood from one human being to another; the Tractatus represents one of the most important works in the history of physiology.

339. Monro, Alexander secundus (1737-1817). De Venis Lymphaticus Valvulosis: et de earum in primus Origine. Edinburgh, 1757; 2nd ed., 1770. The three Alexander Monros held, in turn, the chair of anatomy at the University of Edinburgh for 126 years (1720-1846); in the controversial De Venis Lymphaticus, Monro argued that he, not William Hunter, had first described correctly the general communication of the lymphatic system; in reality, Friedrich Hoffmann (1660-1742), of Halle, preceded both of them with such a description; Monro studied at Edinburgh, Berlin, and Leyden; he wrote also on the nervous system, the physiology of fishes, and on the brain, the eye, and the ear.

340. Nichols, Frank (1699-1779). Compendium Anatomico-OEconomium. London, 1736; further eds. in 1738, 1742. Nichols lectured on anatomy at Oxford and London; James Boswell (in his Life of Johnson) cites him as an example of Lord Bute's "undue partiality to Scotchmen," his lordship having "turned out Dr. Nichols, a very eminent man, from being physician to the King, to make room for one of his countrymen [William Duncan], a man very low in his profession" (James Boswell, Life of Johnson, ed. R.W. Chapman and J.D. Fleeman [London: Oxford University Press, 1970], p. 620).

341. Nicholson, Henrich (1681-1733). Ars Anatomica. London, 1709; an English ed. the same year under the title A Brief Treatise of the Anatomy of Human Bodies.

342. Northcote, William (d.1783?). Anatomy of the Human Body for. . .Naval Practitioners. London, 1772. The writer published no less than four major tracts, ranging from anatomy to pharmacy, between 1770 and 1772.

343. Nourse, Edward (1701-1761). Syllabus totam rem Anatomicam Humanam Complectens. London, 1748. 44pp. The writer, a native of Oxford, served as an apprentice to an assistant surgeon at St. Bartholomew's Hospital, London; in 1725, he received a diploma from the Barber-Surgeons' Hall and eventually gained election as assistant surgeon at St. Bartholomew's (1731) and then (1745) as surgeon there; additional positions included

Anatomy and Physiology   35

         demonstrator of anatomy for the Barber-Surgeons
         (1731) and fellow of the Royal Society (1728); he
         became the first surgeon at St. Bartholomew's
         Hospital to provide regular instruction in anatomy
         and surgery.
344. Peart, Edward (1756-1824). Physiology; or, An Attempt
     to Explain the Functions and Laws of the Nervous
     System. London, 1798. 327pp. The writer, an M.D.,
     published several medical and professional tracts;
     animals and electricity proved high on his list of
     interests.
345. Pole, Thomas (1753-1829). The Anatomical Instructor.
     London, 1790. 304pp. A surgeon, Pole practiced
     his craft at London.
346. Pugh, John. A Treatise on the Science of Muscular
     Motion for Restoring the Power of the Limbs.
     London, 1794. The work includes fifteen plates,
     "with a duplicate set in outline."
347. Redmond, William. The Principles and Constituence of
     Anatomy. London, 1762. 49pp.; 2nd ed., London,
     1763. The writer held the M.D. degree.
348. Ridley, Humphrey (fl.1679-1703). The Anatomy of the
     Brain. London, 1695; a Latin ed. at Leyden in
     1725. The writer earned the M.D. from Leyden in
     1695.
349. Rowley, William (1742-1806). On the Absolute
     Necessity of Encouraging, instead of Preventing or
     Embarrassing, the Study of Anatomy. London, 1795.
     18pp. A native of London and a surgeon in the
     Royal Navy (1760-1763), the writer eventually
     became physician to the St. Marylebone Infirmary,
     London; the majority of his medical publications
     came forth between 1770 and 1792, to be collected
     in 1793 under the title The Rational Practice of
     Physick of William Rowley.
350. Salmon, William (fl.1671-1734). Synopsis Medicinae
     Anatomica. London, 1671; further eds. in 1680,
     1685, 1699. The writer, an M.D., described
     (Allibone 2:1918) as a "noted empiric"; he
     published tracts on medicine, astrology, philology,
     theology, botany, art, and architecture.
351. Simmons, Samuel Foart (1750-1813). Anatomy of the
     Human Body. London, 1780. Born at Sandwich, Kent,
     Simmons settled in London in 1778, where he became
     editor of the London Medical Journal see #2046,
     below) in 1781; he later received an appointment as
     a physician extraordinary to George III.
352. Stedman, John (d.1791). Physiological Essays and
     Observations. Edinburgh, 1769. 140pp. A native of
     Edinburgh, Stedman held the M.D. degree.
353. Tauvry, Daniel (1669-1701). Anatomy according to
     Mechanics. London, 1700. The writer also
     published (1700) an essay on the general subject of
     medicine.
354. Thomson, George (fl.1734-1740). The Anatomy of the
     Human Bones. London, 1734. 299pp. An M.D., the
     writer also published tracts on plants, a threshing
     machine, and teeth.

355. Vaughan, Walter (1766-1828). An Exposition on the Principles of Anatomy and Physiology. 2 vols. London, 1791. A native of Rochester, the writer held the M.D. degree; he authored tracts on a variety of subjects, ranging from the flesh of sheep to the treatment of headaches.
356. Willis, Thomas (1621-1675). Cerebri Anatome, cui accessit Nervorum Descriptio Usus. London, 1644. See, also #276, above. The Cerebri, influenced by Richard Lower (see #338, above) and illustrated by Sir Christopher Wren (1631-1723), proved the most complete and accurate account of the nervous system to that time; Willis classified the cerebral nerves and described the eleventh cranial (spinal accessory) nerve and the hexagonal network of arteries at the base of the brain; thus, came the terms "the nerve of Willis"and "the Willis network."
357. ____. Pathalogiae Cerebri et Nervosi Generis Specimina; in quo agitur Morbis Convulsivis; et de Scorbuto. Oxford, 1667 (not the first ed.); another ed., London, 1668. This work constitutes a significant contribution to the study of nervous diseases.
358. Winslow, James Benigus (1669-1760). An Anatomical Exposition of the Structure of the Human Body. Translated from the French Original by G. Douglas. 2 vols. First English ed., London, 1733. This work appeared initially at Paris in 1732; a Danish teacher of anatomy, Winslow worked to condense and systematize the anatomical knowledge of his day; thus, the Anatomical Exposition became the first work on descriptive anatomy to discard physiological detail and hypothetical explanation that tended to be far removed from the subject; this tract remained a standard textbook for nearly a century.

III

Medicines, Cures, and Healing Agents

359. An Account of the Medical Properties of a Bark, lately procured from South America. London, 1789. 12pp.
360. Adair, James Makittrick (1728-1802). An Essay on Regimen and Air. London, 1799. 208pp. A native of Inverness and an M.D. from Edinburgh (1766), Adair practiced at Antigua, Andover, Guildford, and Bath; he wrote a volume of medical cautions for invalids residing at Bath.
361. Adams, George (1750-1795). An Essay on Electricity. London, 1784. 367pp.; 2nd ed., London, 1785. 476pp.; 3rd ed., London, 1787. 473pp.; 4th ed., London, 1792. 588pp.; 5th ed., London, 1795. 594pp. The writer served as mathematical instrument maker to George III; the author of elementary scientific tracts, he tended to combine science with religion.
362. Alleyne, James. A New English Dispensatory. In Four Parts. London, 1733. 646pp.; another ed. in 1735. The writer held the M.D. degree.
363. Alston, Charles (1683-1760). A Dissertation on Quick-lime and Lime-Water. Edinburgh, 1752. 60pp. Educated at Glasgow, Alston studied medicine under Hermann Boerhaave at Leyden; he later lectured in botany and materia medica at Edinburgh, as well as superintended the botanical gardens there.
364. _____. A Third Dissertation on Quick-lime and Lime-Water. Edinburgh, 1757. 46pp.
365. Anderson, John (d.1804). Medical Remarks on Natural, Spontaneous, and Artificial Evacuation. London, 1787. 122pp.; 2nd ed., London, 1788. 171pp. The writer practiced medicine at Kingston, Surrey, and served as physician to and director of the General Sea Bathing Infirmary at Margate; an M.D. from Edinburgh, he held a fellowship in the Society of Antiquaries.
366. Andree, John (1699?-1785). Observations upon a Treatise on the Virtues of Hemlock. London, 1761. 80pp. An M.D. from Rheims (1739) and a licentiate of the College of Physicians, the writer practiced at London and associated himself with the London Hospital.
367. Archer, Clement (1725-?). Miscellaneous Observations

on the Effects of Oxygen. 2 parts. Bath, 1798. 144pp.; another ed., London, 1798.

368. Awister, John (fl.1760-1770). An Essay on the Effects of Opium. London, 1763. 70pp. An M.D., the writer published various medical tracts between 1763 and 1769.

369. Ball, John (1704?-1779). A New Compendious Dispensatory. London, 1769. 288pp. The writer's various medical works appeared at London between 1758-1771.

370. ____. Pharmacopoeia Domestica Nova. London, 1760. 112pp.

371. Banyer, Henry (fl.1717-1739). Pharmacopoeia Pauperum; or, The Hospital Dispensatory. London, 1717. 128pp.; four eds. through 1739. The writer studied medicine at St. Thomas's Hospital, London, and practiced as a physician at Wisbeach; in 1736 he gained admission as an extraordinary licentiate of the College of Surgeons.

372. Bate, George (1608-1669). Pharmacopoeia Bateana. London, 1688; another ed. in 1700. Bate served as a physician to Charles I, Oliver Cromwell, and Charles II; he became one of the earliest fellows of the Royal Society and lectured on anatomy at the College of Physicians, London; first published in Latin and a full twenty years after its author's death, the Pharmacopoeia appeared again in 1700, in English, under the title Bate's Dispensatory, translated by Dr. William Salmon (see 227, above); the work claims to be a collection of Bate's own prescriptions.

373. Bateman, Charles (fl.1739-1758). An Abstract of a Treatise of the Virtues of Dr. Bateman's Pectoral Drops. London, 1739. 64pp.

374. ____. A Second Letter to an Apothecary at Windsor. London, 1758. 40pp.

375. Becket, John Brice. An Essay on Electricity. Bristol, 1773. 151pp.

376. Beddoes, Thomas (1760-1808), ed. Communications respecting the External and Internal Use of Nitrous Acid. London, 1800. 125pp. See, also, #26, above.

377. ____, and James Watt (1736-1819). Considerations on the Medicinal Use and on the Production of Factitious Airs, and the Manner of Obtaining Them. 3 parts. Bristol, 1794. 32pp.; three eds. through 1796. Watt, the Scottish inventor, gained a permanent niche in history for his steam locomotive (1784); his major interest, of course, focused upon the various applications of steam as a motive force.

378. Berdoe, Marmaduke (fl.1770-1775). An Enquiry into the Influence of Electric-Fluid. Bath, 1771. 183pp. The writer held the M.D. degree.

379. Berkenhout, John (1730?-1801). Pharmacopoeia Medici. London, 1756. 93pp.; 3rd ed., London, 1762. The writer, a naturalist, literary historian, and biographer, attended grammar school at Leeds, studied in Europe, pursued medicine at Edinburgh,

and received (1765) the M.D. from Leyden; he practiced at Isleworth, in Middlesex, traveled to America, and died at Besselsleigh, near Oxford; known for the depth and the breadth of his knowledge, Berkenhout proved his competence in at least five languages.
380. Berlu, John Jacob. <u>The Treasury of Drugs Unlocked, or a Description of All Sorts of Drugs</u>. London, 1690; three eds. through 1738.
381. <u>The Best and Easiest Method of Preserving Uninterrupted Health to Extreme Old Age</u>. London, 1748. 204pp.
382. Blackwell, Elizabeth (1700?-1758). <u>A Curious Herbal</u>. 2 vols. London, 1737-1739. With plates. The writer the wife of a London merchant; under encouragement from Sir Hans Sloane, she painted medicinal plants in fine detail and in their natural colors.
383. Blair, Patrick (d.1728). <u>Pharmaco-Botanologia</u>. London, 1723-1728. See, also, #34 above; the work ends its alphabetical arrangement with the letter "H," presumably the result of the writer's death.
384. Blizard, Sir William (1743-1835). <u>Experiments on the Danger of Copper and Ball Metal in Pharmaceutical and Chemical Preparations</u>. London, 1786. See, also, #35 above; this tract also appeared in the <u>London Medical Journal</u> (see #2046, below) for 1789-1790.
385. Boerhaave, Hermann (1668-1738). <u>Some Experiments concerning Mercury</u>. London, 1734. A translation of a tract by the eminent Dutch physician and botanist; at Leyden, he lectured on the theory of medicine and held professorships there in medicine, botany, and chemistry; patients and students came from throughout Europe to seek his advice and to study with him; the former, no doubt, contributed to his personal fortune, estimated at two million florins.
386. Boulton, Richard (fl.1697-1724). <u>Some Thoughts concerning the Universal Qualities of the Air</u>. London, 1724. 47pp. Educated at Brasenose College, Oxford, the writer resided at Chester; he became known more for his competency as a medical writer than for his skill as a medical practitioner.
387. Bradley, Henry. <u>A Treatise on Mercury</u>. London, 1733. 52pp. In the same year, the writer also produced a tract on the Ancient physicians (see #1871 below).
388. Bradley, Richard (1688-1732). <u>Precautions against Infection</u>. London, 1722(?). 34pp. See, also, #37 above).
389. Bradney, Joseph (fl.1795-1815). <u>The Art of the Apothecary</u>. London, 1796. The writer also published tracts on money and religion.
390. Brest, Vincent (fl.1732-1735). <u>A Dissertation concerning the Use of Crude Mercury in Venereal and Other Inveterate Diseases, and the Best Method of Administering Successfully without Salivation</u>. London, 1735. The writer held the M.D. degree.

391. Brocklesby, Richard (1722-1797). <u>Reflections on Ancient and Modern Musick, with Application to the Cure of Diseases</u>. London, 1749. 82pp. See, also #39 above.
392. Bromfield, William (1712-1792). <u>An Account of the English Nightshades</u>. London, 1757. 84pp. The writer, a physician to George III, wrote, also, tracts on small-pox inoculation and surgery.
393. Brookes, Richard (fl.1721-1763). <u>The General Dispensatory</u>. London, 1753. 408pp; three eds. through 1773. The writer practiced medicine in Surrey, traveled to America and Africa, and compiled gazetteers; his numerous compilations and translations focused upon medicine, surgery, natural history, and geography.
394. Brown, Joseph (fl.1700-1721). <u>Antidotaria, or a Collection of Antidotes against the Plague and Other Malignant Diseases</u>. London, 1721. 39pp. The writer, an accused charlatan, never earned or received the M.D., although he claimed the title of "doctor"; he spent time in prison and in the pillory for attacking (1706) Queen Anne's ministers; see, also, #44-#45 above.
395. Buchan, William (1729-1805). <u>A Letter to the Patentee, concerning the Medical Properties of the Fleecy Hosiery</u>. London, 1790. 20pp.; six London eds. and one American ed. through 1798. See, also, #46 above.
396. Burrows, John (fl.1760-1775). <u>A Dissertation on the Nature and Effects of a New Vegetable Remedy</u>. London, n.d.; a 3rd ed., London, 1767. 76pp. An M.D., Burrows also published a tract on cancer; see, also, #1457 above.
397. Chamberlen, Paul (1635-1717). <u>A Philosophical Essay on the Celebrated Anodyne Necklace</u>. London, 1717. In this seventy-page tract, the writer (hiding behind the persona of an anonymous admirer) recommends to the world his Anodyne Necklace, a string of beads costing five shillings, that he proclaimed would cure everything from children's bad teeth to women suffering during child-bearing labor; Chamberlen did hold the M.D. degree.
398. Chambers, John. <u>A Pocket Herbal</u>. Bury, 1800. 328pp.
399. Chandler, John (1700-1780). <u>Frauds Detected. . . Shewing the Necessity of Some More Effectual Provision against Deceits. . .in Drugs</u>. London, 1748. 34pp. See, also, #988 and #1141 below.
400. Charles, Richard (fl.1785-1788). <u>Observations on Antimonial Preparations</u>. London, 1785. 24pp. The writer practiced surgery at London; see, also #1170 below.
401. Clare, Peter (1738-1786). <u>Miscellaneous Remarks on Mr. Clare's New Method of Applying Mercury</u>. London, 1782. 45pp. A London surgeon, Clare advocated the administration of calomel by friction within the mouth as a remedy for venereal disease; he died at Rugby.
402. Clarke, William (fl.1670-1675). <u>An Essay on Nitre</u>.

Medicines, Cures, and Healing Agents 41

London, 1670; a Latin ed. in 1675. According to the writer, nitre functions as an emetic, purgative, refrigerant, and "febrifuge."

403. Clutton, Joseph (fl.1729-1736). *A True and Candid Relation of. . .Joshua Ward's Pill and Drop*. London, 1736. 114pp. Ward (1685-1761), a London quack and fraudulent politician, had to flee England for his part in the 1715 Jacobite uprising; he engaged in the preparation of pills and drops--most of which proved both ineffective and actually harmful--that earned for him considerable attention from among the satirists (artists and writers) of London.

404. Coatsworth, William. *Pharmacopoeia Pauperum*. London, 1718.

405. Colborne, Robert. *A Complete English Dispensatory*. London, 1753. 348pp.; another London ed. in 1756.

406. Coly, Anthony. *A Dissertation upon Golden Purging Pills*. London, 1671.

407. *The Complete Herbal; or, Family Physician, Giving an Account of All Such Plants as are now in the Practice of Physick*. 2 vols. Manchester, 1787.

408. *A Complete Key to the Dispensary*. London, 1726. 35pp.; four eds. through 1746

409. *Considerations on the Uses and Abuses of Antimonial Medicines in Fevers*. London, 1773. 48pp.; 2nd ed., London, 1773. 48pp. A brittle, metallic substance, usually bluish white in color, antimony also went by the name "monk's bane."

410. Cook, John (fl.1730-1770). *The Natural History of Lac, Amber, and Myrrh*. London, 1770. 31pp.

411. Cowper, James. *A Narrative of the Effects of a Celebrated Medicine Newly Discovered*. London, 1760. 59pp. The writer held the M.D. degree.

412. Crumpe, Samuel (1766-1796). *An Inquiry into the Nature and Properties of Opium*. London, 1793. 304pp.; a German ed. published at Copenhagen in 1796, 216pp. A resident of Limerick and an M.D. from Edinburgh (1788), Crumpe established a reputation from his essays on opium (1793) and on the means for providing employment to the Irish (1793).

413. Culpeper, Nicholas (1616-1664). *Pharmacopoeia Londinensis; or, The London Dispensatory Further Adorned*. London, n.d.; another London ed. in 1702, 382pp. The writer's interests focused upon physic and astrology; he found himself in heated and continual opposition to the Royal College of Physicians.

414. *Cursory Remarks on the New Pharmacopoeia. By Liquor Volatilis Cornu Cervi*. London, 1788. 28pp.

415. Curtis, William (1746-1799). *A Catalogue of the British Medicinal, Culinary, and Agricultural Plants, Cultivated in the London Botanic Garden*. London, 1783. 149pp. Initially apprenticed to an apothecary (his grandfather) in Hampshire, the writer developed an interest in botany before moving on to London to study medicine; he then

became a demonstrator of practical botany in various medical schools, pursued the study of insects, and in 1781 founded the Botanical Magazine.

416. Dale, Samuel (1659?-1739). Pharmacologia seu Manuductio ad Materiam Medicam. London, 1693; 2nd ed., 1710; 3rd ed., 1737; a supplement in 1705. The volume has been described as the first systematic work devoted to pharmacy; Dale practiced (1686) as a physician and apothecary at Braintree, Essex, presumably without degrees or licences in either of those sciences; however, he regularly contributed essays on medicine and biology to the Philosophical Transactions of the Royal Society.

417. Dossie, Robert (1717-1777). The Elaboratory Laid Open; or, the Secrets of Modern Chemistry and Pharmacy. London, 1758. 375pp.; 2nd ed., London, 1768. 456pp. Dossie published tracts on chemistry, surgery, and agriculture.

418. ____. Theory and Practice of Chirurgical Pharmacy. Dublin, 1761. 380pp.; London, 1761. 485pp.

419. Douglas, George (fl.1735-1763). An Essay on Fossil, Vegetable, and Animal Substances Used in Physick. London, 1735. The writer, an M.D., from Edinburgh, also published a tract (1763) on anatomy; compare this title with #434 below.

420. Dover, Thomas (1662-1742). Encomium Argenti Vivi: A Treatise upon the Use and Properties of Quicksilver. London, 1733. 64pp. Born in Warwickshire, Dover at one time had engaged in privateering as a surgeon; after being admitted (1721) a licentiate of the College of Physicians, he practiced medicine at London; he concocted "Dover's Powder," containing opium, ipecacuanha, and sulphate of potash; the record of his discovery, in 1709, of the shipwrecked Alexander Selkirk (1676-1721) emerged as one of the sources that provided Daniel Defoe with the model for his Robinson Crusoe (1719).

421. Duncan, Andrew (1744-1828). An Alphabetical List of the Materia Medica. Edinburgh, 1784. 32pp. Educated at St. Andrew's and Edinburgh (M.D. from the former in 1769), Duncan gained election, on no less than five occasions (beginning 1764), as president of the Royal Medical Society; he traveled to China as a surgeon for the East India Company; the Edinburgh College of Physicians granted him a license in 1770, after which he lectured at Edinburgh (1774-1776) and served there (from 1790) as professor of physiology; he founded a public dispensary and lunatic asylum at Edinburgh, as well as a number of major medical journals.

422. ____. Elements of Therapeutics. 2 vols. Edinburgh, 1773.

423. ____. Heads of Lectures on the Materia Medica. Edinburgh, 1786. 80pp.

424. Dwight, Samuel (1669?-1737). De Vomitione Ejusque Excessu Curando; nec non de Emeticis Medicamentis.

London, 1722. 73pp. A licentiate of the College of Physicians, London, Dwight claimed to have earned a medical degree, but the College never recognized his claim; he apparently established a relationship with Sir Hans Sloane, whom he consulted regarding "difficult" cases.
425. Eaton, Robert (1688?-1728). *An Account of Dr. Eaton's Styptick Balsam*. London, 1723. 71pp.; 2nd ed., London, 1726. 80pp.
426. *The Edinburgh New Dispensatory. . .being an Improvement on the New Dispensatory of Dr.* [William] *Lewis*. Edinburgh, 1786. 720pp.; further editions through 1796. For Lewis, see #465 and #466 below; Charles Webster (see #271 above) and Ralph Irving (see #455 and #456 below) edited the volumes for 1786-1789; Andrew Duncan (see #421 above) for 1790-1794; and John Rotheram (see #502 below) for 1796.
427. *An Essay on the Virtues, Uses, and Effects of Some Valuable Genuine Patent and Public Medicines*. London, 1792(?). 44pp.
428. Ferriar, John (1761-1815). *An Essay on the Medical Properties of the Digitalis Purpurea*. Manchester, 1799. 66pp. The writer studied medicine at Edinburgh (M.D., 1781), then practiced at Stockton-on-Tees and later at Manchester; in 1789 he became physician to the Manchester Infirmary, as well as an advocate of sanitary laws and working conditions for factory children; his interest in literature rivaled his work on medical history.
429. Fox, Edward. *Formulae Medicamentorum Selectae; or, Select Prescriptions*. London, 1777. 404pp.
430. Fuller, Thomas (1654-1734). *Pharmacopoeia Bateana*. London, 1718. Based upon the prescriptions of George Bate; see #372 above; born at Rosehill, Sussex, Fuller graduated M.B. and M.D. from Cambridge and practiced at Sevenoaks, Kent; in all, he published three collections of prescriptions.
431. ____. *Pharmacopoeia Domestica; or, The Family Dispensatory*. London, 1738. 231pp.
432. ____. *Pharmacopoeia Extemporanea; or, a Body of Medicines*. London, 1701. 512pp.; six eds. through 1731.
433. Gataker, Thomas (d.1769). *Observations on the Internal Use of the Solanum, or Nightshade*. London, 1757. 34pp.; four eds. in 1757. A London surgeon, Gataker published medical tracts consistently between 1749 and 1764.
434. Geoffrey, Francis. *A Treatise of the Fossil, Vegetable, and Animal Substances Made Use of in Physick*. London, 1735.
435. Gilchrist, Ebenezer (1707-1774). *On the Use of Sea Voyages in Medicine*. London, 1756. 144pp.; 2nd ed., with Supplement, London, 1757; 3rd ed., 1771; French translation in 1770. The work includes the full analysis of the benefits of exercise at sea and of the sea air, especially as they apply to the cure of consumption; the writer generally limits the focus to short voyages; born at Dumfries,

Gilchrist studied medicine at Edinburgh, London, Paris, and Rheims; he returned to Dumfries and remained to practice and to write; his specialties included investigation and even the revival of the medical treatments practiced by the Ancient physicians.

436. Glass, Samuel (fl.1746-1764). An Essay on Magnesia Alba. Oxford, 1764. 38pp. The writer an Oxford surgeon and a brother of Thomas Glass (see #923 below).

437. Goulard, Thomas. A Treatise on the Effects and Various Preparations of Lead. London, 1775.

438. Graham, James (1745-1794). A New and Curious Treatise of the Nature and Effects of Simple Earth, Water, and Air. London, 1793. 29pp. Born at Edinburgh, the writer studied medicine at the university there, but neither earned nor received the M.D. degree; he practiced at Pontefract, traveled to America (1771-1774), returned to England, and settled at Bristol; his reputation resulted from his "quack" cures, particularly "earth bathing," and from his his religious fervor that bordered upon lunacy.

439. _____. A Short Treatise on the All-Cleansing, All-Healing, and All-Invigorating Qualities of the Simple Earth. Newcastle-upon-Tyne, 1790. 21pp.

440. _____. A Sketch: or, Short Description of Dr. Graham's Medical Apparatus. London, 1780. 92pp.

441. Grant, Alexander. Observations on the Use of Opium. London, 1785. 41pp.

442. Gravere, Julius de. A Treasury of Choice Medicines. London, 1662.

443. Graves, Robert (1673-1849). A Pocket Conspectus of the New London and Edinburgh Pharmacopoeias. Sherborne, 1796. 112pp. Graves' several medical tracts reached publication between 1792 and 1797.

444. Greatrakes, Valentine (1629-1683). A Brief Account of Mr. Valentine Greatrak's [sic], and Divers of the Great and Strange Cures by Him lately performed. Written by Himself in a Letter Addressed to the Hon. Robert Boyle, Esq. Whereunto are annexed the Testimonials of Several Eminent and Worthy Persons of the Chief Matters of Fact therein Related. London, 1666. This work essentially serves as an autobiographical attempt to vindicate the writer's own reputation as a miraculous healer; thus, one discovers more than fifty testimonials from patients and persons of influence; prefixed to the volume rests an engraving of the writer stroking, with both hands, the head of a young boy; an Irishman from Waterford, Greatrakes resided as a country squire and magistrate until, following the Restoration of Charles II, he "discovered" his ability to cure people of the "King's evil" (scrofula); to that exercise he devoted three days of each week.

445. Harris, Thomas. A Treatise on the Force and Energy of Crude Mercury. London, 1732; further eds. in 1734,

further eds. in 1734, 1735.
446. Hawes, William (1736-1808). <u>An Account of the Late Dr.</u> [Oliver] <u>Goldsmith's Last Illness so far as it relates to the Exhibition of James Powders</u>. 3 parts. London, 1774. A native of and practitioner at London, Hawes earned a reputation for his attempts to revive persons apparently dead from drowning or asphyxia; he also founded the Royal Human Society; Goldsmith (1730?-1774), at the outset of his "last" illness, had been administering ipecacuanha to induce vomiting; then, contrary to the advice of his physicians (including Hawes), changed remedies in favor of Robert James' (1703-1776) fever powder; the <u>Account</u>, therefore, attempts to remove any form of "blame" cast upon Hawes and his colleagues who attended the novelist-playwright-poet-essayist during his illness and premature death; for Robert James, see #936 below).
447. Hay, Alexander. <u>Tyrocinium Pharmaceuticum</u>. Edinburgh, 1697.
448. Heberden, William the elder (1710-1801). <u>Antitheriaka. An Essay on Mithridatium and Theriaca</u>. London, 1745. 19pp. Identified by such among the <u>literati</u> as William Cowper, Samuel Johnson, and William Warburton as one of the more eminent and learned among the eighteenth-century English physicians, Heberden studied medicine at Cambridge and London; he also established a reputation as a classical scholar; <u>Mithridatium and Theriaca</u> emerged from his Cambridge lectures on <u>materia medica</u>.
449. Henry, Thomas (1734-1816). <u>An Account of the Medicinal Virtues of Magnesia Alba</u>. London, 1775. 29pp. Born at Wrexham and apprenticed to an apothecary there and to another such later at Oxford, the writer eventually (1764) moved to Manchester; there he acquired a surgery-apothecary business; by 1771, he had devoted himself to almost totally to the study of chemistry; he became a fellow of the Royal Society in 1775, having been recommended by Joseph Priestley; eventually, Benjamin Franklin sponsored Henry's election to membership in the American Philosophical Society.
450. Hill, Aaron (1685-1750). <u>An Account of the Rise and Progress of the Beech-Oil Invention</u>. London, 1715. 112pp. Essentially a collection of popular essays on this suspicious cure by the London playwright, poet, and miscellaneous writer; Hill had absolutely no medical competence or qualifications; after early education at Barnstaple Grammar School and Westminster School, he traveled (c.1700) to Constantinople and the East; he attempted--a quarter of a century before James Oglethorpe--to sponsor a colony at Georgia and involved himself in a literary relationship with Alexander Pope.
451. Hill, Daniel (fl.1795-1815). <u>Practical Observations on the Use of Oxygen, or Vital Air, in the Cure of Diseases</u>. London, 1800. 58pp. The writer held the

M.D. degree and appeared to focus his interests upon the medical application of oxygen.

452. Hill, Sir John (1716-1775). <u>Cautions against the Immoderate Use of Snuff: Founded on the known qualities of the Tobacco Plant. . .and enforced by instances of Persons who have perished. . .of Diseases occasioned by its Use.</u> London, 1759; another ed. in 1761. See, also, #140 above.

453. Howard, John (d.1811). <u>A Treatise on the Medical Properties of Mercury.</u> London, 1782. 120pp. The writer's various medical tracts appeared in print between 1782 and 1811.

454. Ingram, Dale (1710-1793). <u>An Enquiry into the Origin and Nature of Magnesia Alba.</u> London, 1767. 28pp. The writer began his medical practice at Reading in 1733; he spent from 1743 to 1750 on Barbados, then returned to England and practiced midwifery at London; he served, until 1791, as a surgeon at Christ's Hospital, London.

455. Irving, Ralph (fl.1780-1790). <u>The Edinburgh New Dispensatory.</u> Edinburgh, 1786. 720pp.

456. _____. <u>Experiments on the Red and Quill Peruvian Bark.</u> Edinburgh, 1785. 181pp.

457. Ixford, Noah. <u>On Purging.</u> London, 1690.

458. James, Samuel. <u>Observations on the Bark of a Particular Species of Willow, showing its Superiority to the Peruvian in the Cure of Agues.</u> London, 1792. 69pp.

459. Kennedy, Peter (fl.1710-1739). <u>An Essay on External Remedies.</u> London, 1715. 168pp. The writer's medical tracts appeared between 1713 and 1739.

460. Kentish, Richard (fl.1780-1790). <u>Experiments and Observations on a New Species of Bark.</u> London, 1784. 123pp. The writer held the M.D. degree.

461. Kettilby, Mary. <u>A Collection of above Three Hundred Receipts in Cookery, Physick, and Surgery.</u> 2 vols. London, 1718; six eds. through 1746.

462. Knight, Thomas (fl.1725-1750). <u>A Critical Dissertation upon the Manner of the Preparation of Mercurial Medicines, and their Operation on Human Bodies.</u> London, 1734. 64pp. The writer held the M.D. degree.

463. _____. <u>Reflections upon Catholicons, or Universal Medicines.</u> London, 1749. 167pp.

464. Layard, Daniel Peter (1721-1802). <u>Pharmacopoeia in usum Gravidarum Puerperarum.</u> London, 1776. The writer graduated M.D. from Rheims (1742), served at Middlesex Hospital, and eventually practiced medicine within the city of London; he became one of the founders of the British Lying-in Hospital.

465. Lewis, William (1714-1781). <u>An Experimental History of the Materia Medica, or of the Natural and Artificial Substances made use of in Medicine.</u> London, 1761; 2nd ed., 1768; 3rd ed., London, 1784; 4th ed., 2 vols., London, 1791; a German translation in 1771. Lewis received all of his degrees from Oxford (M.D. 1745), practiced medicine in London, and then moved to Kingston-upon-Thames;

he accepted, in 1767, a gold medal from the Society for the Improvement of Arts and Manufactures for an essay on potashes.
466. _____. The New Dispensatory. London, 1753; Edinburgh, 1781; Edinburgh, 1791.
467. Lowndes, Francis (fl.1785-1795). Observations on Medical Electricity. London, 1787. 51pp.
468. _____. The Utility of Medical Electricity. London, 1791. 46pp.
469. Magennis, James. "Medicinal Effects of Digitalis," The Medical and Physical Journal, 2 (1800). See, also, #2051 below; the writer held the M.D. degree.
470. Maywood, Robert. An Essay on the Operations of Mercury. London, 1787. 56pp. The writer held the M.D. degree and practiced in London.
471. Meyrick, William. The New Family Herbal; or, the Domestick Physician. Birmingham, 1790. 498pp.; another ed. at London, 1790.
472. Monk, Francis. Pharmicae Abregee. London, 1702.
473. Monro, Donald (1727-1802). A Treatise on Medical and Pharmaceutical Chemistry and the Materia Medica. 4 vols. London, 1788; 2nd ed., London, 1790. Monro, educated at Edinburgh, received appointment as a physician to the Royal Army; following his election to St. George's Hospital, he served abroad between 1760 and 1763; after returning to St. George's and a lengthy practice, he retired to Argyle.
474. Moore, James Carrick (1763-1834). An Essay on the Materia Medica. London, 1792. 330pp. Born at Glasgow, Moore studied medicine at Edinburgh and London; in 1792, he gained election to membership in the Corporation of Surgeons of London, after which he developed an interest in vaccination.
475. The New British Dispensatory. London, 1781. 173pp.
476. A New Collection of Medical Prescriptions, Distributed into Twelve Classes. London, 1791. 322pp.
477. A New Method for the Improvement of the Manufacture of Drugs. London, 1747. 80pp.
478. Nisbet, William (1759-1822). The Clinical Pharmacopoeia. London, 1800. 377pp. An Edinburgh physician and medical writer, Nisbet, at the beginning of the nineteenth century, settled in London; he had, previously, been elected a fellow of the Royal College of Surgeons, Edinburgh; he wrote on various diseases and composed guides for surgeons and physicians.
479. Norris, Thomas. A Short Essay on the Singular Virtues of an Highly Exalted Preparation of Antimony; or, Dr. Norris's Antimonial Drops. London, 1770. 16pp.
480. Northcote, William (d.1783). Methodus Praescribendi Exemplificata Pharmacopoeiis Noscomicorum. London and Edinburgh, 1772. This work exists, essentially, as a compendium of the pharmacopoeias of the hospitals at London, Edinburgh, Paris, and St. Petersburg, with the formulae employed by the English and Russian fleets and the British Army; a naval surgeon, Northcote wrote, principally, for

the guidance of his fellow naval surgeons, with emphasis upon diseases peculiar to tropical locales; such works tended to underscore the writer's own methods of treatment.

481. Norton, John. An Account of Remarkable Cures performed by the Use of Maredant's Antiscorbutic Drops. London, 1772. 29pp.; further eds. through 1774.

482. O'Ryan, Michael. A Letter on the Yellow Peruvian Bark. London, 1794. 31pp.

483. Payne, Thomas. An Essay on the Use of a New Poultice. London, 1796. The writer practiced surgery at London.

484. Pearson, Richard (1765-1836). A Short Account of the Nature and Properties of Different Kinds of Airs, so far as relates to their Medicinal Use. Birmingham, 1795. 27pp. A native of Birmingham and an M.D. from Edinburgh (1786), Pearson developed an interest in clinical experiments with electricity; after a European tour, he settled at Birmingham, where he became physician to the General Hospital (1792); in 1801, he moved to London, then on to Reading, Sutton Coldfield, and back to Birmingham.

485. Peart, Edward (1756?-1824). On Electricity. London, 1791. Peart practiced medicine at Knightsbridge, then at Butterwick, Lincolnshire; in his written work, he focused upon physical and chemical theory, the greatest portion of which proved unsound and stood far removed from the speculations and practices of his contemporaries.

486. Penrose, Francis (1718-1798). A Treatise on Electricity, wherein its various Phenomena are accounted for, and the Cause of Attraction and Gravitation of Solids Assigned, by Francis Penrose, Surgeon at Bicester, Oxfordshire. Oxford, 1752. Penrose wrote extensively on subjects related to medicine, including magnetism, blood circulation in animals, astronomy, and philosophy; he claimed to have earned the M.D. degree from "a German university."

487. Pharmacopoeia in Usum Nosocomii Bristoliensis. Bristol, 1785. 72pp.

488. Pitt, Robert (1653-1713). The Craft and Frauds of Physick Expos'd. London: Printed for Tim. Childe, 1702. 192pp. The writer taught anatomy at Oxford and received an appointment as physician to St. Bartholomew's Hospital, London (1698-1707); he wrote The Craft and Frauds to demonstrate the inexpensive costs of the "useful" drugs, the worthlessness of the expensive remedies, and the "folly" of indulging more than necessary in physic; the writer provides a clear exposition of the therapeutics of the day, tempered with his own medical observations; Timothy Childe operated two bookshops in St. Paul's Churchyard between 1690 and 1711.

489. Price, James (1752-1783). An Account of Some Experiments on Mercury, Silver, and Gold. Oxford,

1782. This work essentially a report of seven experiments similar with those conducted by the early alchemists; a member of the Royal Society, Price received the M.D. degree from Oxford in 1782, principally for his work in chemistry rather than in medicine; he committed suicide, shortly thereafter and having endured extreme ridicule, by swallowing a glass of "laurel water."

490. Quincy, John (d.1722). Pharmacopoeia Officimalis et Extemporanea; or, A Compleat English Dispensatory; in Four Parts. London, 1718; 4th ed., London, 1722; 12th ed., London, 1749; 14th ed., London, 1774. The work contains a complete account of the materia medica and of therapeutics; a number of the prescriptions remained popular through well into the nineteenth century; Quincy practiced medicine as an apothecary in London; a Dissenter and a Whig, he formed a friendship with Dr. Richard Mead; in addition to studying mathematics and Newtonian philosophy, he received the M.D. degree from Edinburgh in 1712.

491. Radcliffe, John (1650?-1714). Pharmacopoeia Radcliffiana; or, Dr. Radcliffe's Prescriptions, faithfully gathered from the Original Receipts. Oxford, 1716. This work published posthumously; born at Wakefield, Radcliffe studied medicine at Oxford (M.B. 1675, M.D. 1682), began his medical practice in that university town, and then (1684) moved on to London; he treated, among others, Princess Anne of Denmark, William III, the infant Duke of Gloucester (son of Princess Anne), Queen Mary, the Earl of Albermarle, and Prince George of Denmark (Anne's husband); Radcliffe gained the reputation as a competent physician who had achieved skill through actual medical practice, rather than by mere social or political acceptance.

492. _____. Pars Altera; or, The Second and Last Part of Dr. Radcliffe's Prescriptions, faithfully gathered. Oxford, 1716. Published posthumously.

493. Rand, Isaac (d.1743). Horti Medici Chelseiana Index Compendarius. London, 1739. This work essentially an alphabetical Latin listing extending to 214 pages; principally a botanist, Rand, by 1700, had established an apothecary practice in the Haymarket, London; nonetheless, he spent time studying "inconspicuous" plants in and about London, managing to "discover" several species; he rose to the directorship of the Chelsea Botanical Garden, and thus the primary reason for undertaking this 1739 Index.

494. _____. Index Plantarum Officinalium in Horto Chelseiano. London, 1730. This work published under the direction of the Society of Apothecaries, London.

495. Relph, John (d.1804). An Inquiry into the Medical Efficacy of a New Species of Peruvian Bark. London, 1794. 177pp. The writer held the M.D. degree; Peruvian bark (or the balsam of Peru) came

from trees of various species of cinchona; bitter in taste, it appeared to the eighteenth-century physicians as a potent tonic, principally the result of the alkaloids of cinchonia (producing a pale variety), quininia (yielding a yellow version), and their numerous compounds; it served, obviously, as a primitive form of quinine.

496. A Review of the London Dispensatory. Wherein are considered the Inconsistencies of Some Medicines and the Real Merit of Others. London, 1764. 69pp.

497. Reynolds, Thomas. Some Experiments on the Chalybeate Water, Lately Discovered near the Palace of the Lord Bishop of Rochester, at Bromley, in Kent. London, 1756. 69pp. Zachariah Pearce (1690-1774), known for his skill in homiletics and his scholarship, served as bishop of Rochester from 1756 until his death; chalybeate water tended to contain large quantities of iron.

498. Rigby, Edward (1747-1821). An Essay on the Use of the Red Peruvian Bark in the Cure of Intermittents. London, 1783. 107pp. Serving first as an apprentice to a Norwich surgeon, Rigby went on to study medicine at London; he then returned to Norwich and his own practice; after a tour of France (1789), he developed an interest in agriculture and began experiments on his own farm.

499. Robinson, Bryan (1680-1754). Observations on the Virtues and Operations of Medicines. Dublin, 1752. 216pp. An M.D. from Trinity College, Dublin (1711), the writer received appointments as anatomical lecturer (1716-1717) and professor of physic (1745) there; further appointments included fellow of the King's and Queen's College of Physicians in Ireland (1712), member of the Irish Royal College of Surgeons, and medical practitioner at Dublin; he attended Esther Vanhomrigh (Jonathan Swift's "Vanessa") and earned considerable recognition as a writer on mathematics and medicine.

500. Robinson, Nicholas (1697?-1775). A Treatise on the Virtues and Efficacy of a Crust of Bread Early in the Morning. London, 1756. A native of Wales, Robinson graduated M.D. from Rheims before beginning his practice at London; not until 1727 did he receive a license from the London College of Physicians.

501. Rose, Phillip. Iskhaimologia. Being an Historical, Rational, and Practical Account concerning a Celebrated Medicine Commonly Called Styptick. London, 1701. 105pp.

502. Rotherham, John (1750-1804). The Edinburgh New Dispensary. Edinburgh, 1794. Essentially a chemist and natural philosopher, Rotherham eventually attained the chair of natural philosophy at Edinburgh; he had studied at Upsula under Carl Linnaeus and Torbern Olaf Bergman.

503. Rowley, William (1742-1806). An Abstract of the Methods of Curing Diseases of the Eyes, Legs, and

Medicines, Cures, and Healing Agents 51

Breasts, and on the Cure of Cancerous, Scrophulous, and Other Chronic Diseases. London, 1774. 8pp. See, also, #222, above.

504. ____. The Most Cogent Reasons Why Astringent Injections, Caustic Bougies, and Violent Salivations should be banished for ever from Practice. London, 1800. 175pp.

505. Rushworth, John (1664-1736). Two Letters Showing the Great Advantage of Bark in Mortification. London, 1732. A surgeon, Rushworth gained recognition for discovering the effectiveness of chinchona bark in cases of gangrene, a notion that he conveyed to the Company of Barber-Surgeons for the benefit of the profession; he also ranks among the first of the medical practitioners to suggest the establishment of infirmaries and dispensaries in the center of every English county and town.

506. Rutty, John (1698-1775). An Account of the Experiments on Joanna Stephens's Medicine for the Stone. London, 1742. The first medical book published by the Quaker physician; see, also, #226 and #518.

507. ____. Observations on the London and Edinburgh Dispensatories. London, 1775; 2nd ed., London, 1776; another ed. in 1777.

508. Ryan, Michael (1760?-1823). An Essay on Peruvian Bark. London, 1794. An M.D. from Edinburgh and a fellow of the Irish College of Surgeons, the writer practiced medicine at Kilkenny, Edinburgh, and Dublin; he published a number of tracts on asthma and consumption.

509. Saffray, Henry (fl.1770-1790). The Ineffficacy of All Mercurial Preparations in the Cure of Venereal and Scorbutic Disorders. London, 1773; 2nd ed., London, 1776. The writer's theories and disagreements with his contemporaries earned for him a reputation for quackery.

510. Saunders, William (1743-1817). Observations on the Superior Efficacy of the Red Peruvian Bark in the Cure of Agues and Other Fevers. London, 1782. 158pp.; four eds. through 1783. Born at Banff, Saunders graduated M.D. from Edinburgh (1765) and practiced medicine at London; he published tracts on mercury, antimony, mephitic acid, mineral waters, colic, and the liver.

511. See, Thomas. An Essay on Internal Balsam. London, 1665.

512. Seymour, Thomas (fl.1770-1775). Poudre Unique, in the Cure of the Most Desperate Diseases. London, 1772; 2nd ed., London, 1774.

513. Shannon, Robert (fl.1790-1805). Practical Observations on the Operation and Effects of Certain Medicines. London, 1794. 558pp. The writer, an M.D., also published tracts on malt brewing.

514. Short, Thomas (1690?-1772). Medicina Botanica. London, 1745; 2nd ed., 1747; 3rd ed., 1751. A work on herbs and herbals for the general reader; Short

practiced medicine at Sheffield; he studied various cures for dysentery and toured Yorkshire to investigate the mineral springs there.

515. Skeete, Thomas (1757-1789). <u>Experiments and Observations on Quilled and Red Peruvian Bark</u>. London, 1786. 355pp. The British Museum houses a copy of this work; the writer held the M.D. degree.

516. Slare, Frederick (1647?-1727). <u>Experiments and Observations upon Oriental and Other Bezoar Stones</u>. London, 1715. 64pp. The writer attempts to disprove the assumed healing virtues of animal calculi (e.g. bezoar stone), a substance that sold for as high as four pounds per ounce; thus, he cites cases of their failures as healing agents when subjected to medical analysis; born in Northamptonshire, Slare rose to gain entrance into the Royal Society, the Royal College of Physicians, and Oxford University (M.D. 1680); his chemical experiments before the Royal Society attracted notice; he supposedly performed one on phosphorous after dinner at the home of Samuel Pepys (although his name does not appear in the two major editions of the latter's diaries).

517. Spire, John. <u>A Practical Treatise on the Natures of Several Medicines</u>. London, 1698.

518. Stephens, Joanna. <u>A Most Excellent Cure for the Stone and Gravel</u>. London, 1740. 12pp. See, also #506.

519. Storck, Anthony. <u>An Essay on the Medicinal Nature of Hemlock; translated from the Latin</u>. London, 1760.

520. Strother, Edward (1675-1737). <u>Pharmacopoeia Practica</u>. London, 1719. A native of Alnwick, Strother practiced medicine there; in 1720, he graduated M.D. from Utrecht, and a year later he gained a medical license from the London College of Physicians.

521. Swainson, Isaac (fl.1790-1800). <u>An Account of Cures by Velnos' Vegetable Syrup</u>. London, 1790. 151pp.

522. _____. <u>Mercury Stark Naked: Letters to Dr. [Thomas] Beddoes, Stripping that Poisonous Medicine of Its Pretensions</u>. London, 1797. See, also, #26, #376, #377.

523. Taube, William Dove. <u>Tartarologia Brevis: Medicines in the Tartar or Argol, with Its Preparations</u>. London, 1766.

524. Tauvry, Daniel (1669-1701). <u>A Treatise on Medicines</u>. London, 1700.

525. Theobald, John (d.1760). <u>Medulla Medicinae Universae; or, A New Compendous Dispensary</u>. London, 1747. 62pp.; seven eds. through 1771. An M.D., the writer specialized in producing popular medical guides.

526. Thompson, John Weeks. <u>The Poor Man's Medicine Chest; or, Thompson's Box of Antibillious Alterative Pills</u>. London, 1791. 36pp.

527. Tickell, William. <u>A Concise Account of a New Chymical Medicine, entitled Spiritus Aethereus Anodynus</u>. Bath, 1787. 179pp.; 2nd ed., Bath, 1788. 380pp.

528. Trinder, William Martin (fl.1780-1805). <u>An Essay on</u>

Medicines, Cures, and Healing Agents

the Application of Oils to the Human Body. London, 1787. An M.D., the writer published tracts on a variety of subjects, including English grammar, mineral waters, sermons, the New Testament parables, bathing with oils, and military matters.

529. Turnbull, William (1729?-1796). A Letter to Mr. [Peter] Clare on Mercury. London, 1783. Turnbull studied at Edinburgh and Glasgow, later settling in Northumberland and serving as a physician to the Bramborough Infirmary; in 1777, he moved to London; see, also, #401.

530. Vaughan, Walter (1766-1828). Evidence of the Supreme Efficacy of the Yellow Bark. London, 1795. An M.D. from Edinburgh, the writer practiced at Rochester and wrote tracts on anatomy, physiology, and the philosophy of medicine.

531. Wall, Martin (1747-1824). Clinical Observation of the Use of Opium in Low Fevers, with Remarks on the Epidemic [of typhus] Fever at Oxford in 1785. Oxford, 1786; 2nd ed., Oxford, 1786. After earning four degrees from Oxford, Wall studied medicine at St. Bartholomew's Hospital, London; he then continued his work at Edinburgh; while practicing medicine at Oxford, he received an appointment to the Radcliffe Infirmary and served as a reader in chemistry there; in 1785, he gained election as Lichfield professor of clinical medicine.

532. Watson, Sir William (1715-1787). Electricity Applied to Tetanus. London, 1763. Prior to his having been created doctor of physic both at Halle and Wittemberg (1757), Watson had gained attention as an apothecary and for his study of an experiments in botany; he practiced medicine at London, but his interest and labors turned toward electricity and botany; his principal medical writings focus upon various epidemics.

533. Webster, Charles (1750-1795), and Ralph Irving (fl.1780-1790). Edinburgh New Dispensatory. Edinburgh, 1786. See, also, #271, #426, #455; both writers held the M.D. degree from Edinburgh.

534. Wesley, John (1703-1791). A Collection of Receits for the Use of the Poor. Bristol, 1745. A seventeen-page, two-penny tract by the founder and leader of the Methodists; the work intended to disseminate the writer's medical empirics to his followers throughout the British Isles; Wesley's more popular Primitive Physick (1747) actually an expansion of this document; see, above #226.

535. White, Robert (fl.1775-1800). An Analysis of the New London Pharmacopoeia. London, 1792. The writer, an M.D., published tracts on such topics as sea water, surgery, and hydrophobia.

536. White, William (of Bath; fl.1795-1815). Observations and Experiments on Broad-Leaved Willow Bark. London, 1798. 58pp. A Bath surgeon, White also published tracts on billious fever, diseases of the liver, and the intestines.

537. White, William (of York; 1744-1790). Observations on

the Use of Dr. [Robert] James's Fever Powder. London, 1774. 194pp. The writer held the M.D. degree, practiced medicine at York, and published a variety of medical tracts between 1775 and 1782; see, also, #936.

538. Whytt, Robert (1714-1766). An Essay on the Virtues of Lime Water and Soap in the Cure of the Stone. Edinburgh, 1752; 2nd ed., Edinburgh, 1754; 3rd ed., Edinburgh, 1761; French and German translations. Born at Edinburgh, Whytt studied at St. Andrews and Edinburgh before moving on to London; there, he studied medicine and toured the hospitals with William Cheselden (see #301), eventually leaving for France and Holland, as well as to earn the M.D. degree from Rheims in 1736; returning to Edinburgh, Whytt rose to become president of the Royal College of Physicians and to earn appointment as professor of the theory of medicine at Edinburgh.

539. Wilkinson, Charles Hunnings (1763-1850). The Effects of Electricity in Paralytic and Rheumatic Affections. London, 1799. 220pp. An M.D., the writer published tracts on the relationship between physiology and philosophy, the Leyden phial, venereal diseases, and galvanism; he also lectured on experimental philosophy.

540. _____. An Essay on the Leyden Phial. London, 1798. The tract concerns the electrical apparatus that later came to be known as the "Leyden jar."

541. Willis, Thomas (1621-1675). Pharmaceutice Rationalis. Oxford, 1674. After receiving the M.B. degree from Oxford (1646), Willis practiced medicine in that town until 1664, when he removed to London; his experiments in brain dissection led to (then) accurate descriptions of the nervous system, which established his reputation and led to his large practice; he has received credit for the discovery of diabetes mellitus and for his pioneering work on the effects of sugar within the body.

542. Wilson-Philip, Alexander Philip (1770?-1851?). An Experimental Essay on the Manner in Which Opium Acts on the Living Animal Body. Edinburgh, 1795. Wilson-Philip graduated M.D. from Edinburgh; he practiced medicine at Edinburgh, Winchester, Worcester, and London; while engaged in practice, he devoted time to extensive research in physiology and pathology, eventually becoming the first investigator to rely upon a microscope to study inflammation.

543. Withering, William (1741-1799). An Account of the Foxglove [Digitalis] and Some of Its Medical Uses. Birmingham, 1785. An M.D. graduate from Edinburgh (1766), Withering devoted himself to the studies of chemistry, anatomy, and botany; in addition to his medical practice at Stafford, Birmingham, and then London, he engaged in plant collection and chemical research; he also contributed papers on mineralogy to the Philosophical Transactions of the Royal Society; as a result of this Account, the action of

Medicines, Cures, and Healing Agents

digitalis in dropsy and on the heart became generally recognized.

544. ____. <u>A Botanical Arrangement of all the Vegetables naturally growing in Great Britain</u>. 2 vols. Birmingham, 1776. This volume stands as the writer's principal written work, the first of its kind in Great Britain to rely upon the Linnaean binomial nomenclature (the identification of plants by a second, or "trivial" name in addition to the generic label); the popularity of the text held for a century, as witnessed by the publication of the fourteenth edition in 1877.

545. Wood, Loftus (fl.1770-1785). <u>Observations on a New and Easy Method of Curing Disorders by Factitious Air, without the Use of Drugs</u>. London, 1780. 31pp. The writer held the M.D. degree; in addition to his own work in medicine, surgery, and anatomy, he translated the <u>Proceedings</u> (1666-1776) of the Royal Academy of Sciences at Paris.

546. Wright, William (1735-1819). <u>An Account of the Medicinal Plants Growing in Jamaica</u>. London, 1787. Born in Perthshire. Wright studied at Edinburgh before going to sea--first aboard a whaler, then on several naval vessels--as a ship's surgeon; in 1763, he graduated (<u>in absentia</u>) M.D. from St. Andrews, after which he ventured to Jamaica; there, he began an herbarium and engaged in experimentation relative both to botany and medicine; he also advocated cold water treatment for fevers; after brief periods in Edinburgh and London, he returned to Jamaica as a surgeon to an army regiment, then finally returned to and settled in the Scottish capital.

547. Young, George (fl.1750-1760). <u>A Treatise on Opium, founded upon Practical Observations</u>. London, 1753; German translation at Bayreuth in 1760. The writer held the M.D. degree.

548. Young, James (fl.1675-1713). <u>An Essay on the Admirable Virtues of Oleum Terebinthinae</u>. London, 1679. The writer practiced surgery at Plymouth.

549. ____. <u>Currus Triumphalis e Terebintho</u>. London, 1679; Amsterdam, 1698. The original version of #548.

IV

Waters

A. Mineral Water

550. Alexander, William (d.1783). <u>Plain and Easy Directions for the Use of Harrowgate Waters</u>. Edinburgh, 1773. 92pp.; 2nd ed. York, 1780. An M.D., Alexander published his medical tracts at London and Edinburgh between 1767 and 1779.
551. Allen, Benjamin (1663-1738). <u>The Natural History of the Chalybeat and Purging Waters of England, with their Particular Essayes and Uses. To Which are added some Observations on the Bath Waters</u>. London, 1699. The writer's various tracts on mineral waters appeared at London between 1689 and 1711.
552. _____. <u>A Natural History of the Mineral Waters of Great Britain</u>. London, 1711. 104pp. Another version of #551.
553. _____. <u>A Treatise on Mineral Waters</u>. London, 1689.
554. Andree, John (1669?-1785). <u>An Account of the Tilbury Water</u>. London, n.d.; five eds. through 1781. See, also, #366. Situated in Essex, Tilbury had (or has) little or nothing to recommend it in terms of literary, historical, or scientific significance.
555. Ash, John (1723-1798). <u>Experiments and Observations to Investigate by Chemical Analysis the Medicinal Properties of the Mineral Waters of Spa and Aix-la-Chapelle. . .and of the Waters of Boue, near St. Armand</u>. London, 1788. 400pp. Born in Warwickshire, Ash received bachelor, master, and M.D. degrees from Oxford, after which he settled and practiced at Birmingham; in 1787, he moved on to London; he served the College of Physicians as censor and as Harveian orator, Gulstonian lecturer, and Croonian lecturer.
556. Baylies, William (1724-1787). <u>Practical Reflections on the Uses and Abuses of Bath Waters</u>. London, 1757. A native of Worcestershire and an M.D.

Mineral Water (contd.)

graduate of Aberdeen, the writer practiced medicine at Bath and, after a dispute with the principal physicians of that city (1757), he moved to London and received an appointment to the Middlesex Hospital; financial problems caused him to flee to Berlin, where he died; the Reflections had plunged had into a debate with two Bath physicians, a circumstance that ruined his medical practice.

557. ____. Short Remarks on Dr. [Charles] Perry's Analysis Made on the Stratford Mineral Water. Stratford-on-Avon, 1745; another ed. in 1748. See, also, #624.

558. Bevis, John (1693-1771). An Experimental Enquiry concerning the Contents, Qualities, and Medicinal Virtues, of the Two Mineral Waters Lately Discovered at Bagnigge Wells, near London. London, 1760. 61pp.; 2nd ed., enlarged, London, 1767. Although a serious and legitimate student of medicine, Bevis proved that his real interests resided with astronomy, as witnessed by his discovery of the great comet of 1744; the writer held the B.A. and M.A. from Oxford, but no evidence exists that he had prepared for or had earned the M.D. degree; one of the most popular of the eighteenth-century spas, Bagnigge Wells (named for a prominent local family), off King's Cross Road, London, gained fame during the Restoration, when the actress Nell Gwynne entertained Charles II with breakfasts and concerts; in 1757, the place came under the ownership of a tobacconist, Thomas Hughes, who asked Bevis to determine why flowers would not grow in his garden; the latter discovered that the well water contained undue quantities of iron, but a second well yielded water that proved a strong purgative; in 1758, Hughes opened the gardens daily, charged 3d per taste of the water, and then constructed a banquet hall and developed a skittle alley, bowling green, grotto, flower garden, fish pond, fountain, and formal walks; a song published in the London Magazine for 1759 begins,
> Ye gouty old souls and rheumaticks crawl on,
> Here taste these blest springs, and your
>   tortures are gone;
> Ye wretches asthmatick, who pant for your
>   health,
> Come drink your relief, and think not of
>   death.
> Obey the glad summons, to Bagnigge repair,
> Drink deep of its streams, and forget all
>   your care.

The establishment closed in 1841 (see Ben Weintraub and Christopher Hibbert [eds.], The London Encyclopaedia [Bethesda, Maryland: Adler and Adler, 1986] 320).

559. Boyle, Robert (1627-1691). Short Memoirs for the History of Mineral Waters. London, 1684. The

Mineral Water (contd.)

Irish physicist and chemist, among his varied interests, carried forth work on subjects related to medicine; most important, he became one of the first members of the "invisible college," an association of Oxford intellectuals opposed to the prevalent doctrines of scholasticism; that group emerged, as early as 1645, as the Royal Society.

560. Brown, Joseph (fl.1700-1721). An Account of the Wonderful Cures Perform'd by the Cold Baths. London, 1704. 144pp. Brown (or Browne) held the M.D. degree and lectured at London on anatomy and "modern" physick.

561. Carrick, Andrew (fl.1795-1805). Dissertation on the Chemical and Medical Properties of the Bristol Hotwell Water. Bristol, 1797. 167pp. The writer held the M.D. degree.

562. Chapman, Henry. Thermae Redivivae: the City of Bath Described, with Some Observations on those Soveraign Waters, both as to the Bathing in them, and Drinking of them, now so much in Use. London, 1673. This tract runs to twenty-three pages, including title page and two dedications.

563. Charleton, Rice (1710-1789). A Chymical Analysis of the Bath Waters, containing an Account of the Mineral Substances which the Bath Waters bring up with them out of the Earth. Bath, 1750; 2nd ed., Bath, 1775; 3rd ed., Bath, 1776. This title, representing the first part of #565, describes a series a series of experiments to determine the mineral properties of the thermal springs at Bath; essentially, the work follows the chemical system and scientific principles developed by Hermann Boerhaave; educated at Oxford (M.A., M.B., M.D.), Charleton practiced medicine at Bath; he belonged to the London College of Physicians and gained election (1747) as a fellow of the Royal Society.

564. ____. An Inquiry into the Efficacy of Warm Bathing in Palsies. Oxford, 1770. 99pp. Originally published in 1757; the second part of #565.

565. ____. Three Tracts on Bath Waters: 1. A Chemical Analysis of Bath Waters [1750]. 2. An Inquiry into the Efficacy of Bath Water in Palsies [1757]. 3. Histories of Hospital Cases under the Care of Dr. [William] Oliver, with Cases and Notes by the Editor. Bath, 1774. See, also #563, #564, #676.

566. ____. A Treatise on the Bath Waters. Bath, 1754. 74pp.

567. Claramont, Charles. De Aere, locis et et aquis Angliae deque Morbis Anglorum Vernaculis. Dissertatione nec non Observationes Medicae Cambro-Britannicae. London, 1672. The writer held the M.D. degree.

568. Crane, John. An Essay on Nottingham Mineral Water. London, 1790. The writer held the M.D. degree.

569. Davidson, Samuel (fl.1790-1800). The History and Obvious Properties of Wingate Spaw. London, 1792.

Mineral Water (contd.)

84pp.

570. De Castro, Tomasso. On the Use and Abuse of Mineral Waters in England. London, 1756. An Italian text with the title page in English.

571. Denman, Joseph. Observations on the Effects of Buxton Waters. London, 1793. 144pp. The writer held the M.D. degree.

572. Derham, Samuel (1655-1689). Hydrologia Philosophica; or, an Account of Ilmington Waters in Warwickshire, with Directions for Drinking of the Same. Oxford, 1685. A native of Gloucestershire, Derham graduated M.D. from Oxford in 1687; he practiced medicine at Oxford, where he died (suddenly and prematurely) from smallpox; his Hydrologia describes the chalybeate waters at Ilmington and sets forth the writer's own recommendations of that element as a cure for scrofula.

573. Dove, William Taube (fl.1755-1795). A Short Account of Several Excellent Medicines lately discovered in the Argol or Tartar. 2 parts. London, 1755-1757; four eds. through 1766.

574. Elliott, Sir John (1736-1786). An Account of the Nature and Medicinal Virtues of the Principal Mineral Waters of Great Britain and Ireland. London, 1781. 236pp.; 2nd ed., London, 1789. 296pp. The writer, born at Edinburgh and graduated (1759) M.D. from St. Andrews, became a physician to the Prince of Wales.

575. Experimental Observations on the Water of the Mineral Spring near Islington, commonly called New Tunbridge Wells. London, 1773. 42pp. Also known as Islington Spa, New Tunbridge Wells lay opposite Sadler's Wells; its popularity began in 1684, when Robert Boyle analyzed the water there and determined that it contained "medicinal properties"; one eighteenth-century pamphlet praised "the gardens' beauties and the waters' cures for Hysterics, Vapours, Dropsies, and Swellings of the Legs, Rheumatism, Scurvy, Jaundice . . .Want of Digestion, Gravel, Gout, Strangury . . ." (see Ben Weintraub and Christopher Hibbert [eds.], The London Encyclopaedia [Bethesda, Maryland: Adler and Adler, 1986] 414).

576. Eyre, Henry . An Account of the Mineral Waters of Spa. London, 1733. 36pp.

577. _____. A Brief Account of the Holt Waters. . .(near Bath) in Wiltshire. London, 1771. 155pp.

578. Falconer, William (1744-1824). An Account of the Efficacy of the Aqua Mephitica Alkalina in Calculous Disorders and in Various Kinds of Paralytic Disorders. Bath, 1787; 2nd ed., London, 1787; 3rd ed., London, 1789; 4th ed. (with additions), London, 1792; 5th ed., London, 1798. A native of Chester, Falconer earned M.D. degrees from Edinburgh (1766) and Leyden (1767); he served at Chester Infirmary before moving on to Bath, at

Mineral Water (contd.)

which town he gained election to the Bath General Hospital; he achieved considerable reputation as a physician, a scholar, and a writer of miscellaneous prose (particularly in the areas of natural history and theology).

579. _____. An Account of the Use, Application, and Success of the Bath Waters in Rheumatic Cases. Bath, 1795.

580. _____. An Essay on the Bath Waters, in four parts, containing a Prefatory Introduction on the Study of Mineral Waters in General. 2 vols. London, 1770; 2nd ed., 1772. The writer's first published work, dedicated to Dr, John Fothergill (see #112).

581. Floyer, Sir John (1649-1734). An Enquiry into the Right Use of Baths. London, 1697. Later editions published under various titles: The Ancient Pyschrolusia Revived (London, 1702; 1706), A History of Hot and Cold Bathing (London, 1709; 1715; 1722; Manchester, 1794; German ed., Breslau, 1749; Latin eds., Leyden, 1699, and Amsterdam, 1718); see, also, #106.

582. _____. A Letter on Bathing to Dr. Joseph Browne's Account of Cures performed by Cold Baths. London, 1707. See, also, #560.

583. Fothergill, Anthony (1732?-1813). A New Experimental Inquiry into the Nature and Qualities of the Cheltenham Water. Bath, 1785. 71pp.; another ed., Bath, 1788. 122pp. Born in Yorkshire, Fothergill studied medicine at Edinburgh (M.D. 1763), after which he practiced at Northampton; in 1774, he gained appointments as a physician to the Northampton Infirmary and as a licentiate of the College of Physicians; he moved to London in 1780, to Bath in 1784, Philadelphia (1803), and back to London (1812); his interests extended beyond medicine into such areas as chemical analysis.

584. Garnett, Thomas (1766-1802). Experiments and Observations on the Crescent Water at Harrogate. Leeds, 1791. 69pp. This publication reveals the first scientific analysis of the waters at Harrogate, in the North Riding of Yorkshire; a physician and natural philosopher, Garnett studied chemistry and physics prior to completing his medical education at London (M.D. 1788); he contributed a treatise on optics to the Encyclopaedia Britannica, lectured on medicine and philosophy at Manchester and Glasgow, and found the time to publish (1800) a two-volume account of his tour of the Scottish Highlands and the western islands of Scotland.

585. _____. Experiments and Observations on the Horley-Green Spaw. Bradford, 1790.

586. _____. A Treatise on the Mineral Waters of Harrogate. London, 1792. 168pp.; three eds. through 1799. This work an expansion of #584.

587. Gibbes, Sir George Smith (1771-1851). A Treatise on the Bath Waters. London, 1800. 71pp.; 2nd ed.

Mineral Water (cont.)

entitled Comprehending the Medicinal Powers of the Bath Waters in General, and particularly as they relate to the Cure of Dyspepsia, Gout, Rheumatism, and Liver Complaints, Chlorosis, Cutaneous Eruptions, and Palsy. London, 1803; alternate ed., 1812(?). Gibbes graduated M.D. from Oxford in 1799 and began to practice medicine at Bath; a physician to the Bath Hospital, he also served as a physician extraordinary to Queen Charlotte.

588. Graham, James (1745-1794). A New, Plain, and Rational Treatise on the True Nature and Uses of the Bath Waters. Bath, 1789. 48pp. See, also, #438 above.

589. Guidott, Thomas (b.1638; fl. 1698). A Collection of Treatises concerning the City and Waters of Bath. Bath, 1725. 430pp. A translation of #591 below by Henry Chapman (see, also #562); born at Lymington, Hampshire, Guidott studied medicine at Oxford (M.B. 1666); he practiced at Bath and London, his contemporaries labeling him "an ingenious, but vain, conceited, and whimsical physician"; the majority of his publications focus upon waters and bathing.

590. ____. A Discourse of Baths, and the Hot Waters There. Also Some Enquiries into the Nature of the Water at St. Vincent's Rock, near Bristol, and that of Castle Cary. To which is added, A Century of Observations, more fully declaring the nature, property, and distinction of the Baths. With an Account of the Lives and Character of the Physicians of Bath. London, 1676-1677.

591. ____. Observationes in Thermas Bathonienses. London, 1691.

592. ____. Thomae Guidotti. . .De Thermis Britannicis. 2 parts. London, 1691.

593. Haworth, Samuel (fl.1680-1685). A Description of the Dukes Bagnio and Mineral Bath, and Spaw. London, 1683. The writer describes a Turkish bath at Long Acre, at which the attendants practiced "rubbing," poured artificial mineral waters into the ground, and forced the water to issue forth; Haworth claimed to have studied physic, attended Cambridge, and earned the M.D. degree at Paris; however, no evidence of those accomplishments exists; he also produced and sold suspicious and useless tablets and solutions to cure various ailments.

594. Hemming, John. Observations upon the Mineral Waters of Gloucester. London, 1789. The writer did hold the M.D. degree.

595. Hillary, William (d.1763). An Inquiry into the Contents and Medicinal Virtues of Libscomb Spaw Water. London, 1742. 72pp. An M.D., the writer published tracts on a variety of medical subjects between 1735 and 1761.

596. Home, Francis (1719-1813). An Essay on the Contents and Virtues of Dunse-Spaw. Edinburgh, 1751. 216pp. An M.D., the writer served as professor of materia

Mineral Water (contd.)

medica at Edinburgh; in addition to his publications on medicine, he achieved a reputation as the first person to consider agriculture as a science.

597. Horsburgh, William. Experiments and Observations upon the Hartfell Spaw. Edinburgh, 1754. 80pp. The writer held the M.D. degree.

598. Hunter, Alexander (1729-1809). A Treatise on the Nature and Virtues of Buxton Waters. London, 1761. 68pp.; five editions through 1793. A native of Edinburgh and an M.D., the writer settled and practiced at York; in addition to his works on medicine, geography, and agriculture, he published (1776) an edition of John Evelyn's Sylva; or, a Discourse of Forest Trees, and the Propagation of Timber in His Majesty's Dominions (1664).

599. King, John (1696-1728). An Essay on Hot and Cold Bathing. London, 1727. 172pp. Essentially a translator and classical scholar, King did practice medicine successfully at Stamford, Lincolnshire; he never earned the M.D. degree; he also published an English grammar (1716) and wrote an epistle to Dr. John Freind (see #115).

600. Kirwan, Richard (1733-1812). An Essay on the Analysis of Mineral Waters. London, 1799. This work proved valuable in terms of its information and suggested methods; a native of Galway, Ireland, the writer achieved a reputation as a chemist and natural philosopher; he served as president of the Royal Irish Academy, presided over the Dublin Library, founded the Kirwanian Societies, and belonged to the Edinburgh Royal Society; such subjects as mining, bleaching, the chemistry of soils, and the weather occupied his interests and constituted the substances of his various publications.

601. Layard, Daniel Peter (1721-1802). An Account of the Somersham Water in the County of Huntingdon. London, 1767. See, also, #464.

602. Leigh, Charles (1662-1702?). Exercitationes Quinque, de Aquis Mineralibus; Thermis Calidis; Morbis Acutis; Morbis Intermittentib; Hydrope. London, 1697. Leigh graduated M.D. from Cambridge in 1689, practiced medicine at London, moved to Manchester, and then established an extensive medical practice throughout Lancashire; he regularly read papers before the Royal Society and published (1684-1702) in that institute's Philosophical Transactions; he also wrote (published 1705) a history of the Virginia colony.

603. Linden, Diederick Wessel (fl.1745-1770). A Reply to Dr. [Charles] Lucas's Remarks on [Alexander] Sutherland's Treatise on Bath and Bristol Waters. Bath, 1764. See, also, # 606 and #607. The writer held the M.D. degree; he published (at London), between 1751 and 1769, tracts on various aspects of mineral waters.

Mineral Water (contd.)

604. _____. A Treatise on Chalybeat Waters and Natural Hot Baths, with an Appendix on Selter Water, Liquid Shell, and the Glastonbury Waters. London, 1748; 2nd ed., London, 1752; another ed., 1755.

605. Lister, Martin (1638?-1712). De Thermis et Fontibus Medicatis Angliae. London, 1684; Frankfurt-am-Main, 1684; Leipzig, 1684; another ed., London, 1689. Interested principally in the natural sciences, Lister did study medicine in France; he spent time in York investigating natural history and antiquity before moving on to London and receiving an M.D. from Oxford in 1684; in 1660, he had been appointed a fellow of St. John's College, Cambridge.

606. Lucas, Charles (1713-1771). An Analysis of [Dr. John] Rutty's Synopsis of Mineral Waters. London, 1757. An extremely controversial pamphlet, relative to Rutty's own examination of Lucas's analysis of mineral waters (see #226 and #637); born in County Clare, Ireland, Lucas developed an interest in pharmacy, which in turn led him to Dublin politics; thus, the cause of Irish liberty and independence became his principal focus; however, toward the end of his career he turned to medicine, graduating M.D. from Leyden in 1752; after visiting the baths at Spa and Aachen, he proceeded to Bath and conducted experiments on the waters as a cure; Lucas also practiced medicine in London for a brief period before again turning his attention toward politics.

607. _____. Remarks on A[lexander]. Sutherland's Method of Investigating the Bath and Bristol Waters. Bath, 1764. Sutherland (fl. 1755-1765; see # 603, #651, #652) attempted to revive certain theories and doctrines of the Ancients relative to mineral waters as a cure.

608. Lysons, Daniel (1727-1800). A Treatise on Bath Waters, appended to the Author's "Farther Observations on Camphire and Calomel." Bath, 1777. 93pp. Lysons practiced medicine at the Gloucester Infirmary before moving to Bath; in 1780, he gained election as a physician to the Bath General Hospital; his medical treatises appeared regularly between 1769 and 1777; he held the M.D. degree.

609. Madan, Patrick. Observations and Experiments on the Tunbridge Waters. London, 1687.

610. Manning, Martin. De Aquis Mineralibus. London, 1746.

611. Maplet, John (1612?-1670). Epistolae Medicinales Specimen de Thermarum Bathoniensium Effectis, ed. Thomas Guidott, with three plates. London, 1694. This work dedicated to the leading contemporary physicians; Maplet practiced at Bath in the summer and in Bristol during the winter; he graduated M.D. from Oxford in 1647 and immediately thereafter traveled about Europe as tutor to the third Earl of

Mineral Water (contd.)

Falkland; Guidott (b. 1638; fl.1668-1705) held the M.D. and published a number of tracts upon the effects of the waters at Bath and Islington; his collected works appeared at Bath in 1725; see, also, #589.

612. Meade, William (fl.1785-1805). A Dissertation upon Mineral Water. Edinburgh, 1790; the original text written in 1790 in Latin; The writer, an M.D. from Dublin, resided in that city.

613. Medley, John. Tentamen Hydrologicum; or, an Essay upon Matlock-Bath, in Derbyshire. Nottingham, 1730. 92pp. Whatever natural baths lay in this area gave way--in terms of historical note--to Masson Mills (a mile south of Matlock Bath), a six-story red-brick cotton textile mill, one of Great Britain's earliest and finest factories owned by Sir Richard Arkwright (1732-1792).

614. Meighan, Sir Christopher (fl.1740-1760). A Treatise on the Nature and Power of Bareges's Baths and Waters in the Cure of Wounds. London, 1742. 146 pp.; a new ed. at London, 1764. 222pp.

615. Moncreiff, John. An Inquiry into the Medicinal Qualities and Effects of the Aerated Alkaline Water. Edinburgh, 1794. 205pp.

616. Monro, Alexander the elder (1697-1767). A Treatise on Mineral Waters. 2 vols. London, 1760. See #1009.

617. Monro, Donald (1720-1802). A Treatise on Mineral Waters. 2 vols. London, 1770. This work provides an account of all English, Scottish, and Irish mineral and bath waters; see, also, #473 above.

618. Nessel, Edmund. An Essay on Waters of the Spa. London, 1715. The writer held the M.D. degree.

619. Nicholls, William (1664-1712). God's Blessing on the Use of Mineral Waters. London, 1702. 22pp. The writer (his name also spelled Nichols) served as a fellow of Merton College, Oxford (1684); rector of Selsey, Sussex (1691); a learned divine (but not a medical "professional"), he published a number of theological works between 1698 and 1712.

620. Nott, John (1751-1825). Of the Hotwell Waters near Bristol. Bristol, 1793. 94pp. Born at Worcester, Nott studied surgery at Birmingham, London, and Paris; he resided at Paris (1775-1777), London (1777-1783), and then traveled as a surgeon to the East India Company; initially, he acquired an interest in Persian studies, and not until 1789 did he seek admittance to the London College of Physicians; eventually, he settled in Bristol, where he wrote poetry, prose fiction, medical tracts, and scholarly textual studies.

621. Oliver, William (1658-1716). A Practical Dissertation on Bath Waters, to which is added a Relation of a very extraordinary Sleeper near Bath. Bath, 1707. 136pp.; five eds. through 1764. A native of Cornwall, Oliver studied physic at Leyden, but then departed to participate in the European wars; he

Mineral Water (contd.)

spent the period 1702-1709 at London and Bath; from there he served as physician to the hospital at Chatham and then to the Royal Hospital at Greenwich.

622. Owen, William. An Account of the Nature, Properties, and Uses of All the Remarkable Mineral Waters of Great Britain. London, 1769. This compilation contains brief descriptions of more than ninety British mineral spas, a number of them not being (during the eighteenth century) generally known.

623. Pearson, George (1751-1828). Observations and Experiments for Investigating the Chymical History of the Tepid Springs of Buxton. 2 vols. London, 1783; another ed., London, 1785. This work resulted from the writer's six-year residence at Doncaster, during which he demonstrated that nitrogen appeared to be the gas rising from the waters at Buxton; Pearson studied chemistry and medicine at Edinburgh (M.D. 1773), then continued his work at St. Thomas's Hospital, London; later (1775-1777), he toured France, Germany, and Holland before settling at Doncaster; in 1787, he became a physician to St. George's Hospital, where he lectured on chemistry, the practice of physic, and the materia medica.

624. Perry, Charles (1698-1780). An Enquiry in the Nature and Principles of the Spaw Waters. To Which is subjoined a Cursory Inquiry into the Nature and Properties of the Hot Fountains at Aix-la-Chapelle. London, 1734. Perry, born at Norwich, graduated (1727) M.D. from Cambridge; after a period of travel (1739-1742) throughout Europe, as well as the experience of publishing narratives relative to those journeys, he settled in to the practice of medicine.

625. "Philander, Eugenius." A Quaere concerning Drinking Bath-Water Resolved. London, 1673.

626. Pierce, Robert (1622-1710). Bath Memoirs, or, Observations in Three-and Forty Years' Practice at the Bath. Bristol, 1697; 2nd ed. retitled History and Memoirs of the Bath Cures Wrought by the Waters . . . [with an] Account of King Baldud, the Founder. London, 1713. A native of Somerset and an M.D. graduate from Oxford in 1661, Pierce practiced first in Somerset and then at Bath; his patients included members of the military and the nobility; he appears to have been the first English medical writer to note the occurrence of acute rheumatism as a sequel to scarlet fever and to describe the lympho-sarcoma of the pericardium; Raphael Holinshed, in his Chronicles (1587), identified Baldud as the father of King Lear.

627. Plot, Robert (1640-1696). De Origine Fontium Tentamen Philosophicum. In Praelectione Habita Coram Societate Pholosophica nuper Oxonii Instituta ad Scientiam Naturalem Promovendam. Oxford, 1685.

Mineral Water (contd.)

Plot's interests in chemistry and antiquity brought him into associations with the Royal Society, the Ashmolean Museum, and Oxford University.

628. Pratt, Edward (fl.1680-1690). A Treatise on Metallic and Mineral Waters. London, 1684. The writer held the M.D.degree and wrote, in addition, tracts on surgery.

629. Pugh, Benjamin (fl.1748-1785). A description of the Mineral Waters of Baloruc, Languedoc, from the French of M. Pouzaire. Chelmsford, 1785. The writer also published tracts on midwifery and on the climate of Italy.

630. Pugh, Robert (fl.1666-1676). Bathoniensium et Aquisgranensium Thermarum Comparatio. London, 1676. The writer served as an officer in the Royal Army; he appears to have had no real interest in medicine.

631. Quinton, John (fl.1707-1734). De Thermis; or, Of Natural and Artificial Baths. The writer practice medicine at London.

632. ____. A Treatise of Warm Waters, and of the Cures Lately Made at Bath. Oxford, 1733-1734.

633. Randolph, George (1708-1764). An Enquiry into the Medicinal Virtues of Bristol Waters. Oxford, 1745. 114pp. The writer held the M.D. degree.

634. ____. An Enquiry into the Medicinal Virtues of Bath Waters. London, 1752. 65pp. A companion to #633.

635. Rutty, John (1698-1775). An Argument of Sulphur or No Sulphur in Waters Discussed, with a Comparison of the Waters of Aix-la-Chapelle, Bath, and Bristol. 3 parts in one volume. Dublin, 1762. Rutty proved to have been only one of several contributors to these arguments; see, also, #226.

636. ____. An Essay towards a Natural, Experimental, and Medicinal History of the Mineral Waters of Ireland. Dublin, 1757.

637. ____. An Examination of [Charles Lucas's] Analysis of Rutty on Mineral Waters. See, also, #606.

638. ____. A Methodical Synopsis of Mineral Waters, Comprehending the Most Celebrated Medicinal Waters, both Cold and Hot, of Great Britain, Ireland, and Other Parts of the World. Dublin, 1757. This volume comprises a series of inquiries and experiments conducted over a number of years; it includes notices of 113 mineral springs in Ireland alone; the work created considerable controversy between Rutty and Charles Lucas (see #606 and #637) that extended over three years, specifically focusing upon the presence of sulphur in water; the account of the debate may be found in the Dublin Quarterly Journal of Medical Science 3:561, 7:476.

639. Saunders, William (1743-1817). A Treatise on the Chemical History and Medical Powers of Some of the Most Celebrated Mineral Waters. London, 1800. 2nd ed., London, 1806. 483pp. See, also, #510.

640. Shaw, Peter (1694-1763). An Enquiry into the

Mineral Water (contd.)

Contents, Virtues, and Use of the Scarborough Spaw Waters. Scarborough, 1734. See, also, #234.

641. _____. Experiments and Observations upon Mineral Waters, with Notes. London, 1731; 2nd ed., London, 1743. This work a translation of an original German text written by Dr. Friedrich Hoffmann (1660-1742), professor of medicine at Halle and a physician to Frederick I of Prussia.

642. Shebbeare, John (1709-1788). A New Analysis of the Bristol Waters; together with the Cause of Diabetes and Hectic, and their Cure, as it results from these Waters. London, 1740; reissued in 1760. See, also, #235; related somewhat to consumption, hectic fever caused flushed cheeks and hot dry skin.

643. Short, Thomas (1690?-1772). An Essay towards a Natural and Medicinal History of the Principal Mineral Waters of Cumberland, Northumberland, Durham, Lancashire, Staffordshire, Shropshire, Worcestershire, Gloucestershire, Warwickshire, Northamptonshire, Leicester, and Nottinghamshire: particularly those of Neville-Holt, Cheltenham, Weatherslack, Hartlepool, Astrop, and Cartmel. To Which is added a Discourse on Cold and Tepid Bathing and a Table of All the Warm Waters in England and most of the Cold Baths from Carlisle to Gloucester and Oxford. Sheffield, 1740. See, also, #514.

644. _____. A General Treatise on Various Cold Mineral Waters in England, but more particularly those of Harrowgate, Thorp-Arch, Dorset-Hill, Wigglesworth, Neville-Holt, and others of a like Nature; with their Principles, Virtues, and Uses. London, 1765.

645. _____. The Natural, Experimental, and Medicinal History of the Mineral Waters of Derbyshire, Lincolnshire, and Yorkshire. London, 1734.

646. Smith, Hugh (1736-1789). A Treatise on the Use and Abuse of Mineral Waters. London, n.d.; four eds. through 1780. The writer, an M.D., practiced at London; his biography appeared in a 1791 edition of his Formulae Medicamentorum Concinnatae.

647. Smith, Joseph (fl.1786-1798). Observations on the Nature, the Use and Abuse of the Cheltenham Waters. Cheltenham, 1786. 67pp.; a new ed. in 1798.

648. Soame, John. Hampstead Wells: or, Directions for the Drinking of those Waters. London, 1734. 110pp. The writer held the M.D. degree; Hampstead Wells dated from the Restoration, becoming popular for its mineral waters (sold also at London public and coffee houses); it catered to the rich and the poor alike, but had grown quite disreputable by the end of the eighteenth century (see Ben Weintraub and Christopher Hibbert [eds.], The London Encyclopaedia [Bethesda, Maryland: Adler and Adler, 1986] 358).

Mineral Water (contd.)

649. Stevens, J.N. (fl.1755-1760). *Observations on the Medical Qualities of Bath Waters.* Bristol, 1758. The writer held the M.D. degree.
650. Stubbs, Henry (1632-1676). *Directions for Drinking the Bath-Water.* London, 1679. This work published posthumously and attached to an edition of John Hall's *Observations on English Bodies; or, Cures in Desperate Diseases* (1657); a native of Lincolnshire, a scholar at Westminster School, and a student at Oxford, Stubbs practiced physic and engaged in political writing; he also evidenced strong interests in Latin and Greek studies and in mathematics; he practiced at Jamaica (1661-1665), then at London, Stratford, Warwick, and Bath.
651. Sutherland, Alexander (fl.1755-1765). *An Attempt to Ascertain the Virtues of Bath and Bristol Waters.* London, 1764. The writer held the M.D. degree.
652. _____. *The Nature and Qualities of Bristol Water, with Reflections on Bath Waters.* Bristol, 1758.
653. Trinder, Rev. William Martin (fl.1780-1805). *Chemical Experiments on the Barnet Well Water.* London, 1800. 14pp. See, also, #528.
654. _____. *An Inquiry into Mineral Waters in Essex.* London, 1783.
655. Walker, Joshua (fl.1780-1790). *An Essay on the Waters of Harrowgate and Thorp-Arch, in Yorkshire.* London, 1784. The writer, a native of Leeds, held the M.D. degree.
656. Wall, John (1708-1776). *Experiments and Observations on the Malvern Waters.* Worcester, 1756. 14pp.; three eds. through 1763. Born at Powick, Worcestershire, the writer received the M.D. from Oxford in 1759; he practiced at Worcester from 1736 to 1776; his written tracts focus principally upon fevers, and he devoted his leisure hours to painting.
657. Willan, Robert (1757-1812). *Observations on the Sulphur Water of Croft, near Darlington.* London, 1782. 56pp.; 2nd ed., 1786; a "new" ed. in 1815. Willan, a native of Yorkshire, studied medicine at Edinburgh (M.D. 1780), attended medical lectures at London, and settled to practice at Darlington; after moving to London, he practiced and taught at the Public Dispensary; he became the first physician in England to classify skin diseases and to label them by name; as a result, in 1790, the Medical Society of London honored him with the Fothergillian Medal.
658. Williams, John (fl.1771-1774). *A Treatise on the Medicinal Virtues of the Mineral Waters of the German Spa.* London, 1773. The writer held the M.D. degree and wrote extensively on mineral waters as cures, as well as upon the gout, the governments of Scandinavian nations, and that of the United Provinces (Denmark, Sweden, Russia, and Poland).

Mineral Water (contd.)

659. _____. A Treatise on the Medicinal Virtues of the Waters of Aix-la-Chapelle and Borset. London, 1772.
660. Willich, Anthony Florian Madinger (fl.1790-1800). A Comparative View of the Bristol Hot-Well Water. London, 1798. The writer held the M.D. degree; in 1799, he published, in the Medical and Physical Journal (see #2051) and "interesting" paper on flannel worn next to the skin.
661. Wilson, Edmund. Spadacrene Dunelmensis; or, an Account of the Spaw near Durham. London, 1675. The writer held the M.D. degree.
662. Worthington, James. An Account of Experiments on the Spa at Mount Sion, near Liverpool. London, 1773.
663. Wynter [also Winter], John (fl.1720-1730). Cyclus Metasyncriticus; or, an Essay on Chronical Diseases and the Medicinal Waters of Bath and Bristol. London, 1725.
664. _____. Of Bathing in the Hot Baths at Bathe [sic], with regard to Palsie and some Diseases in Women. London, 1728.

B. Common Water

665. Buchan, William (1729-1805). Cautions concerning Cold Bathing. London, 1786. A native of Ancrum, Scotland, the writer held the M.D. degree; see #46.
666. Butler, Thomas. A Safe, Easy, and Expeditious Method of Procuring Any Quantity of Fresh Water at Sea. London, 1755. 43pp. The writer, an M.D., proposed to add a quart of strong soap lye to fifteen gallons of salt water to produce, by distillation, twelve gallons of fresh water.
667. Directions for Preparing Aerated Medicinal Waters, by Means of the Improved Glass Machines Made at Leith Glass Works. Edinburgh, 1787. 12pp. This booklet issued by the Edinburgh Glass-House Company at Leith.
668. Experiments Lately made by several Eminent Physicians on the Surprising and Terrible Effects of Almond-Water and Black-Cherry Water. London, 1741. 62pp.
669. Floyer, Sir John (1649-1734). The History of Cold Bathing: Both Ancient and Modern. In Two Parts. London, 1699; further eds. through 1844. See, also, #106 and #581-#582.
670. Hancocke, William. Febrifugum Magnum, Morbitigum Magnum. London, 1726.
671. Lewis, Polydore. An Essay on Common Water. London, 1790. The writer held the M.D. degree.
672. Lucas, Charles (1713-1771). An Essay on Waters, in Three Parts, treating, first, of Simple Waters, second, of Cold Waters, and third, of Natural Baths. 3 vols. London, 1756-1758; French translation at Liege, 1765; German translation by J.C. Zeiher, 3 vols., Altenburg, 1768-1769. This work has been identified as perhaps the most

Common Water (contd.)

significant discussion on the part of eighteenth-century physicians devoted to the waters at Bath and on the Continent; see, also, #606-#607.

673. Meighan, Sir Christopher (fl.1740-1760). Bath Waters in the Cure of Wounds. London, 1742; another ed. in 1764.

674. Observations on the Efficacy of Cold Bathing in the Cure of Nervous, Bilious, Scrofulous, and Other Chronic Diseases. Dublin, 1786. 73pp.

675. Observations on the Use of Bathing; Warm and Cold; and the Diseases it will cure without a Doctor. London, 1759. 43pp.

676. Oliver, William (1695-1764). A Practical Essay on the Use of Warm Bathing in Gouty Cases. Bath, 1751. 68 pp.; three eds. through 1764. Born at Ludgvan, Cornwall, Oliver studied at Cambridge (M.D. 1725) and completed his medical education at Leyden; he practiced medicine at Plymouth and then settled at Bath (1725-1764); a principal promoter of the Royal Mineral Water Hospital at Bath, he served that institution as physician and surgeon; he gained a reputation from his production of the "Bath Oliver biscuit," which he made from wheat flour.

677. Percival, Thomas (1740-1804). A Treatise on Water. London, 1768. Born at Warrington, Lancashire, Percival studied at Edinburgh, London, and Leyden; he practiced medicine at Warrington and Manchester; however, his principal interests and efforts concerned the improvement of sanitary conditions at Manchester, changes in the factory system, and the promotion of culture in that city.

678. Quinton, John (fl.1707-1734). An Essay on Warm Bath Water. Oxford, 1733-1734. See, also, #214.

679. Rotherham, John (1750?-1804). A Philosophical Inquiry into the Nature and Properties of Water. Newcastle-upon-Tyne, 1770. 132pp. See, also, #426, #502.

680. Short, Thomas (1690?-1772). A Rational Discourse on the Inward Uses of Water. London, 1725. See, also #514.

681. Smith, John (1648-?). The Curiosities of Common Water. London, 1723. 76pp.; ten eds. through 1740. A miscellaneous writer more than a medical practitioner, Smith dabbled in mathematics (Stereometrie [London, 1673]) and painting (The Art of Painting [London, 1676], The Art of Painting in Oyl [London, 1723], Painting in Water Colours [London, 1680]).

682. Smollett, Tobias George (1721-1771). Essay on the External Use of Water. London, 1752. The Scottish novelist, historian, and physician sought, in this piece, to prove that, for hydropathic purposes, the mineral waters at Bath had little advantage over any other water; he wrote the tract during the period of his medical practice at Bath and Chelsea and with the intention of revealing to the public

Common Water (contd.)

the unhealthy conditions in the former city; the writer had received the M.D. from Marischal College, Aberdeen, in 1750.

683. Wilson, Andrew (1718-1792). <u>Bath Waters: A Conjectural Idea to Their Nature and Qualities, in Three Letters. To which is added Putridity and Infection unjustly imputed to Fevers</u>. London, 1788. Wilson studied medicine at the University of Edinburgh (M.D. 1749); he then practiced at Newcastle and London; in addition to his tracts on medicine, he published, anonymously, pamphlets on philosophy.

C. Vapor

684. Denman, Thomas (1733-1815). <u>A Letter to Dr. Richard Huck on. . .Vapour Baths</u>. London, 1768. 14pp. Denman studied medicine at St. George's Hospital, London, and then entered the naval service as a surgeon (1757-1763); he graduated M.D. from Aberdeen in 1764 and practiced at Winchester and London; after obtaining a position as a surgeon aboard the royal yacht, he lectured on midwifery and became associated with the Middlesex Hospital; in 1783, he gained admittance as a licentiate in midwifery to the College of Physicians. Richard Huck (or Huch; d.1785; fl.1765-1785) held the M.D. degree and served as a physician to the Royal Army; in 1767, he published several essays on common water and vapor in the annual <u>Medical Observations and Inquiries</u>.

685. Playfair, James. <u>A Method of Constructing Vapour Baths</u>. London, 1783. 19pp.

686. Smyth, James Carmichael (1741-1821). <u>The Effect of the Nitrous Vapour in Preventing and Destroying Contagion</u>. London, 1799. 234pp. The Scottish born writer studied at Edinburgh and Leyden, then entered the Royal Army as a physician; in 1780, he served as the principal medical officer of the French prison at Winchester; there he developed successfully a method of arresting contagion through vapors from mineral acids; in 1802, he received appointment as physician extraordinary to George III.

687. Symons, John (fl.1765-1770). <u>Observations on Vapour-Bathing</u>. Bristol, 1766. 103pp.

D. Sea Water

688. Anderson, John (d.1804). <u>A Preliminary Introduction to the Act of Sea-Bathing</u>. Margate, 1795. 28pp. See, also, #365.

689. Kentish, Richard (fl.1785-1790). <u>An Essay on Sea-Bathing and the Internal Use of Sea Water</u>. London, 1787. An M.D., Kentish published several medical tracts between 1785 and 1787.

Waters   73

            Sea Water (contd.)

690.   Reid, Thomas (1739-1802). <u>Directions for Warm and
       Cold Sea-Bathing</u>. London, 1795. 75pp.; another ed.
       in 1798. An M.D., Reid also published tracts on
       pulmonary diseases.
691.   Russell, Richard (1687-1759). <u>A Dissertation
       concerning the Use of Sea Water in Diseases of the
       Glands</u>. Oxford, 1753. 398pp.; five eds. through
       1769. A native of Lewes, Sussex, Russell graduated
       M.D. from Rheims in 1738; he practiced at Ware and
       Reading; his published works focus upon sea water
       and the diseases and treatment of the glands.
692.   Rymer, James (fl.1775-1822). <u>A Sketch of Great
       Yarmouth, with Some Reflections on Cold Bathing</u>.
       London, 1777. This work written while the author
       served as a surgeon to the sloop <u>Alderney</u>, then
       anchored at Great Yarmouth; a native of Scotland,
       Rymer studied anatomy and medicine at Edinburgh;
       after removing to London, he sailed with several
       ships as surgeon; upon leaving the naval service in
       1782, he practiced medicine at Reigate (Surrey) and
       Ramsgate (Kent).
693.   Speed, John (1703-1781). <u>De Aqua Marina Commentarius</u>.
       London, 1754. 33pp.; another ed., Oxford, 1755.
       The writer held the M.D. degree.
694.   Tonstall, George. <u>A Description of the Waters of
       Scarborough Spaw</u>. London, 1670.
695.   White, Robert (fl.1775-1800). <u>The Use and Abuse of
       Sea Water</u>. London, 1775; 3rd ed., London, 1791.
       See, also, #535.

       E.   Tar Water

696.   Berkeley, George, Bishop of Cloyne (1684-1753).
       <u>Farther Thoughts on Tar-Water</u>. London, 1752. Born
       at Kilkenny and educated at Trinity College,
       Dublin, Berkeley came to London in 1713; he formed
       associations with the noted <u>literati</u> of his day:
       Pope, Steele, Addison, Swift, <u>et al</u>; he became dean
       of Derry (1724) and Bishop of Cloyne (1734-1752),
       after which he retired to to Oxford and died there;
       Berkeley remains a principal figure of eighteenth-
       century philosophy, literature, and theology; see
       #698.
697.   _____. <u>Siris, a Chain of Philosophical Reflections and
       Inquiries Respecting the Virtues of Tar-Water in
       the Plague</u>. Dublin, 1744. 261pp.; two other eds.
       in 1744; further eds. in 1746 and 1748; also
       translations to French, German, Dutch, and
       Portuguese.
698.   _____. <u>Three Letters to Thomas Prior and a Letter to
       the Rev. Dr. [Stephen] Hales on the Virtues of Tar
       Water</u>. London, 1720; further eds. in 1744, 1746,
       1747. Berkeley's attraction to tar water came as
       the result of an attack of nervous colic; following
       the appearing of this tract and <u>Siris</u> (#697), tar
       water became a popular medicine and tonic for

Tar Water (contd.)

almost every human disorder, as well as a supposed guard against infection and even old age; it consisted, simply, of an infusion of tar into cold water; concerning Hales and Prior, see #699 and #701.

699. Prior, Thomas (1682?-1751). An Authentic Narrative of the Success of Tar-Water, in Curing a Great Number and Variety of Distempers. London, 1746. 192pp. A native of Queen's County, Ireland, Prior studied at Trinity College, Dublin; he eventually founded the Dublin Society and devoted his labors to the promotion of material and industrial works among the Irish Protestants.

700. Reeve, Thomas (d.1790; fl.1744-1789). An Essay on the Cure of the Epidemical Madness of Drinking Tar Water. London, 1744. 66pp.

701. Reid, Andrew (d.1767?). A Letter to Dr. [Stephen] Hales on Tar Water. London, 1747. Born in Fifeshire, Reid went to London in 1720 and became involved in a variety of literary and scientific interests; he had not received formal education in medicine, nor did he practice that profession. The Rev. Stephen Hales (1677-1761), perpetual curate of Teddington, Middlesex, gained fair recognition as a philosopher and as an advocate of temperance (see, also, #698).

702. Remarkable Cures Perform'd by Tar-Water; Collected out of the Gentleman's Magazine. London, 1745. 24pp. The Gentleman's Magazine had been in publication since 1731.

F. Drowning

703. Cullen, William (1712-1790). A Letter to Lord Cathcart concerning the Recovery of Persons Drowned and Seemingly Dead. Edinburgh, 1775. See, also, #79; Cullen addressed this essay to William Schaw Cathcart, tenth Baron Cathcart (1721-1776), a representative peer of Scotland in the House of Lords.

704. Curry, James (fl.1790-1815). Popular Observations on Apparent Death from Drowning. Northampton, 1792. 113pp. The writer held the M.D. degree.

705. Fothergill, Anthony (1732?-1813). A New Inquiry into the Suspension of Vital Action in Cases of Drowning and Suffocation. Bath, 1795. 189pp. See, also, #111.

706. Fuller, John (d.1825). Hints Relative to the Recovery of Persons Drowned and Apparently Dead. London, 1784. 32pp. The writer proposes transfusion from the carotid artery of a sheep as a means of resuscitation; Fuller practiced surgery at Ayton, Berwickshire, then shifted his interests to agriculture, county history, and statistical reporting; in 1789, he received the M.D. from St. Andrews through the influence of a number of

Drowning (contd.)

Edinburgh physicians and surgeons.
707. Jackson, Rowland (d.1787? fl.1740-1750). <u>A Physical Dissertation on Drowning</u>. London, 1746. 80pp.; Dublin, 1747. 69pp.; 2nd ed., London, 1747. 80pp. An M.D., the writer published several medical tracts between 1747 and 1748.
708. Johnston, Alexander (1716?-1799). <u>A Treatise on Drowned Persons</u>. London, 1773. The writer held the M.D. degree.
709. Macpherson, Robert. <u>A Dissertation on the Preservative from Drowning</u>. London, 1783. 129pp.

V

General Surgery, Wounds, Dissection, Embalming, Rupture, Testicles

A. General Surgery

710. Abernethy, John (1764-1831). Surgical and Physiological Essays. Part I: On Lumbar Abscess; Part II: On Matter Perspired. . . by the Skin; Part III: Injuries of the Head. London, 1793-1797. An eminent London surgeon, the writer rose to the height of his profession, principally through his lectures at St. Bartholomew's Hospital, London; ultimately, he founded the medical school associated with that ancient institution.
711. Aitken, John (d.1790). An Address to the Chirurgo-Obstetrical Society. Edinburgh, 1786. 15pp. See, also, #288.
712. ____. Essays and Cases in Surgery. London, 1775. 241pp.
713. ____. Essays on Fractures and Luxations. London, 1790. 173pp.; 2nd ed., London, 1800. 173pp.
714. ____. Systematic Elements of the Theory and Practice of Surgery. Edinburgh, 1779. 574pp.
715. Alanson, Edward (1747-1823). Practical Observations upon Amputation. London, 1779. 64pp.; 2nd ed., London, 1782. 296pp.; French ed., Paris, 1784. 208pp.; German ed., Gotha, 1785. 172pp. Alanson's published tracts on various aspects of surgery appeared, generally, between 1771 and 1782.
716. Antrobus, Thomas. "An Amputation of a Leg, without any Subsequent Haemorrhage," Medical Observations and Inquiries 2 (1762) 152ff. The writer practiced as a surgeon at Liverpool.
717. Arnott, James (fl.1795-1816). Remarks on the Present Mode of Chirurgical Attendance in the Royal Infirmary of Edinburgh. Edinburgh, 1800. 14pp. Arnott (also Arnot) practiced surgery at Edinburgh; his published works on surgery appeared, principally, between 1800 and 1816.
718. Atkins, John (1685-1757). A Treatise on Chirurgical Subjects. London, 1729(?). 47pp. See, also, #1842. As a ship's surgeon, the writer traveled extensively to Guiana, Brazil, and the West Indies; thus, his travel narratives gained him more

General Surgery (contd.)

attention than did his medical publications.

719. Aylett, George (d.1792). A Genuine State of a Case in Surgery. London, 1759. 35pp. The writer published tracts on surgery at London between 1744 and 1759.
720. Batting, John. Chirurgical Facts relating to Wounds and Contusions of the Head. Oxford, 1760. 100pp.
721. Becket, Thomas. Chirurgical Remarks. London, 1709.
722. Becket, William (1684-1738). A Collection of Chirurgical Tracts. 2 vols. London, 1740. Born at Abingdon, Berkshire, the writer developed, in London, a reputation as a surgeon and antiquary; in 1718, he gained election as a fellow of the Royal Society, followed by his membership in the Society of Antiquaries; he practiced as a surgeon at St. Thomas's Hospital, Southwark.
723. ____. Practical Surgery, Illustrated and Improved, with Remarks on the Most Remarkable Cases, Cures, and Discussions in St. Thomas's Hospital. London, 1738(?). 294pp.; another ed., London, 1740. 294pp.
724. Bell, Benjamin (1749-1806). A System of Surgery. 6 vols. Edinburgh, 1782-1787; seven eds. through 1801; French and German translations. A valuable yet popular work in its day, Bell's System gained attention from its writer's promotion of a scheme for saving the skin from every operation; Bell, born at Dumfries, studied medicine at Edinburgh and at Paris; he served as surgeon to the Royal Infirmary at Edinburgh (1772-1801), as well as to Watson's Hospital; in addition, he developed a deep interest in agriculture.
725. Bell, Sir Charles (1774-1842). A System of Dissections. 2 vols. Edinburgh, 1798-1799. Born at Edinburgh, Bell became one of the leading proponents of human anatomy during the first half of the nineteenth century; he achieved recognition as the discoverer of the distinct functions of the nerves; Bell's System, with the writer's own drawings and illustrations, represents his earliest major contribution to surgery and human anatomy, it having been published during his tenure as a medical student at Edinburgh; he issued an Appendix in 1800.
726. Bernard, Christopher. Observations on the Present State of Chirurgery. London, 1703.
727. Boulton, Richard (fl.1697-1724). A System of Rational and Practical Surgery. London, 1713. 352pp. See, also, #386.
728. Bromfield, William (1712-1792). Chirurgical Cases and Observations. 2 vols. London, 1773. The writer practiced and taught surgery at London; in addition to being one of the planners of the Lock Hospital London, for the treatment of venereal diseases (not to be confused with the more noted Lock Hospital, Southwark, which closed its doors in 1760), he practiced surgery both there and at St. George's Hospital.

Surgery, Wounds, Dissection 79

General Surgery (contd.)

729. Browne, John (1642-1700?). <u>A Complete Description of Wounds, both General and Practical</u>. London, 1678. The writer served as a surgeon at St. Thomas's Hospital, London; his tracts on surgery appeared at London between 1678 and 1703.
730. ____. <u>The Surgeon's Assistant</u>. London, 1703. 183pp.
731. Butter, William (1726-1805). <u>Dissertatio Medica et Chirurgica de Arteriotamia</u>. Edinburgh, 1761. A native of the Orkney Islands and an M.D. graduate from Edinburgh, Butter practiced at Derby and then at Edinburgh; he wrote a number of tracts on fevers, coughs, arterial surgery, and the diseases of the blood.
732. ____. <u>An Improved Method of Opening the Temporal Artery</u>. London, 1783. 213pp.
733. Cheston, Richard Browne (fl.1765-1785). <u>Pathological Inquiries and Observations in Surgery</u>. Gloucester, 1766. 144pp.
734. Cooke, James (1614-1694?). <u>Mellificium Chirurgiae; or, The Marrow of Chirurgery, Anatomy, and Physick</u>. London, n.d.; six eds. through 1717; a <u>Supplement</u> at London in 1655.
735. <u>Cystitomia Hypogastrica; or, the Method of Performing the High Operation. . .Collected from the Writings of. . .Francis Rosset. . .John Douglas. . .William Cheselden</u>. London, 1724. 28pp. For Douglas, see #315; for Cheselden, see #301.
736. Davy, Sir Humphry (1778-1829). <u>Researches, Chemical and Philosophical; chiefly concerning Nitrous Oxide, or Dephlogisticated Nitrous Air, and its Respiration</u>. London, 1799; 2nd ed., London, 1800. 580pp. This work stands as an example of what the writer, himself, termed an immature hypothesis, "the dreams of misemployed genius [he being only twenty-one years of age at the time] which the light of experiment and observation has never conducted to truth" (see <u>DNB</u>). Davy, the noted natural philosopher and chemist, achieved recognition, of course, not for any contribution to medicine, but for what he did to advance the knowledge of chemistry and galvanism.
737. Dease, William (1752?-1798). <u>An Introduction to the Theory and Practice of Surgery</u>. 2 vols. London, 1780. Born at Lisney, County Cavan, Dease studied medicine at Dublin and Paris; he then settled at Dublin to practice surgery; in 1785, he became the first professor of surgery of the College of Surgeons, Dublin, and advanced to the presidency of that institution in 1789; he published tracts on a variety of medical topics, from midwifery to venereal diseases.
738. Douglas, James (1675-1742). <u>The History of the Lateral Operation</u>. London, 1726. 88pp. See, also, #312.
739. Douglas, John (d.1743). <u>A Syllabus of Chirurgical Operations</u>. London, 1727. 38pp. See, also, #315.

General Surgery (contd.)

740. Dunn, Edward (fl.1720-1725). A Compendious and New Method of Performing Chirurgical Operations. London, 1724. 215pp.

741. Earle, Sir James (1755-1817). The Chirurgical Works of Percival Pott, with a Life. 3 vols. London, 1790. Born at London, Earle received his medical education at St. Bartholomew's Hospital, London, where he served as principal surgeon from 1784 to 1815, succeeding Percival Pott (1713-1788; see #770); known for his skill in lithotomy (removal of stone from the urinary bladder), Earle also introduced improved treatments of hydrocele (see #1215).

742. Farmer, John (d.1770?). Select Cases in Surgery, Collected in St. Bartholomew's Hospital. London, 1757. 28pp.

743. Fordyce, Sir William (1724-1792). Fragmenta Chirurgica et Medica. London, 1784. 102pp. Born at Aberdeen, Fordyce left his studies at Edinburgh to join the Royal Army, then (1748) engaged against the French; he served as an army surgeon until 1750, returning to London and entering upon general practice there; a royal mandate created him (1770) M.D. from Cambridge; in 1786, he obtained an appointment as a licentiate of the Royal College of Physicians; the Society of Arts awarded him a gold medal for his research on rhubarb for medical application.

744. Gooch, Benjamin (d.1780?). Cases and Practical Remarks in Surgery. London, 1758. 184pp.; enlarged ed. published under the title of A Practical Treatise on Wounds and Other Chirurgical Subjects; to which is prefixed a Short Historical Account of Surgery and Anatomy. 2 vols. Norwich, 1767; an appendix came forth under the title, Medical and Chirurgical Observations. London, 1773. As far as evidence can be gathered, Gooch practiced medicine at Shottisham, Norfolk, and gained appointment as a consulting surgeon to the Norfolk and Norwich Hospital.

745. Handley, James (fl.1705-1725). Colloquia Chiurgica; or, the Whole Art of Surgery. London, 1705. 192pp.; five eds. through 1743. The writer also published works upon anatomy, animal agriculture, and the plague.

746. Hill, James (fl.1770-1780). Cases in Surgery. Edinburgh, 1772. 263pp.

747. Ingram, Dale (1710-1793). Practical Cases and Observations in Surgery. London, 1751. 245pp. See, also, #454.

748. Justamond, John Obadiah (d.1786). Surgical Tracts. London, 1789. 394pp. The writer served as a surgeon in the Royal Army; his primary interest and labors, however, focused upon a translation of the private life of Louis XV of France (1781) and translations of Abbe Raynal's histories (1776-

Surgery, Wounds, Dissection 81

General Surgery (contd.)

1784).
749. Kirkland, Thomas (1721-1798). An Inquiry into the Present State of Practical Surgery. 2 vols. London, 1783-1786. An M.D. graduate of St. Andrews (1769), Kirkland practiced medicine at Ashley-de-la-Zouche, Leicestershire; he held membership in the Royal Medical Society (both in London and Edinburgh).
750. Lara, Benjamin. A Dictionary of Surgery; or, the Young Surgeon's Pocket Assistant. London, 1796; a two-volume ed. published at Leipzig, 1779-1800.
751. Latta, James (fl.1790-1795). A Practical System of Surgery. 3 vols. Edinburgh, 1794-1795. The writer practiced surgery at Edinburgh.
752. Le Dran, Philippe (1685-1770). The Operations in Surgery of Mons. Le Dran. Trans[lated] Thomas Gataker [d.1769]. With Remarks, Plates. . .and a Sett of Instruments by William Cheselden. London, 1749; 2nd ed., London, 1752. Le Dran achieved recognition for having improved the surgical technique of lithotomy; his Traie des Operations de Churgurie (Paris 1742) had been edited by William Cheselden (see, also, #301) prior to Gataker's translation; see, also #120.
753. Manning, Henry (fl.1770-1780). Modern Improvements in the Practice of Surgery. London, 1780. 423pp. The writer held the M.D. degree.
754. Mason, Henrich (fl.1753-1765). An Extract from an Old Treatise of Surgery. London, 1754. The original "old tract" written by one Dr. Wurguis.
755. Middleton, John (fl. 1725-1735). A Short Essay on the Operation of Lithotomy. London, 1727. 72pp.
756. Mihlis, Samuel (fl.1745-1755). The Elements of Surgery. London, 1746. 324pp.; 2nd ed., London, 1764. 368pp. The writer also published a volume of lectures (or translations thereof) on physiology (2 vols., London, 1753).
757. Monro, Hugh. A Compendious System of Theory and Practice of Modern Surgery. London, 1792. The writer practiced surgery at London.
758. Moore, James Carrick (1763-1834). A Dissertation on the Process of Nature in Filling up of Cavities, Healing of Wounds, and Restoring Parts which have been Destroyed. London, 1789. 76pp. See, also, #474.
759. _____. A Method of Preventing or Diminishing Pain in Several Operations of Surgery. London, 1784. 50pp.
760. Moyle, John (d.1714). Chyrurgic Memoirs. London, 1708. 128pp. The writer, a career naval surgeon, retired (1690) on a pension that allowed him to write about his naval and medical experiences; he published at least four such volumes between 1686 and 1708.
761. _____. The Experienced Chirurgion. London, 1703. 320pp.
762. Mynors, Robert (1739-1806). Practical Thoughts on

General Surgery (contd.)

Amputations. Birmingham, 1783. 91pp. Mynors practiced surgery at Birmingham from 1775 to 1806; his published work focused upon amputations and head surgery.

763. Neal (also Neale), George. Memoirs of the Royal Academy of Surgery at Paris; translated from the Original. 3 vols. London, 1758.

764. Nisbet, William (1759-1822). The Clinical Guide; or, A Concise View of. . .Surgery. Edinburgh, 1793. 436pp.; 2nd ed., Edinburgh, 1799; 3rd. ed., Edinburgh, 1800. See, also, #478.

765. Parker, Henry. The Ligature Preferable to Agaric in Securing the Blood-Vessels after Amputation. London, 1755. 18pp.

766. Pearson, John (1758-1826). Principles of Surgery. Part I. London, 1788; another ed. in 1808. This work prepared for those students attending the writer's lectures on surgery; two parts had been planned, but only the first reached the publisher; born at York, Pearson studied surgery at Morpeth, Leeds, and London; at the last-named city, he entered St. George's Hospital as a pupil of John Hunter; he served as a surgeon to an army regiment and then received an appointment to the Lock Hospital, where he remained from 1781 to 1818; in addition, he formed associations with the public dispensary in Carey Street, London, as well as the Royal Society, the Linnean Society, the Royal College of Surgeons of Ireland, and the Royal Medical Society of Edinburgh.

767. Perkins, Benjamin Douglas (1774-1810). The Efficacy of Perkins' Patent Metallic Tractors on the Human Body. London, 1798; another ed., London, 1800. 135 pp. Perkins spent the major portion of his adult life as a bookseller in New York City; however, he did reside for a period in London, during which time he promoted and attempted to sell a "metallic tractor" invented by his father, Elisha Perkins, M.D.

768. _____. The Influences of Metallic Tractors on the Human Body. London, 1798. 98pp. This work a variant edition of #767.

769. Pharmacopoeia Chirurgica; or, Formulae for the Use of Surgeons; including. . .all the Principal Formulae of the Different Hospitals. London, 1794. 130pp.; four eds. through 1799.

770. Pott, Percival (1714-1788). The Chirurgical Works. 4 vols. London, 1771; 4 vols. London, 1775; 3 vols., London, 1790. Pott succeeded William Cheselden (see #301) as the most significant English surgeon of the eighteenth century; born at London, he became, eventually, assistant surgeon, then senior surgeon, at St. Bartholomew's Hospital, London; in 1764, he gained election to the Royal Society.

771. _____. Some Few General Remarks on Fractures and Dislocations. London, 1765; 3rd ed., London, 1769.

Surgery, Wounds, Dissection 83

General Surgery (contd.)

In this piece, Pott described the abduction fracture of the leg bones near the ankle--a trauma that he, himself, had suffered and which eventually became known as "Pott's Fracture"; the writer emphasizes the urgency for an immediate setting of the fracture, while stressing the need to relax the muscles for a successful setting.

772. Pratt, Edward (fl.1680-1690). <u>Chirurgus Methodicus</u>. London, 1689.
773. <u>The Present State of Chyrurgery</u>. London, 1703. 28pp.
774. Pye, Samuel. <u>Some Observations on the General Methods of Lithotomy</u>. London, 1724. The writer practiced surgery at Bristol; this tract written in direct opposition to the "high" operation, which Pye had attempted unsuccessfully.
775. Ranby, John (1703-1773). <u>Chirurgical Observations</u>. London, 1740. A member of the Barber Surgeons Company and of the Royal Society, Ranby held appointments as a surgeon-in-ordinary to the King's household and sergeant-surgeon to George II; he succeeded in promoting Parliamentary action in separating the Corporation of Surgeons from the Company of Barbers; further, he gained appointment as surgeon to to the Chelsea Hospital (1752), succeeding William Cheselden (see #301).
776. Reid, Alexander (1586-?-1641). <u>Chirurgorum Comes, or the Whole Practice of Chirurgery, begun by the learned Dr. Reid and completed by a member of the College of Physicians in London</u>. London, 1687. Essentially a collection of Reid's surgical tracts; the volume also also contains a treatise on midwifery and another piece on "plastic operations; Reid studied at Aberdeen and prepared for surgical practice in France; he served as a surgeon both in North Wales and at London.
777. Rushworth, John (1664-1736). <u>A Letter to the Mrs.</u> [masters] <u>or Governors of the Mystery and Commonality of Barber Surgeons</u>. Northampton, 1731. The writer lived and practiced medicine at Northampton; he achieved recognition for discovering the efficacy of cinchonia bark in cases of gangrene; see, also, #505.
778. _____. <u>A Proposal for the Improvement of Surgery; offered to the Masters of the Mystery of Barbers and Surgeons at London</u>. London, 1732. A variation of #777; within the context of #777-#778, the term "mystery" refers to a service or an occupation.
779. Rymer, James (fl.1775-1822). <u>An Introduction to the Study of Pathology on a Natural Plan, containing an Essay on Fevers</u>. London, 1775. See, also, #692.
780. Salmon, William (1644-1713). <u>Ars Chirurgica</u>. 2 vols. London, 1699. The work stands, essentially, as a treatise on general surgery; Salmon established a medical practice of questionable repute near the Smithfield Gate of St. Bartholomew's Hospital, London; simply, he treated patents who could not

General Surgery (contd.)

gain admission to the hospital, selling to them his own drugs, casting horoscopes, and professing a knowledge of alchemy; his published works range from almanacs to tracts on religion and practical physic; see, also, #227.

781. Sharp, Samuel (1700?-1778). A Critical Inquiry into the Present State of Surgery. London, 1750. 294pp. 2nd ed., 1750; 3rd ed., 1754; 4th ed., 1761; translations in French (1751), Spanish (1753), German (1756), Italian (1774). The volume contains thirteen brief chapters on hernia, lithotomy, amputation, concussion on the brain, tumors of the gall bladder, extirpation of the tonsils, and hydrocele; Sharp served for seven years as an apprentice to William Cheselden (see #301) at St. Thomas's Hospital, London; he also studied in France before returning to London and to eventual election as a surgeon at Guy's Hospital; in addition, he lectured on surgery at Covent Garden.

782. ____. A Treatise on the Operations of Surgery. London, 1739. 224pp.; 2nd ed., 1739; 3rd ed., 1740; 4th ed., London, 1743; 6th ed., 1751; 8th ed., 1761; 9th ed., 1769; 10th ed., London, 1782; French translation at Paris, 1741.

783. Shirley, John (fl.1678-1682). A Short Compendium of Chirurgery. London, 1768; 2nd ed., 1783. The writer held the M.D. degree.

784. Smith, George (fl.1725-1735). Institutiones Chirurgicae; or, Principles of Surgery. London, 1732. 396pp. The writer also published tracts on distilling (1725) and fermentation (1729).

785. Stuart, Alexander (fl.1702-1740). New Discoveries and Improvements in the Most Considerable Branches of Anatomy and Surgery. London, 1738. 55pp. The writer, an M.D., published, between 1702 and 1738, essays on medicine and antiquity in the Philosophical Transactions of the Royal Society.

786. Tomlinson, Francis (fl.1675-1690). Chirurgical Treatises. London, 1676; another ed., London, 1686. The writer served as a principal surgeon to Charles II; his surgical Treatises considered "a very respectable performance in its time" (Allibone 3:2431).

787. Turner, Daniel (1667-1741). Apologia Chyrurgica, a Vindication of the Nobel [sic] Art of Chirurgery. London, 1695. Born at London, Turner became a member of the Barber Surgeons' Company and practiced surgery at London; his publications exist, essentially, as records of his own cases.

788. ____. The Art of Surgery. 2 vols. London, 1722; 2nd ed., 2 vols., London, 1725; six eds. through 1741.

789. Underwood, Michael (1736-1820). Surgical Tracts on Ulcers of the Legs. London, 1783. 158pp.; 2nd ed., London, 1788; another ed. in 1789. Born in Surrey, Underwood studied medicine at St. George's Hospital, London, and at Paris; for a number of

Surgery, Wounds, Dissection   85

       General Surgery (contd.)

              years he practiced surgery in London, then turned
              his attention to midwifery and formed an
              association with the British Lying-in Hospital.
790.   Victor, Benjamin (d.1778). Memoirs of the Life of
              Barton Booth, Esq.; With His Character. To which
              are added Several Poetical Pieces. . .To which is
              likewise annex'd, The Case of Mr. Booth's last
              Illness, and what was observ'd (particularly with
              regard to the Quick-Silver found in his Intestines)
              upon Opening of His Body, in the Presence of Sir
              Hans Sloan, by Mr. Alexander Small, Surgeon.
              London, 1733. 58pp. The value of this volume to
              the history of medicine in the eighteenth century
              lies in the section entitled "The Case of Mr.
              Booth" (pp.19-25), in which the writer sets forth
              the specifics of an autopsy of the subject,
              including the prescriptions administered to him
              during his last illness; Booth (1681-1733), an
              Irish-trained actor, rose to become manager of
              Drury Lane Theatre, London.
791.   Warner, Joseph (1717-1801). Cases in Surgery, with
              Introductions, Operations, and Remarks; to which is
              added an Account of the Preparation and Effects of
              the Agaric of the Oak in Stopping of Bleeding,
              after some of the most capital Operations. London,
              1754; 2nd ed., 1754; 3rd ed., London, 1760; 4th
              ed., London, 1784; French translation at Paris,
              1757. Warner's reputation as a surgeon emerges
              from this volume; the cases range throughout the
              domain of surgery and represent the opinions of the
              writer's contemporaries; Born on Antigua, in the
              West Indies, Warner studied surgery at Guy's
              Hospital, London, under Samuel Sharp (see #781); in
              1744 he joined the Royal Army in Scotland; becoming
              a surgeon at Guy's Hospital (1745-1780), he also
              lectured on anatomy there; eventually, he received
              appointment as an examiner for the Corporation of
              Surgeons, London.
792.   Wathen, Jonathan (fl.1762-1782). Instruments for
              Fractures. London, 1767; 2nd ed., 1768; 3rd ed.,
              London, 1781. A surgeon, the writer published
              translations of Hermann Boerhaave's Latin lectures
              (1763) and tracts on venereal diseases.
793.   Weldon, Walter (fl.1790-1810). Observations on
              Compound Fractures. Southampton, 1794. The writer
              practiced surgery at Southampton and London.
794.   ____. Observations on the Different Modes of
              Puncturing the Bladder in Cases of Retention of
              Urine. Southampton, 1793. 171pp.
795.   White, Charles (1728-1813). An Account of the Topical
              Application of Sponge in the Stoppage of
              Haemmorrhage. London, 1762. Born at Manchester,
              White studied medicine at London and Edinburgh;
              returning to the city of his birth, he helped to
              found the Manchester Infirmary, an institution that
              he served from 1752 to 1790; he also participated

General Surgery (contd.)

in establishing the Manchester Literary and Philosophical Society; competent in general medicine, surgery, and midwifery, he achieved a reputation for rescuing midwifery from its state of extreme primitivism to a rational, humane, and respected practice.

796. _____. Cases in Surgery. London, 1770.
797. White, Robert (fl.1775-1800). The Present Practice of Surgery. London, 1786. See, also, #535.
798. Wilmer, Bradford (fl.1770-1795). Cases and Remarks in Surgery and the Bronchocele. London, 1779. The writer practiced surgery at Stony-Stratford (Northamptonshire), then at Coventry.
799. Wiseman, Richard (1622?-1676). Several Chirurgical Treatises. London, 1676; 2nd ed., London, 1686; 3rd ed., 1696; 4th ed., 1705; 5th ed., 2 vols., London, 1719; 6th ed., 2 vols., London, 1734; a pirated edition published by Samuel Clement, London bookseller with a shop at St. Paul's Churchyard, and containing copies of the 1676 and 1686 editions, appeared in 1692. Born in London, Wiseman served as both a naval and army surgeon; he then practiced surgery at London (at St. Thomas's Hospital and also as an independent practitioner) and even managed a tour of service with the Spanish navy; through his writing, Wiseman elevated the profession of surgery to that of equality with physicians; Samuel Johnson, for his Dictionary of 1755, selected examples from Wiseman's work as accurate "surgical nomenclature."
800. Young, James (fl.1675-1705). Observations in Surgery and Anatomy. London, 1687; another ed., London, 1692. Young practiced surgery at Plymouth; he published tracts on injuries to the brain and various medicinal cures, as well as contributed (beginning c.1702) essays to the Philosophical Transactions of the Royal Society.

B. Wounds

801. Bell, John (1763-1820). Discourses on the Nature and Cure of Wounds. Edinburgh, 1795. Along with Pierre Joseph Desault (1744-1795)--the French surgeon, anatomist, and founder of the first school of clinical surgery in France--and John Hunter (1728-1793), Bell involved himself with the founding of the modern surgery of the vascular system; the Discourses represents one of the writer's most significant contributions to the study of surgery in general and, particularly, to a knowledge of surgery for wounds of the arteries.
802. Clark, Thaddeus. An Account of a Remarkable Case of the Tetanus. Norwich, 1794. 30pp.
803. Jurin, James (1684-1750). An Expostulary Address to John Ranby, Esq.,. . .occasioned by His Treatise on Gunshot Wounds. Born in London and educated at

Wounds (contd.)

Cambridge, Jurin taught at the grammar school at Newcastle-upon-Tyne; in 1709, he entered Leyden as a medical student, but resigned and returned to Cambridge, where he earned his M.D. in 1716; admitted as a candidate of the College of Physicians, London, in 1718, he received, shortly thereafter (1719) his appointment as a fellow; the year previous (1718), he had gained election as a fellow of the Royal Society, serving from 1721 to 1727 as its secretary; an appointment as a physician to Guy's Hospital, London, followed; he has been recognized as one of the most learned medical practitioners of his day. See, also, #804.

804. Ranby, John (1703-1777). The Method of Treating Gun-Shot Wounds. London, 1744; 2nd ed., 1760; 3rd ed., 1781. See, also #775, #803.

805. Rattray, Sylvester (fl.1650-1666). Prognosis Medica ad usum Praxeos facili Methodo Digesta. Glasgow, 1666. A native of Angus, Scotland, Rattray proclaimed that he possessed degrees both in medicine and theology; he published, between 1658 and 1666, at least three medical tracts, each in Latin.

806. Whateley, Thomas (d.1821). Practical Observations on the Cure of Wounds and Ulcers on the Legs. London, 1790. 352pp. A London surgeon, the writer published tracts on venereal diseases, urethra, the nose, and the tibia.

807. Wiseman, Richard (1622?-1676). A Treatise of Wounds. London, 1672. See, also, #799.

C. Dissection

808. Hannes, Sir Edward (d.1710). An Account of the Dissection of the Duke of Gloucester. London, 1700. The writer had attended, on 30 July 1700, the death of William, Duke of Gloucester (b.1689, the young son of Princess Anne), and shortly thereafter published his Account; an anonymous satirical poem, Doctor Hannes, Dissected, in a Familiar Epistle by Way of Nosce Teipsum (London, 1700), ridiculed that narrative; a poet and miscellaneous prose writer, Hannes read chemistry at Oxford and received both the M.B. (1691) and M.D. (1695) from that institution; he also served as a physician to Queen Anne.

809. Lettsome, John Coakley (1744-1815). Hints Respecting Human Dissection. London, 1795. 27pp. See, also, #160.

810. Lyser, Michael (d.1660). The Art of Dissecting the Human Body. London, n.d.; a later ed., London, 1740. 276pp.

811. Millington, Sir Thomas (1628-1704), et. al. The Report of the Physicians and Surgeons Commanded to Assist at the Dissecting the Body of His Late Majesty. London, 1702. 5pp. This terse narrative

Dissection (contd.)

concerns the death of William III (1650-1702), who had been in frail health; yet, his demise resulted directly from a broken collarbone: he had fallen from his horse during an afternoon gallop in Richmond Park. Millington, a native of Newbury, Berkshire, attended Westminster School, Trinity College, Cambridge (A.B. 1649, M.A. 1657), and Oxford (M.D. 1659); an original member of the Royal Society and a fellow of the College of Physicians, he also became Sedleian professor of natural philosophy at Oxford (1675-1704); he served as a physician to William III and Mary, and later to Queen Anne.

812. Thomson, George (fl.1734-1740). <u>The Art of Dissecting Human Bodies; from the Latin of Lyserus</u>. London, 1740. See, also #354.

813. Umfreville, Edward. <u>Lex Coronatoria; or, The Office and Duty of Coroners</u>. 2 vols. London, 1761; another ed. at Bristol in 1822.

D. Embalming

814. Greenhill, Thomas (1681-1740?). <u>Nekrokedeia; or, The Art of Embalming; wherein is shewn the right of Burial, the Funeral Ceremonies, especially that of Preserving Bodies after the Egyptian Method. Part I</u>. London, 1705. Parts II and III never published; although the work lacks originality and reveals little beyond superficial investigation into the subject, it proved generally useful to the writer's contemporaries; a London surgeon whose formal education cannot be readily identified, Greenhill appears to have secured his reputation to this single literary effort, written when he had not yet reached his twenty-fourth year.

815. Kirkpatrick, James (d.1770). <u>Some Reflections on the Causes and Circumstances that may retard or prevent the Putrification of Dead Bodies</u>. London, 1751. 40pp. An M.D., the writer published a variety of medical tracts between 1751 and 1769.

E. Rupture

816. Andree, John (fl.1779-1799). <u>Account of an Elastic Trochar. . .for Tapping the Hydrocele</u>. London, 1781. 41pp. The writer served as an apprentice in surgery at the London Hospital; subsequently, he lectured on anatomy, gained an appointment as a surgeon to the Magdalen Hospital, and practiced surgery at London; he also served as a surgeon to the Finsbury Dispensary (1784) and to St. Clement Danes workhouse (1784); his publications focus upon surgery.

817. Blakey, William (1711?-?). <u>An Essay on the Manner of Preserving Children and Grown Persons from Ruptures</u>. London, n.d.; five eds. through 1793.

Surgery, Wounds, Dissection

Rupture (contd.)

An M.D., the writer had received an appointment to the College of Surgeons at Paris.

818. _____. Observations concerning Ruptures. London, 1764.
819. Boles, Katherine. An Answer to a Book, entitled, The History of Ruptures, by Robert Houstoun. London, 1726. 64pp. See #825.
820. Brand, Robert. The True Method of Reducing Ruptures. London, 1771. 47pp.
821. Brand, Thomas (fl.1775-1790). Chirurgical Essays on the Causes and Symptoms of Rupture. London, 1782. 108pp. The writer practiced surgery at London; his published tracts appeared between 1778 and 1788.
822. _____. Chirurgical Essays on the Cure of Ruptures. London, 1784. 119pp.; 2nd ed., London, 1785.
823. Douglas, John (d.1743). A Treatise on the Hydrocele. London, n.d.; another ed. at London, 1755. 222pp. The writer served as a surgeon to the Westminster Infirmary; see, also, #833.
824. Else, Joseph (d.1780). An Essay on the Cure of the Hydrocele. London, 1770. 68pp.; 2nd ed., London, 1772. 72pp. Else practiced surgery at London.
825. Houston, Robert (fl.1720-1725). A History of Ruptures and Rupture Curers. London, 1726. 240pp. An M.D., the writer also published essays in the Philosophical Transactions of the Royal Society; see, also #819.
826. Humpage, Benjamin (fl.1785-1795). An Essay on the Rupture Called Hydrocele. London, 1788. 38pp.
827. Pott, Percival (1713-1788). An Account of a Particular Kind of Rupture. London, 1757; three eds. through 1769; later eds. bound with #828. The work includes the first description of congenital hernia; see, also, #741.
828. _____. A Treatise on Ruptures. London, 1756; three eds. through 1769; later eds. bound with #827. This volume stands as a classic work on hernia; Pott refutes the majority of the old theories concerning the causes of the problem, as well as denounces the methods of treatment based upon those speculations.
829. Turnbull, William (1729?-1796). Rules for Ruptures. London, 1788; another ed., London, 1798. The writer studied medicine at Edinburgh and Glasgow, then settled at London; see, also #529.
830. Wilmer, Bradford (fl.1770-1775). Practical Observations on Hernia. London, 1788. See, also, #798.

F. Testicles (see, also, #816, #823, #824, #826)

831. Bell, Benjamin (1749-1806). A Treatise on the Hydrocele. . .and Other Diseases of the Testes. Edinburgh, 1794. 295pp. See, also, #724.
832. Howard, John (d.1811). Observations on the Method of Curing the Hydrocele, by Means of a Seton. London,

Testicles (contd.)

1783. 56pp. See, also, #453.
833. Justamond, John Obadiah (d.1786). Remarks on Mr. [John] Douglass's Treatise on the Hydrocele. London, 1758. 148pp. See #823; also, #748.
834. Keate, Thomas (1745-1821). Cases of the Hydrocele. London, 1788. 60pp. Keate studied medicine at St. George's Hospital, London; he succeeded John Hunter as surgeon-general of the army (1793), became an examiner of the College of Surgeons (1802, 1809, 1818), and served as a surgeon to the Prince of Wales and to Chelsea Hospital.
835. Warner, Joseph (1717-1801). An Account of the Testicles. . .and the Diseases to which they are Liable. London, 1774; 2nd ed., London, 1775; a German translation in 1775. See, also, #791.

VI

Plague/Epidemic, Fever, Scarlet Fever, Yellow Fever, Small Pox, Cow Pox, Inoculation, Venereal Diseases

A. Plague/Epidemic

836. Baker, John (1708-1749). A Defense of a Late Treatise entitled, An Inquiry into. . . the Present Epidemick Fever. Sarum, 1743. 12pp. See #837.
837. ———. An Inquiry into the Nature, Cause, and Cure of the Present Epidemick Fever. London, 1742. 128pp. See, also, #836, #838.
838. The Best Preservative against the Plague. With a Short Account of the State of This Nation. London, 1721. 51pp. This tract combines medical advice with political argument. For a fairly clear notion in terms of specific diseases and numbers of deaths from the plague within the various London parishes, the reader would do well to consult M. Dorothy George, London Life in the XVIIIth Century (New York: Alfred A. Knopf, 1926) 405-410.
839. Blackmore, Sir Richard (1650-1729). Discourse on the Plague and Malignant Fevers. London, 1720. This piece represents but one of at least seven medical tracts written by the London poet, physician, political essayist, critic, and satirist; his reputation has arisen more from his literary efforts and his associations with the literati of the day than from his contributions to the history of medicine; Blackmore received the M.A. and B.A. from Oxford, while his M.D. came to him by way of Padua.
840. Borthwick, George (fl.1772-1796). The Method of Preventing and Removing the Causes of Infectious Diseases. Cork, 1784. 47pp. The writer held the M.D. degree.
841. Bradley, Richard (1688-1732). The Virtue and Use of Coffee, with Regard to the Plague. London, 1721. 34pp. See, also #37.
842. Brown, Joseph (fl.1700-1721). A Practical Treatise of the Plague. London, 1720. 79pp.; 2nd ed., London,

Plague/Epidemic (contd.)

1720. 79pp. The work includes a prefatory epistle to Dr. Richard Mead, as well as an address to the members and the president of the Royal College of Physicians (to which the writer did not belong); this piece proved to have been Brown's first published tract; see, also, #44.

843. Brownrigg, William (1711-1800). Considerations on the Means of Preventing the Communication of Pestilential Contagion, and the Methods by which it is Conveyed from Place to Place and from One Person to Another. London, 1771. 40pp. This work came forward as a reaction to outbreaks of plague on the Continent in 1771, but its effect and popularity diminished when the contagion failed to reach the British Isles; Brownrigg, a physician and chemist from Cumberland, studied medicine at London and Leyden (M.D. 1737); he practiced and conducted research (chemical and medical) at Whitehaven, but he never published his work to the extent that he should have; also, in 1772, he associated himself with several of Benjamin Franklin's experiments and with projects sponsored by the Royal Society.

844. Bruce, Alexander. An Inquiry concerning the Cause of the Pestilence, and the Diseases in Fleets and Armies. Edinburgh, 1759. 154pp.

845. Byrd, William (1674-1744). A Discourse concerning the Plague, with Some Preservatives against It. London, 1721. 40pp. See, also, #838.

846. Colebatch, Sir John (1670-1729). A Scheme for Proper Methods to be taken should it please God to visit us with the Plague. London, 1721. 21pp. See, also, #66. The writer defends his theory that diseases in the system arise principally from an excess of alkalis in the blood and the (so-called) humors; in practice, he liberally administered acids to his patients.

847. Davies, Richard (d.1762). An Essay concerning Pestilential Contagion. London, 1748. 72pp.; 2nd ed., London, 1757. 72pp. The writer held the M.D. from Cambridge (1748) and practiced medicine at Shrewsbury and Bath; his election as a fellow of the Royal Society came in 1738.

848. Distinct Notions of the Plague, with the Rise and Fall of Pestilential Contagion. By the Examiner. London, 1722. 131pp. See, also, descriptive note in #838.

849. Doctor [Richard] Mead's Short Discourse [1720] Explain'd. Or, His Account of Pestilential Contagion and Preventing Exploded. London, 1722. 103pp. See #869.

850. Fothergill, John (1712-1780). A Sketch of the Late Epidemick Disease. . .in London. London, 1775. 4pp. See descriptive note in #838, as well as #112.

851. The Free-Thinker. Considerations on the Nature,

Plague, Fever, Inoculation, Diseases 93

Plague/Epidemic (contd.)

Causes, Cure, and Prevention of Pestilence. London, 1721. 198pp.
852. Gataker, Thomas (d.1769). Observations on Venereal Complaints. London, 1754. 66pp.; 2nd ed., London, 1755. 43pp. Both versions in the form of the epistolary address. See, also, #120.
853. Gibson, Edmund (1669-1748). The Causes of the Discontents in Relation to the Plague, and the Provisions against It. London, 1721. 14pp. A native of Bampton, Westmoreland, Gibson entered Queen's College, Oxford, in 1686; taking Holy Orders, he rose to become rector of Lambeth (1703), archdeacon of Surrey (1710), Bishop of Lincoln (1715), and Bishop of London (1723); the majority of his written works tend to focus upon theological issues and antiquarian subjects; thus, this essay represents a number of his purely occasional pieces.
854. Grant, William (d.1786). A Short Account of the Present Epidemic Cough and Fever. London, 1776. 30pp. See, also, the descriptive note in #838. An M.D., Grant published various medical tracts between 1771 and 1782.
855. Handley, James (fl.1705-1725). A Description of the Plague. London, 1721. See, also, #745.
856. Henderson, William (fl.1784-1813). A Few Observations concerning the Plague. London, 1789. 79pp. The writer held the M.D. degree; he also published (1813) an essay relative to Sir Humphry Davys' observations on chlorine.
857. Hendley, William (1691?-1724). Loimologia Sacra: or, A Discourse shewing that the Plague never proceeds from any first Natural Cause, but is sent immediately from God. . . . With and Appendix, wherein the Case of flying from a Pestilence is briefly consider'd. London, 1721. 88pp. This work came to be considered only on the periphery of medical study or analysis; Hendley, ordained curate of Aylesford, Kent, and elected to the lectureship of St. James, Clerkenwell, participated in the Bangorian controversy (1717: attacking Church authority) and advocated the development of charity schools.
858. Hird, William (fl.1750-1785). Remarks upon Pestilence. London, 1753. 96pp. The writer, an M.D., published medical tracts between 1751 and 1781.
859. Hodges, Nathaniel (1629-1688). Loimologia, sive Pestis Nuperae apud Populum Londinensem Grassantis Narratio Historica. London, 1672; and English edition came forth at London in 1720 under the title, Loimologia, or an Historical Account of the Plague in London, in 1665, with Precautionary Directions; to which is added an Essay on the Causes of Pestilential Diseases. Hodges received the M.D. from Oxford; see, also, #142.

Plague/Epidemic (contd.)

860. Huxham, John (1694-1768). Observationes de Aero et Morbis Epidemicis. 3 vols. London, 1731; further eds. 1739, 1752, 1771; an English ed. (London, 1759) under the title, Observations of the Air and Epidemic Diseases from the Year 1728-1737 (and bound with Huxham's A Short Dissertation on the Devonshire Colic). The writer's description of the stomach disorders accompanying the drinking of cider led to Sir George Baker's discovery of lead poisoning; see, also, #334.

861. Johnstone, James (1730-1802). Historical Dissertation on the Malignant Epidemic Fever of 1756. London, 1758. 68pp. A native of Annan, Scotland, Johnstone practiced medicine at Kidderminster, near Birmingham, and later at Worcester; between 1760 and 1795, he contributed medical tracts to the Philosophical Transactions of the Royal Society.

862. Kemp, William (fl.1650-1670). A Treatise on the Nature, Cure, Signs, and Causes of the Pestilence. London, 1665.

863. Kennedy, Peter (fl.1710-1738). A Discourse on Pestilence. London, 1721. 38pp. See,also, #459.

864. Kephale, Richard. Medela Pestilentiae. London, 1665.

865. Lyons, John. A Prevention of the Plague. London, 1743. 23pp.

866. Manningham, Sir Richard (1690-1759). A Discourse concerning the Plague. London, 1758. 84pp. Born at Eversley, Hampshire, and educated (LL.B. and M.D.) at Cambridge, Manningham practiced midwifery in London and established himself at the head of his profession; a licentiate of the College of Physicians and knighted (1721) by George I, his name achieved additional recognition through representation in Laurence Sterne's Tristram Shandy (1759-1767).

867. _____. The Plague No Contagious Disease. London, 1744. 70pp.

868. May, William (fl.1785-1795). Observations on Epidemic Fever. London, 1790. The writer held the M.D. degree.

869. Mead, Richard (1673-1754). A Short Discourse concerning Pestilential Contagion, and the Methods to be used to Prevent It. London, 1720; seven eds. within the first year following publication; 8th ed., London, 1722; 9th ed., London, 1744. This work came to be written because of a plague at Marseilles in 1719 and a concern by the British government that the disease would spread to London; Mead advocated proper facilities in which to isolate the sick, as opposed to the usual general quarantine or fumigation; the volume did come under attack by George Pye (see #873) and others (see #849) who advocated quarantine and fumigation; see, also, #176.

870. Musgrave, Samuel (1732-1780). An Essay on the Nature and Cure of the (so-called) Worm-Fever. London,

Plague/Epidemic (contd.)

1776. 32pp. A native of Washfield, Devonshire, Musgrave studied at Oxford and at universities in Holland and France; in 1760, he gained election as a fellow of the Royal Society and eventually (1763) earned the M.D. from Leyden; he resided for a year (1764) in France before settling at Exeter as a physician to the Devon and Exeter Hospital; moving on to Plymouth in 1768, he involved himself in political affairs; after receiving the M.D. from Oxford in 1775, Musgrave removed himself to London, became a fellow of the College of Physicians (1777), and received appointment as Gulstonian lecturer and censor (1779); he also achieved a reputation as a Greek scholar and as the possessor of a large personal library.

871. Observations on the Present Epidemic Fever, Deduced from Plain Facts, Confirmed by Experience, and Illustrated by Suitable Cases. London, 1741. 62pp. See, also, descriptive note in #838.

872. Pringle, John. A Rational Inquiry into the Nature of the Plague. London, 1722. 24pp. The writer, an M.D., should not be confused with Sir John Pringle (1707-1782; see #954), the eminent and influential London physician, who would, of course, have been only fifteen years of age in 1722; see, also, DNB 16:388.

873. Pye, George (fl.1715-1725). Two Discourses on the Plague; wherein Dr. [Richard] Mead's Notions are Considered and Refuted. London, 1721. The writer held the M.D. degree; see #869.

874. Quincy, John (d.1722). Essays on Pestilential Diseases. London, 1721. A collection of essays by the London apothecary concerning such subjects as ague, fevers, gout, leprosy, and the king's evil (scrofula); the volume substantiates the criticism against Quincy's limited knowledge of medicine, although he did demonstrate an ability to prescribe "reasonable" remedies; thus, according to his own statements, dried millipedes proved valid for "tuberculosis lymphatic glands," but the "royal touch" would serve only "on a deluded imagination" and it deserved to be "banished with the superstition and bigotry that introduced it"; see, also, #490.

875. Rainey, John (fl.1715-1725). A Treatise on Pestilential Diseases. London, 1720. The writer held the M.D. degree.

876. Rogers, Joseph (fl.1730-1735). An Essay on Epidemical Diseases and Statical Experiments. Dublin, 1734. 312pp. The work focuses upon events at Cork.

877. Rose, Phillip (fl.1720-1725). A Theorico-Practical, Miscellaneous, and Succinct Treatise of the Plague. London, 1721. 56pp. The writer also published tracts on the art of printing and on reading verse.

878. Rosewell, Thomas (1630-1692). The Causes and Cure of the Pestilence. London, 1665. A native of

Plague/Epidemic (contd.)

Dunkerton, near Bath, Rosewell entered the ministry and served as domestic chaplain to a number of titled families; nothing in his background indicates knowledge, preparation, or practice of medicine; after his ejection from the rectory of Sutton Mandeville in 1662 for nonconformity, he spent the next dozen years defending himself against charges of high treason.

879. Russell, Patrick (1726-1805). A Treatise of the Plague. 2 vols. London, 1791. Born at Edinburgh and an M.D. graduate of the University there, Russell eventually succeeded (1753) his brother Alexander (1715?-1768; see #224) as physician to the English factory at Aleppo, in Syria; this Treatise resulted from and focuses upon three epidemics at Aleppo between 1760 and 1762, as well as the methods of inoculation practiced in that part of the world; in addition to his practice of medicine, Russell developed strong interests in botany and zoology.

880. Samber, Robert (1633-1729). A Treatise of the Plague. By Eugenius Philalethes, Jun. London, 1721. 32pp. A miscellaneous writer, Samber will be best remembered for his Roma Illustrata; or, a Description of the most Beautiful Pieces of Painting, Sculpture and Architecture at and near Rome. London, 1722; a copy of that work resides in Horace Walpole's library (see Allen T. Hazen, A Catalogue of Horace Walpole's Library [New Haven and London: Yale University Press, 1969], 1:110).

881. Simpson, William (fl.1665-1680). A Short Discourse of the Plague. London, 1665. The writer achieved a modest reputation for his tracts describing Scarborough and other spa towns, published between 1669 and 1679.

882. Simms, James (1741-1820). Observations on Epidemic Disorder, with Remarks on Nervous and Malignant Fevers. London, 1773; 2nd ed., London, 1776; German translation at Hamburg, 1775; French translation at Avignon, 1778. Simms graduated M.D. from Leyden in 1674 and practiced medicine first in County Tyrone, Ireland, and then at London; he served the General Dispensary in Aldersgate Street and the Surrey Dispensary; for twenty-two years he presided over the Medical Society of London.

883. Smyth, James Carmichael (1741-1821). An Account of the Experiment. . .To Determine the Effect of the Nitrous Acid in Destroying Contagion. London, 1796. 75pp. See, also, #686.

884. Strother, Edward (1675-1737). Practical Observations on the Epidemical Fever. London, 1729. See, also, #258.

885. Thomson, George (b.1620; fl.1648-1679). Loimotomia: A Consolatory Advice, and Some Brief Observations concerning the Present Pest. London, 1665. Essentially, the writer considers the conduct of

Plague/Epidemic (contd.)

those members of the College of Physicians who fled London during the Great Plague; Thomson graduated M.D. from Leyden in 1648, then proceeded to London and the practice of medicine there; he appears to have devoted considerable effort to observing both causes and symptoms of plague.

886. Willis, Thomas (1621-1675). A Plain and Easy Method for Preserving (by God's Blessing) those that are Well from the Infection of the Plague or any Contagious Disease, in City, Camp, Country, Fleet, &c.; and for Curing such as are Infected with it. London, 1691; 2nd ed., London, 1722. This work written in 1660, but published posthumously by the physician's amanuensis, James Henning; see, also, #276.

887. Wintringham, Clifton the elder (1689-1748). Commentarium Nologicum Morbos Epidemicos et Aeris Variationes in Urbe Eboracensi, Losique Vicinis, 1715-1725. London, 1727; 2nd ed., London, 1733. See, also, #280.

888. ____. An Essay on Contagious Diseases, more particularly on the Small Pox, Measles, Putrid, Malignant, and Pestilential Fevers. York, 1721.

889. ____. A Treatise of Epidemic Diseases. York, 1718.

B. Fever

890. Alderson, John (1758-1829). An Essay on the Nature and Origin of the Contagion of Fevers. Hull, 1788. 58pp. Alderson served as a physician to the Hull Infirmary; he practiced physic at Hull and became the principal physician of that town; his written work focused upon fever and paralysis.

891. Balfour, Francis (fl.1769-1812). A Treatise on Sol-Lunar Influence in Fevers. Calcutta, 1784; 2nd ed., London, 1795; 3rd ed., Cupar, 1815; 4th ed., Cupar, 1816; a German translation with a preface by one "Herr Luth," at Strasburg, 1786. The writer sets forth his theory that fevers arise from the direct influence of the moon, reaching their critical stage with the coming of the full moon; an Anglo-Indian medical officer, Balfour earned the M.D. degree from Edinburgh, served the East India Company at Bengal as a surgeon, and practiced at Edinburgh following his retirement from the foreign service; he also belonged to the Bengal Asiatic Society and contributed the results of his research on the Arabic language to that organization.

892. Ball, John (1704?-1779). A Treatise of Fevers. London, 1758. 243pp. See, also, #19.

893. Beddoes, Thomas (1760-1808). Observations on the Nature and Cure of Calculus, Sea Scurvy, Consumption, Catarrh, and Fever: together with Conjectures upon Several Other Subjects of Physiology and Pathology. London, 1793. 172pp.; an American ed. at Philadelphia, 1797. As indicated

Fever (contd.)

by its title, this work served as a handbook of procedures for various ailments; Beddoes, known principally for his work with inhalation therapy, was a native of Shiffnall, Shropshire; he assumed, in 1785, the lectureship in chemistry at Oxford; his wide interests extended to politics, education, political economy, biography, and even to poetry.

894. Browne, Andrew (fl.1690-1715). An Essay on the New Cure of Fevers. Edinburgh, 1691. A native of Scotland, the writer practiced medicine at Edinburgh.

895. ____. Vindication of [Thomas] Sydenham's Method of Curing Continual Fevers. London, 1700.

896. Chalmers, Lionel (1715?-1777). An Essay on Fevers. London, 1768. 96pp. A native of Scotland, the writer emigrated to South Carolina in 1736, and he practiced medicine in that colony for more than forty years; however, he published his essays and books at London.

897. Charsley, William. An Essay to Investigate the Cause of the General Mortality of Fevers. London, 1793. The writer held the M.D. degree; see, also, the descriptive note in #836.

898. Cheyne, George (1671-1743). A New Theory of Acute and Slow-Continued Fevers. Edinburgh, 1702; London, 1702; further London eds. in 1715, 1722, 1724. Cheyne composed this tract in haste and without consulting sources; he then published it anonymously; it constitutes the writer's contribution to a controversy involving Dr. Archibald Pitcairn (see, also, #55), then professor of medicine at the University of Edinburgh, and that theorist's "ratromathematical" system of medicine in the treatment of fevers; see, also, #55, as well as #952.

899. Chisolm, Colin (1755-1825). An Essay on the Malignant Pestilential Fever. London, 1795. 279pp.; Philadelphia, 1799. 308pp. Chisholm served as a naval surgeon before commencing medical practice at Bristol; he died at London; a contributor of essays to a number of medical periodicals, he also managed to achieve, in 1808, election as a fellow of the Royal Society.

900. Clark, John (1744-1805). Observations on Fevers. London, 1780. 398pp.; another ed., London, 1792. 398pp. Clark studied divinity and medicine at Edinburgh; in 1768, he obtained an appointment as a surgeon's mate with the East India Company, a position that he held until 1775; he then practiced medicine at Newcastle and graduated M.D. from St. Andrews; his interest on behalf of the sick poor led to his founding of the Newcastle Dispensary.

901. Clutton, Joseph (fl.1725-1740). A Short and Certain Method of Curing Continu'd Fevers. London, 1735. 133pp.; three eds. through 1748. The writer published medical essays between 1729 and 1736.

Fever (cont'd.)

902. Cockburn, William (1669-1739). The Danger of Improving Physick: with an Account of the Present Epidemick Fever. London, 1730. 39pp. Cockburn had initially secured his professional reputation (as well as his financial position) through his "cure" for dysentery; the thirty-nine page Danger constitutes a response to those academics and physicians who opposed that "secret remedy"; particularly, the writer challenged the attacks by Dr. John Freind in that physician's History of Physick (1725); see, also #1883.

903. Cole, William (1635-1716). Novae Hypotheseos ad Explicanda Febrium Intermittentium Symptomata Hypotyposis. London, 1694; Amsterdam, 1698; Geneva, 1696 and 1697; Lyons, 1737. An M.D. from Oxford (1666), Cole practiced medicine at Worcester before moving on to London in 1692; the extent to which his published works appeared in translation on the European continent attests to his overall reputation as a medical writer; he concerned himself more with theory and hypothesis rather than with actual medical observation and practice.

904. Cross, Francis. De Febre Intermittente. Oxford, 1668.

905. Currie, James (1756-1805). Medical Reports on the Effects of Water, Cold and Warm, as a Remedy in Fever and Febrile Diseases, whether applied to the Surface of the Body or used as a Drink; with Observations on the Nature of Fever and on the Effects of Opium, Alcohol, and Inanition. Liverpool, 1797; 2nd ed., 1799; 3rd ed., 2 vols., 1804; 4th ed., 1805. The writer maintains that the early stage of fever should be treated by pouring cold water over the body; in later stages, the body temperature should be reduced by bathing with tepid water; in all stages of fever, "abundant" quantities of cold water will prove beneficial; Currie includes case studies (actual observations) and quotes passages from old medical books to support his thesis; after spending some time in America, the Scottish-born Currie returned to Edinburgh, studied medicine there, assumed practiced at Liverpool, and then moved on to Bath; he involved himself with the study of the effects of cold bathing and expended his spare moments upon the movement to abolish the slave trade.

906. Curry, John (d.1780). An Essay on Ordinary Fevers. London, 1743; another ed. at Dublin, 1773. An Irish physician and historian, the writer drew the critical attention of the poet Thomas Moore (1779-1852), who referred to him in his verse as "honest Currie."

907. _____. Some Thoughts on the Nature of Fevers. Dublin, 1774; London, 1774. 94pp.

908. Descherny, David (b.1730?; fl.1750-1763). An Essay on Fevers. London, 1760. The writer, an M.D., also

Fever (contd.)

published essays on the stone (1753), small pox (1760), and the gout (1760).

909. Dickinson, Caleb. An Enquiry into the Nature and Causes of Fever. Edinburgh, 1785. 192pp. A volume with this title and imprint exists in the National Library of Medicine; Allibone (1:501) cites "Dickson, Caleb, M.D. Fever, Lon., 1585, 8vo."

910. Drake, James (1667-1707). Orationes Tres: De Febre Intermittente, de Variolis et Moribillis, et de Phermacia Hodierna. London, 1742. 52pp. See, also, #316.

911. Drummond, Alexander M. Febribus. Edinburgh, 1770.

912. Dwight, Samuel (1669?-1737). De Febribus Symptomaticis. . .deque cum Earum Curatone. London, 1731. Dwight dedicated this volume to Sir Hans Sloane; see, also, #424.

913. Etherington, Rev. George (fl.1755-1765). General Cautions in the Cure of Fevers. London, 1760. 116pp. This work stands as merely a collection from the tracts of a number of contemporary physicians, but primarily from the pen of John Huxham; according to the London Monthly Review (23 [1760], 281), "such a compilation, however judicious, can avail but little in supplying the want of a regular medical education."

914. Fordyce, George (1736-1802). A Dissertation on Simple Fever. London, 1794. 238pp.; further London eds. in 1795, 1798, 1799, 1800. See, also, #104.

915. _____. A Second Dissertation on Tertian Intermittent Fever. London, 1795.

916. _____. A Third Dissertation on Continued Fever. 2 parts. London, 1798-1799.

917. Fordyce, John (fl.1750-1760). Historia Febris Miliaris. London, 1758. 106pp. The writer held the M.D. degree.

918. Fordyce, Sir William (1724-1792). A Letter to Sir John Sinclair on the Virtues of Muriatic Acid in Curing Putrid Diseases. London, 1790. 34pp. See, also, #743. The Right Honourable Sir John Sinclair (1754-1835), a native of County Caithness, Scotland, became, in 1755, a member of the Faculty of Advocates; he served in Parliament for thirty years (1780-1818), practiced law, and stood as a philanthropist who promoted projects for the benefit of agriculture and medicine.

919. _____. A New Inquiry into the Causes, Symptoms, and Cure of Putrid and Inflammatory Fevers, with an Appendix on the Hectic Fever and on the Ulcerated Sore Throat. London, 1773. 228pp.; 4th ed., London, 1777; a German ed. at Leipzig in 1774.

920. Franks, John (fl.1790-1799). A Treatise on Typhus Contagion. London, 1799. The writer also published tracts on animal life and death.

921. Fuller, Thomas (1654-1734). Exanthematalogia; or, an Attempt to give a Rational Account of Eruptive Fevers. London, 1730. 439pp. See, also, #430.

Fever (contd.)

This work represents another attempt of the writer-physician to provide medical assistance to the poor.

922. Gibson, John (fl.1768-1799). A Treatise on Continual, Intermitting, Erupting, and Inflammatory Fevers. London, 1769. 330pp. Possessed of a degree in medicine, Gibson wrote on a variety of subjects, ranging from fruit gardens to bilious diseases.

923. Glass, Thomas (1709-1786). Twelve Commentaries on Fevers. London, 1752. 302pp. Born at Tiverton, Glass studied medicine at Leyden (M.D. 1731); he practiced at Tiverton and Exeter, at the latter town he received appointment as a physician of the Devon and Exeter Hospital.

924. Grainger, James (1723?-1767). Historia Febris Anomalae Batavae, Annorum 1746-1748. Edinburgh, 1753. 196pp. A native of Dunse, Grainger served for a time as an army surgeon in Scotland and Germany; afterward, he practiced as a physician in London, then on St. Christopher's in the West Indies, where he died in 1767; he also wrote verse:
> Youth, you're mistaken, if you think to find
> In shades a medicine for a troubled mind;
> Wan Grief will haunt you whereso'er you go,
> Sigh in the breeze, and in the streamlet flow.

"Solitude. An Ode" (1755)

925. Grant, William (d.1786). An Enquiry into the Nature, Rise, and Progress of the Fevers Most Common in London. London, 1771. 463pp. See, also #854, and the descriptive note in #838.

926. _____. An Essay on the Pestilential Fever of Sydenham. London, 1775.

927. _____. A Short Account of a Fever and Sore Throat. London, 1777. 47pp.

928. Griffith, Moses (1724-1785). Practical Observations on the Cure of Hectic and Slow Fevers. London, 1776. 92pp.; other eds. in 1795, 1799. The writer held the M.D. degree.

929. Hawkbridge, John. A Treatise on Fevers. York, 1764. 55pp.

930. Heysham, John (1753-1834). An Account of the Gaol Fever. . .at Carlisle. London, 1782. 59pp. Born at Lancaster and educated by Quakers, the writer studied medicine at Edinburgh (M.D.1777); he practiced at Carlisle (1778-1834) and gained a reputation for his statistical observations relative to births, marriages, deaths, and diseases; he also studied the causes and effects of jail fever.

931. Huggenson, John (fl.1730-1740). A Short and Certain Method of Curing Continued Fevers. London, 1735.

932. Hussey, Garret (fl.1780-1785). A Physical Inquiry into the Cause and Cure of Fevers. Dublin, 1779. 275pp. The writer has been identified as an M.D., while his Inquiry received acknowledgement as "an

Fever (contd.)

attempt to revive the old doctrine of Error Loci" (Allibone 1:926).

933. Huxham, John (1694-1768). An Essay on Fevers and Their Various Kinds. London, 1739; further eds. in 1750, 1757, 1764, 1767, 1769; 8th ed., Edinburgh, 1779. See, also #334. This principal publication by the eminent physician and theorist contains an historical introduction to the Ancient physicians and a description of the types of and treatments for simple, intermittent, and nervous fevers, small pox, pleurisy, inflammation of the lungs, and bronchitis.

934. Jackson, Robert (1750-1827). An Outline of the History and Cure of Fever. Edinburgh, 1798. 396pp. The writer served as a physician in the British Army; his publications appeared, principally, between 1798 and 1817; his tract on army discipline reached three editions by 1845.

935. ____. A Treatise on the Fever of Jamaica. London, 1791; Philadelphia, 1795; a German ed. at Leipzig, 1796. The writer recommends that fevers be treated by "cold affusion," a remedy gained from his experience as an assistant to a doctor at Savanna-la-mer, Jamaica, between 1774 and 1780; a Scotsman, Jackson served with the army in Jamaica, Europe, America, and Scotland; he eventually rose to the position of inspector-general of army hospitals.

936. James, Robert (1703-1776). A Dissertation on Fevers. London, 1748. The writer recommends his own method of cure, for which he had been granted a patent the year previous to publication; James received the B.A. from Oxford (1726) and the M.D. by Royal mandate from Cambridge in 1728; before coming to London, he had practiced Sheffield, Lichfield, and Birmingham; he not only achieved a reputation from his numerous publications, but gained lasting recognition (at least from medical historians and scholars) for his fever powder and for the events surrounding the death of the poet-playwright-novelist-essayist Oliver Goldsmith.

937. Jones, Robert (fl.1781-1789). A Treatise on Nervous Disorders. Salisbury, 1789. The writer did possess the M.D. degree.

938. Kennedy, Peter, of Aylesbury. An Account of a Contagious Fever Which Prevailed lately at Aylesbury. Aylesbury, 1785. 52pp. Aylesbury lay in Buckinghamshire.

939. Kirkland, Thomas (1721-1798). An Essay towards an Improvement in the Cure of Those Diseases which are the Causes of Fevers. London, 1767. See, also, #749 and Archibald Maxwell's Answer (#950).

940. ____. A Reply to Mr. [Archibald] Maxwell's Answer to His Essay on Fevers; wherein the Utility of the Practice of Suppressing Them is further Exemplified. London, 1769. See,also, #950.

Plague, Fever, Inoculation, Diseases 103

Fever (contd.)

941. Lettsome, John Coakley (1744-1815). Reflections on the General Treatment and Cure of Fevers. London, 1772. 67pp. See, also, #160.
942. Lind, James (1716-1794). Two Papers on Fevers and Infection. London, 1763. 119pp. Born in Scotland and apprenticed to an Edinburgh surgeon, Lind served as a surgeon with the navy at Minorca, Guinea, and the West Indies; after receiving the M.D. (1748) from Edinburgh, he practiced (1748-1758) in the Scottish capital; one of the earliest physicians to write on sea scurvy, he eventually rose to become treasurer of the Edinburgh College of Physicians (1757-1758) and received an appointment as a physician to the Naval Hospital at Haslar (1758-1794)
943. Lipscomb, George (1773-1846). An Essay on the Nature and Treatment of a Putrid Malignant Fever. Warwick, 1799. 95pp. A native of Buckinghamshire, Lipscomb received his early medical education from his father, a Royal Navy surgeon; he then went forth to London for further, formal study; after an appointment (1792) as a house surgeon of St. Bartholomew's Hospital, he received (1806) the M.D. from Aberdeen; his interests focused upon history, political economics, and statistics, as well as on medicine; thus, he became known more as a county historian than as a medical practitioner or writer.
944. Lobb, Theophilus (1678-1763). Medical Practice in Curing Fevers Correspondent to Rational Methods. London, 1735. Born at London and educated for the Nonconformist ministry, Lobb moved (1706) to Shaftesbury, Dorset, and began to practice medicine there; in 1722, he proceeded to Witham, Essex, and during that year managed to obtain an M.D. from Glasgow; beginning in 1740, after his election as a licentiate of the Royal College of Physicians, London, he devoted himself entirely to the practice of physic; a year prior to his death, Lobb received a patent for "a tincture to preserve the blood from dizziness" and another for "a saline scorbutic acrimony."
945. _____. Rational Methods of Curing Fevers. London, 1734.
946. Lysons, Daniel (1727-1800). An Essay upon the Effects of Camphire and Calomel in Continual Fevers. London, 1771. 80pp. See, also, #608.
947. _____. Practical Essays upon Intermitting Fevers, Dropsies...and the Operation of Calomel. Bath, 1772. 214pp. Calomel, or mercurous chloride, functioned as a general purgative.
948. Manningham, Sir Richard (1690-1759). The Symptoms, Nature, Causes, and Cure of the Febricula, or Little Fever. London, 1746. 112pp.; four eds. through 1760. See, also, #866.
949. Mason, Simon (fl.1745-1756). The Nature of an Intermitting Fever and Ague Consider'd. London,

Fever (contd.)

1745. 296pp. See, also, #175.
950. Maxwell, Archibald (fl.1760-1770). <u>An Answer to [Thomas] Kirkland's Essay towards an Improvement in the Cure of Those Diseases which are the Cause of Fevers</u>. London, 1758. 67pp. See #939, #940.
951. Parker, Thomas (fl.1790-1800). <u>A Practical Treatise on Fever</u>. London, 1796. 90pp.
952. Pitcairne, Archibald (1652-1713). <u>Dissertation de Curatione Febrium, quae per Evacuationes Instituiter</u>. Edinburgh, 1695. Born at Edinburgh and educated there and at Paris, Pitcairne combined the studies of mathematics and medicine; after obtaining the M.D. degree from Rheims (1680), he practiced medicine at Edinburgh and published on blood circulation, mathematics, and fevers; he also wrote anonymous pamphlet attacks and satirical verse directed against the Scottish Kirk, as well as more serious poems and translations in Latin.
953. Poole, Richard (fl.1790-1795). <u>An Account of Fever in Somersetshire in 1792</u>. The writer practiced surgery at Sherburne, in the East Riding of Yorkshire.
954. Pringle, Sir John (1707-1782). <u>Observations on the Nature and Cure of Hospital and Jayl Fevers, in a Letter to Dr.</u> [Richard] <u>Mead</u>. London, 1750. Pringle studied at Edinburgh, Amsterdam, and Leyden (M.D. 1730); he then returned to Edinburgh to lecture on metaphysics and moral philosophy and to practice medicine; after serving with the Royal Army under the Duke of Cumberland in Flanders and Scotland, Pringle settled in London; there, he gained royal favor, association with the Royal Society, and eminence as a scientist; above all, he contributed significantly to the reform of medical practice in the military and to the improvement of sanitation; in terms of jail fever (a form of typhus), Pringle demonstrated its kinship with hospital fever.
955. Quinton, John (fl.1707-1734). <u>De Thermis</u>. London, 1726. The writer did hold the M.D. degree and practiced surgery at London.
956. Richardson, Alexander M. (fl.1765-1770). <u>The Modern Practice of Physick in Fevers and Measles</u>. London, 1768.
957. Riddel, John (fl.1780-1890). <u>An Essay on Continued Fevers</u>. Glasgow, 1788.
958. Riollay, Francis (1748-1797). <u>The Study of Fevers</u>. London, 1788. This volume arose from the three Gulstonian lectures on fever delivered by the writer in 1787; published with a preface in Latin, the essays detail classical, medieval and extant doctrines relative to fevers, but do so without clinical illustrations or personal observations; Riollay, born in Brittany, studied at Trinity College, Dublin, and at Oxford; he practiced and lectured at London, wrote on the gout, and

Plague, Fever, Inoculation, Diseases

Fever (contd.)

commented upon Hippocratic doctrines.
959. Roberts, John (fl.1780-1785). <u>Observations upon Fever</u>. London, 1781.
960. Robertson, Robert (1742-1829). <u>An Essay on Fevers</u>. London, 1790. 286pp. A native of Scotland, the writer obtained appointment as a surgeon on a whaling ship, after which he entered (1760) the Royal Navy as a surgeon's mate; he served in Portugal, Newfoundland, Ireland, Cornwall, the West Indies, and Africa; the University of Aberdeen conferred upon him the M.D. (1779), and later (1793) he became a physician to the Greenwich Hospital.
961. _____. <u>Observations on Jail, Hospital, or Ship Fever</u>. London, 1783; 318pp.; another ed., London, 1784.
962. Rowley, William (1742-1806). <u>The Causes of the Great Number of Deaths amongst Adults and Children in Putrid, Scarlet Fevers, and Ulcerated Sore Throats Explained</u>. London, 1793. 47pp. See, also, descriptive note in #838, and #222.
963. Simpson, William (fl.1665-1679). <u>A History of the Present Fever</u>. London, 1678. The writer achieved some recognition for his studies of the various spas in the north of England.
964. Slaughter, Henricus. <u>Dissertatio Medica Inauguralis, de Febre Puerperale</u>. Edinburgh, 1780. 29pp. A copy of this thesis for the M.D. degree (Edinburgh) resides in the British Museum.
965. Stevens, J.N. (fl.1755-1760). <u>A Practical Treatise on Fevers</u>. London, 1760. 510pp. An M.D., the writer also wrote upon diseases of the head and neck, as well as on the waters at Bath; see, also, #649.
966. Sudel, Nicholas (fl.1690-1700). <u>An Essay on Kentish and All Other Agues</u>. London, 1699.
967. Talbor, Sir Robert (fl.1672-1682). <u>Observations on the Cause and Cure of Agues</u>. London, 1672.
968. _____. <u>A Treatise on the Secret and Curing of Agues and Fevers</u>. London, 1682.
969. Turner, John (fl.1708-1713). <u>De Febre Britannica Anni 1712 Schediasma</u>. London, 1713. 7pp.
970. Vaughan, William (fl.1670-1675). <u>Disputatio Medica de Febre Continuata</u>. London, 1671.
971. Warren, Martin (fl.1730-1735). <u>Dr. Warren's Epistle to His Friend, of the Method and Manner of Curing the Late Raging Fevers</u>. London, 1733. 79pp.
972. White, John (fl.1710-1715). <u>De Recta Sanguinis Missione: or, New and Exact Observations of Fevers</u>. London, 1712. The writer held the M.D. degree.
973. White, Richard (fl.1755-1765). <u>Animadversions on the Increase of Fevers and Other Diseases</u>. London, 1760. See, also, the descriptive note in #836.
974. Wigan, John (1696-1739). <u>De Curandi Febribus Continuis, Liber; from the Original of Longinus</u>. London, 1718. A native of Kensington, Middlesex, Wigan received the M.D. from Oxford (1727) before serving (1733-1737) as physician to the Westminster

Fever (contd.)

Hospital, London; he died at Jamaica, where he had been practicing medicine; his reputation as a writer arose from his translations and editions of the Ancients.

975. Wilson-Philip, Alexander Philip (1770?-1851?). A Treatise on Febrile Diseases. 4 vols. Winchester, 1799-1804. See, also, #542.

976. Withers, Thomas (fl.1772-1794). Dissertatio Inaug. de Febribus Continuis Medendis. Edinburgh, 1772. This constitutes the writer's M.D. thesis from Edinburgh; he also published a number of tracts on asthma and on medical education.

C. Scarlet Fever

977. Clark, Thaddeus (fl.1790-1800). A Treatise on the Scarlatina Anginosa. Norwich, 1795. 48pp.

978. Cotton, Nathaniel (1705-1788). Observations on a Particular Kind of Scarlet Fever that Lately Prevailed in and about St. Albans. London, 1749. 22pp. This volume represents the only medical publication by the London poet and physician; his cultivated, pious, and didactic verse proved extremely popular; see, also, the descriptive note in #836.

979. Withering, William (1741-1799). An Account of the Scarlet Fever and Sore Throat, or Scarlatina Anginosa. Birmingham, 1778; 2nd ed., Birmingham, 1793. See, also, #543.

D. Yellow Fever

980. Blicke, Sir Charles (1745-1815). An Essay on the Bilious or Yellow Fever of Jamaica, Collected from the MSS. of a Late Surgeon. London, 1772. 71pp. In his preface, the writer (or editor?) states that he abridged the original and simplified its style; the volume advances the treatment of fever by bleeding, purging, warm baths, fresh air, and acid drinks; it includes testaments from some twenty writers, reference to an expedition to Carthagena, and a discussion of the exportation of water from the Bristol hot wells to Jamaica; Blicke received his medical education at St. Bartholomew's Hospital (London) and practiced surgery there; this Essay stands as his only identifiable published work.

981. Bryce, James (fl.1792-1809). An Account of the Yellow Fever. Edinburgh, 1796. 97pp. The writer also published a tract on the cow pox (1802, 1809).

982. Holliday, John ((fl.1790-1800). A Short Account of the Origin, Symptoms, and Most Approved Method of Treating the Putrid Bilious Yellow Fever. London, 1795; another ed. published at Boston in 1796. Allibone (1:866) cites another John Holiday (1730-1801) who wrote a biography of William, Earl of Mansfield (1797) and published (1800) a poem

Plague, Fever, Inoculation, Diseases

Yellow Fever (contd.)

entitled The British Oak.

E. Small Pox

983. Aberdour, Alexander (fl.1790-1795). Observations on the Small Pox and Inoculation. Edinburgh, 1791. 83pp.
984. Baker, Sir George (1722-1809). An Inquiry into the Merits of a Method of Inoculation of the Small Pox, which is now Practised in Several of the Counties of England. London, 1766. See, also, #17.
985. Baylies, William (1724-1787). Facts and Observations Relative to the Inoculation of the Small Pox at Berlin. Edinburgh, 1781. See, also, #556. The work concerns the writer's experiences and practices as a physician to Frederick the Great; the writer originally composed the volume in French and published it at Dresden in 1776.
986. Blackmore, Sir Richard (1650-1729). A Treatise on the Small Pox. London, 1723. See, also, #839.
987. Bromfield, Sir William (1712-1792). Thoughts Arising from Experience concerning the Present Peculiar Method of Treating Persons Inoculated for the Small Pox. London, 1767. 88pp.; Dublin, 1767. 87pp. Bromfield lectured at London on anatomy and surgery. See, also, #728.
988. Chandler, John (1700-1780). A Discourse concerning Small-Pox, occasioned by Dr. [Richard] Holland's Essay. London, 1729. Chandler, a London, apothecary, served with the firm of Smith and Newsome, King Street, Cheapside; see, also, #998.
989. Deering, George Charles (1695?-1749). A Method of Treating the Small Pox. London, 1737. The writer, who claimed a medical degree from Leyden, did study anatomy and botany at Paris; upon his return to England, he concentrated his energies upon the study of botany.
990. Descherny, David (b.1730?; fl. 1760-1763). Some Observations on the Small-Pox. London, 1760. See, also, #908.
991. Fowle, William (fl.1780-1800). An Essay on the Use of Mercury in the Small-Pox. London, 1793. The writer, an M.D., spent some time in the West Indies; he practiced medicine there and at London.
992. Franklin, Richard (fl.1720-1725). Dissertatio de Variolis; or, a Discourse concerning the Small Pox. 22pp.
993. Frewen, Thomas (1704-1791). Some Reasons Given against an Opinion that a Person infected with Small Pox may be cured by Antidote. London, 1759. 39pp. The writer, an M.D., published a number of medical treatises between 1749 and 1780; he practiced as a surgeon and apothecary at Rye, then as a physician at Lewes; one of the first among the English physicians to adopt inoculation to small pox, Frewen experimented with over 350 cases.

Small Pox (contd.)

994. Glass, Thomas (d.1786). <u>A Letter to Dr.</u> [Sir George] <u>Baker, on the Means of Procuring a Distinct and Favourable Kind of Small Pox</u>. London, 1767. 72pp.; a second <u>Letter</u> in 1767. 55pp. See #984 and, also, #923.
995. Haygarth, John (1740-1827). <u>An Inquiry how to prevent the Small Pox</u>. Chester 1784. 223pp; 2nd ed., Chester, 1785. A native of Yorkshire, Haygarth practiced physic at the Chester Infirmary (1767-1798) and then moved on to Bath; his major contribution to medicine concerned treating fever patients in separate wards or even in separate hospitals; further, he became one of the earliest of physicians to distinguish the different types of fevers by their periods of incubation.
996. <u>   . A Sketch of a Plan to Exterminate the Causal Small-pox, and to Introduce General Inoculation</u>. 2 vols. London, 1793. The idea of this volume, although innovative at the outset, soon became obsolete following Edward Jenner's discovery of vaccination.
997. Hillary, William (d.1763). <u>A Rational and Mechanical Essay on the Small-Pox</u>. London, 1735. 184pp.; 2nd ed., London, 1740. A pupil of Hermann Boerhaave at Leyden, where he graduated M.D. in 1722, Hillary practiced medicine at Ripon, Bath, the Barbados, and London; he devoted his energies to systematic observations of the weather and to studies of the prevalent diseases.
998. Holland, Richard (1688-1730). <u>An Essay on the Nature and Cure of the Small Pox</u>. London, 1728. 162pp.; further eds. in 1740, 1741 (2 vols.), 1746. The writer held the M.D. degree; see, also #988.
999. Holwell, John Zephaniah (1711-1798). <u>An Account of the Method of Inoculation for the Small-Pox in the East Indies</u>. London, 1767. 40pp. The writer studied surgery at Guy's Hospital, London, went to Calcutta as a surgeon's mate, and became a medical officer aboard several ships; he practiced surgery at Calcutta, returned to England, and embarked on a medical career in his native country; eventually, returned to India as governor of Bengal; his written work focuses largely upon historical, scholarly, and antiquarian subjects related to East India.
1000. Jurin, James (1684-1750). <u>A Letter to the Learned Caleb Cotesworth. . .containing a Comparison between the Mortality of the Natural Small Pox and that given by Inoculation</u>. London, 1723. 31pp. See, also, #803.
1001. Lampard, John (fl.1680-1690). <u>A Treatise on the Small Pox</u>. London, 1685.
1002. Langrish, Browne (d.1759). <u>Plain Directions in Regard to the Small-Pox</u>. London, 1758. 35pp.; 2nd ed., London, 1759. 58pp. See, also, #159.
1003. Lynn, Walter (1677-1763). <u>An Essay towards a more</u>

Small Pox (contd.)

easie and safe Method of Cure in the Small Pox. London, 1714. A native of Northamptonshire, Lynn graduated B.A. and M.B. from Oxford; he practiced music, wrote about medicine, and engaged in attempts to construct a steam engine.

1004. ____. Some Reflections upon the Modern Practices of Physick in Relation to the Small Pox. London, 1715. 27pp.

1005. Lynn, William (1753-1837). The Singular Case of a Lady Who Had the Small Pox during Pregnancy. London, 1776. 19pp.

1006. Mackenzie, James (1680?-1761). A Short and Clear Account of. . .Inoculating the Small Pox. Edinburgh, 1760. 31pp. An M.D. who practiced at Worcester, Mackenzie also published a history of health (1759), an essay on Luxation of the Thigh (1756), and a collection of Essays and Meditations (1762).

1007. Maitland, Charles (1668-1748). An Account of Inoculating the Small Pox. London, 1722. 35pp.; 2nd ed., London, 1723.

1008. Mead, Richard (1673-1754). De Variolis et Moribillis. London, 1747; eds. in English and German followed. See, also #176. According to the Lives of British Physicians (London, 1830, p.159), "The purity and elegance of [Latin] style exhibited in this work have attracted the admiration of scholars" (see Allibone 2:1257).

1009. Monro, Alexander the eldest (1697-1767). An Account of the Inoculation of Small Pox in Scotland. Edinburgh, 1764. Monro received his medical education at Edinburgh (M.D.) and studied further (principally in anatomy) at London; he then went to Leyden, enrolling as a pupil of Hermann Boerhaave, before returning to Edinburgh as professor of anatomy and surgery to the Surgeons' Company; in 1720, he became the first professor of anatomy at the University of Edinburgh, lecturing on that discipline annually for the next thirty-nine years.

1010. Mudge, John (1721-1793). Dissertation on Inoculated Small-Pox; or, an Attempt toward an Investigation of the real Causes which render the Small Pox by Inoculation so much more mild and safe than the Same Disease when produced by the Ordinary Means of Infection. London, 1777. The writer attempts to improve upon the work of Richard Mead (see #1008); born at Bideford, Devonshire, Mudge studied medicine at Plymouth Hospital, gained admission to the Royal Society, and received the Copley Medal for a tract on telescopes; he also formed associations with Sir Joshua Reynolds and Samuel Johnson.

1011. Phillips, Daniel (1668?-1748). A Dissertation of the Small Pox. London, 1702. 119pp. The text of this volume printed both in Latin and English.

1012. Roe, Charles (fl.1775-1785). An Essay on the Natural

Small Pox (contd.)

Small Pox. London, 1780.
1013. Some, David (fl.1730-1750). *The Case of Receiving the Small-Pox by Inoculation*. London, 1750. 43pp. The writer also published a collection of funeral sermons (1736).
1014. Strother, Edward (1635-1737). *Experimental Measures how to manage the Small Pox and Plague*. London, 1721. See, also, #258.
1015. Thompson, Thomas (fl.1740-1773). *An Inquiry into the Small Pox*. London, 1752. An M.D. who practiced at London, Thompson published additional pieces on gout, midwifery, and medical consultations.
1016. Wagstaffe, William (1685-1725). *A Letter to Dr.[John] Freind Showing the Danger and Uncertainty of Inoculating the Small-Pox*. London, 1722. Wagstaffe studied medicine at London before finally receiving, in 1714, the M.D. from Oxford; he gained appointments as censor to the College of Physicians (1720), reader on anatomy to the Barber-Surgeons Company, and as a physician to St. Bartholomew's Hospital, London.
1017. Walker, Robert (fl.1785-1795). *An Inquiry into the Small-Pox, Medical and Political*. London, 1790. 499pp. The writer held the M.D. degree; this tract came under attack in Alexander Aberdour's *Observations on the Small Pox and Inoculation*, published in the following year (see #983).
1018. Watson, Sir William (1715-1787). *An Account of a Series of Experiments instituted with a View of Ascertaining the Most Successful Method of Inoculating the Small Pox*. London, 1768. Watson determined that preparatory drugs had no effect upon the small pox, that matter from natural or inoculated small pox produced the same result, and that children under three years of age ought not to be inoculated. See, also, #532.
1019. Wheler, John (fl.1760-1765). *A Treatise on Small-Pox and Fevers; wherein is demonstrated the Salutary Effects of a Medicine known by the name of Sexton's Powder*. London, 1761. 35pp.
1020. Woodward, John (1665-1728). *The State of Physick and of Diseases; with an Inquiry into the Late Increases of Them, but more particularly of the Small-Pox*. London, 1718; a Latin translation at Zurich in 1720. See, also, #211. Both a physician and a geologist, Woodward, a native of Derbyshire, studied philosophy, anatomy, and physic under Dr. Peter Barwick (see #22); he gained election as professor of physic at Gresham College (1692) and eventually founded the professorship of geology at Cambridge.

F. Cow Pox

1021. Barry, John Milner (1768-1822). *A Treatise on the Cow-Pox*. Cork, 1800. A native of Kilgobbin, Cork,

Plague, Fever, Inoculation, Diseases   111

          Cow Pox (contd.)

               Barrie graduated M.D. from Edinburgh in 1792; he
               practiced medicine at Cork until his death; his
               reputation arose from his having introduced
               vaccination into Cork, as well as from founding the
               Cork Fever Hospital and House of Recovery and
               lecturing on agriculture at the Royal Cork
               Institute.
1022. Fermor, William (fl.1795-1805). Reflections on the
          Cow-Pox and Small-Pox. Oxford, 1800. 47pp.
1023. Jenner, Edward (1749-1823). Further Observations on
          the Varioloae Vaccinae, or Cow-pox. London, 1799.
          See, also, #1048. In 1800, Jenner continued to
          publish the results of his observations and
          research, producing two additional titles: A
          Continuation of Facts and Observations relative to
          the Variolae Vaccinae, or Cow-pox and A Complete
          Statement of Facts and Observations relative to the
          Cow-pock; see, also #1026.
1024. Paytherus, Thomas (fl.1795-1800). A Comparative
          Statement of Facts and Observations relative to the
          Cow-Pox. London, 1800. 43pp.
1025. Pearson, George (1751-1828). An Inquiry concerning
          the History of the Cow-Pox. London, 1798. 116pp.
          Born at Rotherham, in the south of Yorkshire,
          Pearson studied medicine and chemistry at Edinburgh
          (M.D. 1773), then moved down to London for further
          study at St. Thomas's Hospital; at St. George's
          Hospital, London, he lectured on chemistry, materia
          medica, and the practice of physic; in 1799, he
          established the first vaccine pock institution at
          London for the army and the navy.
1026. Woodville, William (1752-1805). A Comparative
          Statement of Facts and Observations relative to the
          Cow-Pox, published by Doctors [Edward] Jenner and
          [William] Woodville. London, 1800. Woodville, a
          Quaker, studied medicine at Edinburgh (M.D. 1775);
          after further study in Europe, he returned to
          England and practiced medicine at Papcastle,
          Cumberland, then moved on to Denbigh and London;
          his interest in botany led to investigations into
          medicinal plants; in 1791, he gained election to
          the small pox and inoculation hospitals at St.
          Pancras, and thus he developed an additional
          interest in the various remedies for small pox;
          see, also, #1023.

          G. Inoculation: see, also, specified titles under
                           "E. Small Pox"

1027. Baylies, William (1724-1787). Facts and Observations
          relative to the Inoculation of the Small Pox at
          Berlin. Edinburgh, 1781. See, also, #556 and
          #985.
1028. Blake, John (fl.1770-1775). A Letter to a Surgeon on
          Inoculation. London, 1771. 81pp.
1029. Bolaine, Nathaniel (fl.1750-1755). Some Remarks on

Inoculation (contd.)

Inoculation. London, 1754.
1030. Brady, Samuel (fl.1720-1725). Some Remarks upon Dr. [William] Wagstaffe's Letter to Dr. [John] Freind . . .against Inoculating the Small Pox. London, 1722. 40pp. See #1016.
1031. Burges, James (fl.1750-1755). An Account of the Preparation and Management Necessary to Inoculation. London, 1754. 44pp.; 2nd. ed., London, 1754.
1032. Chandler, Benjamin (1737-1786). An Essay towards an Investigation of the Present. . .Method of Inoculation. London, 1767. 47pp. The writer practiced surgery at Canterbury, also finding the time to publish tracts on inoculation, apoplexy, and palsy; in 1783, he gained admittance as an extra-licentiate of the London College of Physicians.
1033. Cox, Daniel (d.1759?). A Letter to a Friend on the Subject of Inoculation. London, 1757. 52pp. Cox received the M.D. from St. Andrews in 1742; in 1746, he gained an appointment as a physician to the Middlesex Hospital; he published tracts on fevers, bleeding, and purging.
1034. Creaser, Thomas (fl.1795-1805). A Treatise on Vaccine Inoculation. London, 1800; 2nd ed., London, 1803.
1035. Dimsdale, Thomas (1712-1800). The Present Method of Inoculating for the Small Pox. London, 1767. 160pp.; eight eds. through 1779. Emerging from Quaker ancestry, the writer studied medicine at St. Thomas's Hospital, London, and then practiced at Hertford; he joined the army of the Duke of Cumberland during the Jacobite uprising of 1745; in 1761, he received the M.D.; his experimentation and research with inoculation achieved for him world-wide recognition, particularly in Russia and Austria. in fact, Catherine II, the "great" Empress of Russia, created him a Baron of the Empire for his success in inoculating the Grand Duke and her.
1036. ____. Remarks on a Letter. . .upon General Inoculation by John Coakley Lettsom. London, 1779. 16pp. See #1052; see, also, #160.
1037. ____. Thoughts on General and Partial Inoculations. London, 1776. 70pp.
1038. ____. Tracts on Inoculation. London, 1781. 249pp. The volume contains essays written by Dimsdale between 1767 and 1781.
1039. A Dissuasive against Inoculating for the Small Pox. London, 1751. 54pp.
1040. Dodd, William (1729-1777). Some Observations on Vaccination. London, 1800. 122pp. This title illustrates the full range of interests by the writer, who had no formal training in medicine, nor did he practice that craft; a native of Bourne, Lincolnshire, Dodd received Holy Orders in 1753 and proceeded to earn a reputation as one of the most elegant pulpit orators in London; he became a

Inoculation (contd.)

>prebendary of Brecon and as a tutor to the future Earl of Chesterfield; he held lavish personal tastes and aspired to high Church office, which he failed to achieve; in 1777, he forged Lord Chesterfield's name to a bond and found himself convicted of forgery; his execution at Tyburn occurred on 27 June 1777; Samuel Johnson wrote a number of his letters and sermons (see, particularly, W. Jackson Bate, Samuel Johnson [New York and London: Harcourt Brace Jovanovich, 1977] 523-524).

1041. Dunning, Richard (fl.1795-1810). Some Observations on Vaccination. London, 1800. 122pp. Between 1801 and 1806, the writer published a number of tracts on the cow pox.

1042. Fraser, Thomas (fl.1755-1780). Observations on Inoculation in Antigua. London, 1778. The writer describes events that occurred in 1755 and 1756; in 1762, he published a piece on "Olium Ricini" in Medical Observations and Inquiries.

1043. Frewen, Thomas (1704-1791). The Practice and Theory of Inoculation. London, 1749. 61pp. See, also, #994.

1044. A General Method of Inoculation. . .in the Counties of Kent and Sussex. London, 1767. 18pp. This tract supposedly written by one "Hostis Monopolarum."

1045. Houlton, Robert (fl.1755-1801). Indisputable Facts relative to the Suttonian Art of Inoculation. Dublin, 1768. 32pp. See #1065 and #1066. The writer also published sermon tracts between 1765 and 1767.

1046. Howgrave, Francis (fl.1723-1727). Reasons against the Inoculation of the Small Pox. London, 1724. 72pp.

1047. Inoculation Made Easy. Containing a Full and True Account of the Method Practiced in the County of Essex. London, 1766. 11pp.

1048. Jenner, Edward (1749-1823). An Inquiry into the Cause and Effects of the Variolae Vaccinae, a Disease Discovered in Some of the Western Counties of England, particularly Gloucestershire, and known by the name of the Cow-Pox. London, 1798. A classic among the medical tracts of the eighteenth century, this seventy-five page volume (with colored plates and dedicated to Dr. Caleb Hillier Parry [1755-1822], a Bath physician and writer) describes the writer's investigations relative to the protective power of cow pox against small pox; in addition to the plates, Jenner included twenty-three descriptions of actual cases; credited with the discovery of vaccination, Jenner served as a surgeon's apprentice at Sudbury, Suffolk, before going off to London as a pupil in residence to John Hunter; after a term as an assistant to Sir Joseph Banks (1743-1820), the eminent naturalist, he began his formal medical studies at St. George's Hospital, London, after which he developed a large

Inoculation (contd.)

practice in midwifery and surgery; the M.D. from St. Andrews came to him in 1792; after 1794, following his own serious illness from typhus, Jenner pursued with intensity those studies and investigations that led to his lasting reputation within the pages of medical history; see, also, #1023.

1049. Jurin, James (1684-1750). An Account of the Success of Inoculating for the Small Pox. London, 1774; further eds. in 1725, 1726, 1727. See, also, #803.

1050. Kirkpatrick, James (d.1770). The Analysis of Inoculation. London, 1754. 288pp.; 2nd ed., London, 1761. 429pp. See, also, #815.

1051. Langton, William (fl.1765-1770). An Address to the Public on the Present Method of Inoculation. London, 1767. 38pp. The writer held the M.D. degree.

1052. Lettsom, John Coakley (1749-1815). A Letter to Sir Robert Baker. . .upon General Inoculation. London, 1778. 13pp. See, also, #160.

1053. Lywythlan, Evan David (fl.1765-1770). Some Observations on Dr. [Giles] Watts on Inoculation. London, 1768. See, also, #1069-#1071.

1054. Massey, Edmund (d.1765). A Sermon against the Dangerous and Sinful Practice of Inoculation. London, 1722. 16pp.; 2nd ed., London, 1722. 30pp. Massey, a London churchman, published his sermon texts between 1721 and 1736.

1055. Massey, Isaac (fl.1720-1730). A Short and Plain Account of Inoculation. London, 1722. 22pp.; 2nd ed., London, 1723; further eds. through 1727.

1056. Mather, Cotton (1663-1728). An Account of the Method and Success of Inoculating the Small Pox in Boston. London, 1721. 22pp. Although the New England divine, pulpit orator, and ecclesiastical historian belongs to the annals of American letters, this tract on inoculation managed to attract a wide reading audience in London; see, also, #1058.

1057. May, Nicholas the younger (fl.1770-1775). Impartial Remarks on the Suttonian Method of Inoculation. London, 1771. 199pp. See #1065 and #1066.

1058. Neal, Daniel (1678-1743). A Narrative of the Method and Success of Inoculating the Small-Pox in New England, by Mr. Benjamin Colman; with a Reply to the Objections made against it from Principles of Conscience, in a Letter from a Minister at Boston. To Which is prefixed an Historical Introduction. London, 1722. A London Dissenter and historian, Neal had no professional involvement with the practice of medicine; this Narrative emerged from the efforts of Lady Mary Wortley Montagu (1689-1762) to introduce the practice of inoculation into England; physicians and clergy, particularly (see, for instance, #1054), objected to that method, but Neal rose to its defense; in his introduction to this volume, he assumes the role of objective

Inoculation (contd.)

historian who would permit the world to determine the benefits from or the shortcomings of inoculation; Benjamin Colman (1673-1747), the minister of the Brattle Street (Congregational) Church, Boston, and an outspoken defender of inoculation (some seventy years prior to Edward Jenner's work), published this Narrative at Boston in 1721 (reprinted in London in 1722); Neal's "Historical Introduction" appears only in the London edition; see, also, #1056.

1059. Nettleton, Thomas (1683-1742). An Account of the Success of Inoculating the Small Pox. London, 1722. 12pp. An M.D., Nettleton practiced medicine at Edinburgh and Halifax; his A Treatise on Virtue and Happiness (1729) reached seven editions by 1774.

1060. The New Practice of Inoculating the Small-Pox Consider'd. London, 1722. 40pp.

1061. Percival, Thomas (1740-1804). Observations on the Inoculation of Children. London, 1786. See, also, #204.

1062. Robinson, Bryan (1680-1754). The Cure of Five Children who were Inoculated in Dublin. Dublin, 1725. 8pp. See, also, #499.

1063. Ruston, Thomas (1739?-1804). An Essay on Inoculation for the Small Pox. London, 1767. 74pp.; three eds. through 1768. The writer held the M.D. degree.

1064. Sparham, Legard (fl.1720-1725). Reasons against the Practice of Inoculating the Small Pox. London, 1722. 30pp.; three eds. in 1722.

1065. Sutton, Daniel (1735-1819). A Narrative of the Trial of Daniel Sutton, for Preserving Lives by Inoculation. London, 1767. The satiric quality of the piece appears most obvious from its title.

1066. ____. The Inoculator; or, the Sutton System of Inoculation. London, 1796. 160pp.

1067. Watkinson, John (fl.1775-1780). An Examination of a Charge brought against Inoculation. London, 1777. 46pp. The writer, an M.D., also conducted and published A Philosophical Survey of the South of Ireland (1777).

1068. Watson, Sir William (1715-1787). An Account of a Series of Experiments Instituted with a View of Ascertaining the Most Successful Method of Inoculating the Small-Pox. London, 1768. 58pp. Born at London, the writer was created (1757) doctor of physic by the University of Halle and of Wittemberg; he then practiced physic at London and received (1762) an appointment as a physician to the Foundling Hospital there; his interests extended to botany and experiments with electricity (the latter exercise bringing him into contact with Henry Cavendish and Benjamin Franklin; see, also, #532.

1069. Watts, Giles (fl.1754-1767). A Letter to Dr. [Thomas] Frewen on Inoculation. London, 1755. See, also,

Inoculation (contd.)

#1043.
1070. ____. A Second Letter to Dr. [Thomas] Frewen on Inoculation. London, 1756. See, also, #1043 and #1069.
1071. ____. A Vindication of the New Method for Inoculating. London, 1767. See, also, #1053.
1072. Williams, Perrott (fl.1720-1725). Some Remarks upon Dr. [William] Wagstaff's Letter against Inoculating the Small-Pox. London, 1725. 35pp. See #1016. The writer held the M.D. degree; he published a number of medical tracts in the Philosophical Transactions of the Royal Society (1723).
1073. Woodville, William (1752-1805). A History of the Inoculation of the Small-Pox in Great Britain. London, 1796. This work represents the first part of a projected two-volume treatise; the second volume never appeared, principally because of Edward Jenner's discovery of vaccination from the cow pox; see, also, #1026 and #1048.
1074. ____. Report of a Series of Inoculations for the Variolae Vaccinae, or Cow-Pox; with Remarks and Observations on the Disease considered as a Substitute for the Small Pox. London, 1799. Woodville, who at first opposed vaccination, eventually came to embrace both the concept and the practice.

H. Venereal Disease

1075. Andree, John the younger (fl.1779-1799). Observations on the Theory and Cure of the Venereal Disease. London, 1779. 146pp.; 2nd ed. published under the title, An Essay on the Theory and Cure of the Venereal Gonorrhoea. London, 1781. 85pp. See, also, #816.
1076. Armstrong, Charles (fl.1780-1815). An Essay on the Symptoms and Cure of the Virulent Gonorrhoea. London, 1783. 44pp. The writer held the M.D. degree; his medical tracts appeared at London between 1783 and 1812.
1077. Armstrong, John (1709-1779). A Synopsis of the History and Cure of Venereal Diseases. London, 1737. 519pp. See, also, #12.
1078. Becket, James (fl.1760-1770). A New Essay on the Venereal Disease. London, 1765. 114pp.; four eds. through 1769. The writer held the M.D. degree and published a volume of his professional tracts in 1765.
1079. Beddoes, Thomas (1760-1808), ed. A Collection of Testimonies respecting the Treatment of the Venereal Disease by Nitrous Acid. London, 1799. 277pp. See, also, #26.
1080. ____, ed. Reports, Principally concerning the Effects of Nitrous Acid in the Venereal Disease. Bristol, 1797. 101pp. This work essentially an earlier and shorter version of #1079.

Venereal Disease (contd.)

1081. Bell, Benjamin (1749-1806). <u>A Treatise on Gonorrhoea Virulenta, and Lues Venerea</u>. 2 vols. Edinburgh, 1793; Dublin, 1793; Philadelphia, 1795; 2nd ed., 2 vols., Edinburgh, 1797. See, also, #724.

1082. Blair, William (1766-1822). <u>Essays on the Venereal Disease</u>. 2 vols. London, 1798-1800. A native of Essex, Blair became a respected surgeon; however, he also managed to involve himself in distributing copies of Bibles and with prison reform; his publications focused upon the improving the health of soldiers (1798) and anthropology (1803); in 1806, he joined the debate over vaccination with a tract entitled <u>The Vaccine Contest, or Mild Humanity, Reason, Religion, and Truth against fierce, unfeeling Ferocity, overbearing Insolence, mortified Pride, false Faith, and Desperation; being an exact outline of the Arguments and interesting Facts added by the principal Combatants on both sides respecting the Cow-Pox Inoculation</u>.

1083. Brest, Vincent (fl.1732-1735). <u>A Dissertation concerning . . .Crude Mercury in Venereal. . . Diseases</u>. London, 1735. See, also, #390.

1084. Brown, Richard (fl.1725-1735). <u>A Letter. . .giving an Account of the Montpellier Practice in Curing the Venereal Disease</u>. London, 1730. 24pp.

1085. Buchan, Alexander Peter (1764-1824). <u>Enchiridion Syphiliticum; or, Directions for the Conduct of Venereal Patients</u>. London, 1797. 64pp. Born near Pontefract, Wales, and educated at Edinburgh, Buchan studied anatomy at London and received the M.D. from Leyden in 1793; he practiced at London and associated himself with the Westminster Hospital.

1086. Buchan, William (1729-1805). <u>Observations concerning the Prevention and Cure of the Venereal Disease</u>. Dublin, 1796. 144pp.; two London eds. in 1796 and 1797. See, also, #46.

1087. Butter, William (1726-1805). <u>A Treatise on the Venereal Rose</u>. London, 1799. 78pp. See, also, #731.

1088. Cam, Joseph (fl.1715-1732). <u>A Practical Treatise: or, Second Thoughts on the Consequences of the Venereal Disease</u>. London, 1724. 90pp.; four eds through 1729.

1089. ____. <u>A Short Account of the Venereal Disease</u>. London, 1717. 52pp.

1090. Chapman, Samuel (fl.1750-1770). <u>An Essay on the Venereal Gleet</u>. London, 1751. 41pp. The writer practiced surgery at London.

1091. Clare, Peter (1738-1786). <u>A New and Easy Method of Curing the Lues Venerea</u>. London, n.d.; three eds. through 1780. See, also, #401.

1092. ____. <u>A Practical Treatise on the Gonorrhoea</u>. London, 1786. 48 pp.; five eds. through 1789.

1093. Clubbe, John (fl.1775-1790). <u>An Essay on the Virulent Gonorrhoea</u>. London, 1786. 77pp. The writer

Venereal Disease (contd.)

practiced surgery at London.

1094. ____. *An Inquiry into the Nature of the Venereal Poison*. Ipswich, 1782. 80pp.

1095. Clutterbuck, Henry (1767-1856). *Remarks on Some of the Opinions of the Late Mr. John Hunter respecting the Venereal Disease*. London, 1799. 72pp. See #1110. Born at Marazion, Cornwall, and apprenticed to a surgeon at Truro, Clutterbuck came to London to study at the United Borough Hospitals; in 1790, he gained admission to the College of Surgeons and practiced at Walbrook (London); eventually, he became a popular lecturer and a serious writer of medical tracts, a large portion of which he published between 1794 and 1807.

1096. Cockburn, William (1669-1739). *The Symptoms, Nature, Cause, and Cure of a Gonorrhoea*. London, 1713. 188pp.; four eds. through 1728. See, also, #65.

1097. Cribb, William ((fl.1770-1775). *Consideration on the Use of Injections in the Gonorrhoea*. London, 1773. 68pp.

1098. Deacon, Henry (fl.1785-1790). *A Compendious Treatise on the Venereal Disease*. London, 1789. 132pp.

1099. Dease, William (1752?-1798). *Observations on the Different Methods of Treating the Venereal Disease*. Dublin, 1779. 131pp. See, also, #737.

1100. *A Dissertation on the Origin of the Venereal Disease; proving that it was not brought from America, but began in Europe*. London, 1751. 92pp.

1101. Douglas, John (d.1743). *A Dissertation on the Venereal Disease*. 3 vols. London, 1737-1739. See, also, #315.

1102. Duncan, Andrew (1744-1828). *Observations on the Operation and Use of Mercury in the Venereal Disease*. Edinburgh, 1772. 175pp. See, also, #421.

1103. Ellis, William (fl.1770-1775). *An Essay on the Cure of the Venereal Gonorrhoea*. London, 1771; 2nd ed., London, 1773. 40pp.

1104. Foot, Jesse (1744-1826). *Observations upon the New Opinions of John Hunter, in his late Treatise on the Venereal Disease*. 3 vols. London, 1786-1787. See, also, #1110. Foote practiced surgery at London; in addition to a number of medical tracts, he published biographies of Dr. John Hunter (1794), A.R. Bowes (1810), the Countess of Strathmore (1810), and the actor and playwright Arthur Murphy (1811).

1105. Fordyce, Sir William (1724-1792). *A Review of the Venereal Disease*. London, 1767. 95pp.; five eds. through 1785. See, also, #743.

1106. Godfrey, C.B. (fl.1795-1800). *An Historical and Practical Treatise on the Venereal Disease*. London, 1797. 146pp.

1107. Higgs, Joseph (fl.1750-1760). *A Practical Essay on the Cure of Venereal, Scorbutic, Arthritic. . .and Cancerous Disorders*. London, 1755. 40pp.

1108. Houlston, William (fl.1790-1795). *Sketches of Facts*

Venereal Disease (contd.)

and Opinions respecting the Venereal Disease. London, 1792. 47pp.; 2nd ed., London, 1794. 95pp.

1109. Howard, John (d.1811). Practical Observations on the Natural History and Cure of the Venereal Disease. 3 vols. London, 1787-1794. See, also, #453.

1110. Hunter, John (1728-1793). A Treatise on the Venereal Disease. London, 1786; five eds. through 1810; revisions in England and America between 1818 and 1853. The younger brother of William Hunter, John Hunter rose to prominence as a surgeon and anatomist; he studied at St. George's Hospital, London, practiced as a surgeon in London, and began to lecture on anatomy and dissection; by 1788, he had risen to the head of his profession; see, also, #1095, #1104.

1111. Innes, James Dunbar (fl.1780-1785). A Treatise on the Venereal Disease. London, 1783. 100pp.

1112. Key, George (fl.1745-1755). A Dissertation on the Effects of Mercury on Human Bodies in the Cure of the Venereal Disease. London, 1747. 79pp.

1113. Mooney, Matthew (fl.1755-1760). A Treatise on the Nature and Cure of the Venereal Disease. London, 1756.

1114. Neale, Thomas (fl.1750-1760). A Practical Treatise on the Venereal Disease and the Art of Bleeding. London, 1755; another ed., London, 1756. 260pp.

1115. Nevill, James (fl.1750-1755). A Description of the Venereal Gonorrhoea. London, 1754. 115pp.

1116. Nicholson, James Francis (fl.1715-1720). An Essay on Modern Syphilis. London, 1718.

1117. Nisbet, William (1759-1822). First Lines of the Theory and Practice in Venereal Diseases. Edinburgh, 1787. 453pp. See, also, #478.

1118. Norman, John (fl.1755-1760). A Compendious and Easy Method of Curing the Virulent Stillicidium commonly call'd Gonorrhoea. London, 1756. 36pp.

1119. Pearson, John (1758-1826). Observations on the Effects of Various Articles of the Materia Medica on the Cure of Lues Venerea. London, 1800. 188pp. A native of York, Pearson studied surgery at Morpeth and the Leeds General Infirmary; in 1780, he went to London as a student at St. George's Hospital, after which he received appointments as a house surgeon and surgeon to the Lock Hospital (1782-1818) and to the public dispensary in Carey Street; he became a fellow of the Royal Society and of the Linnean Society, an honorary member of the Royal College of Surgeons of Ireland, and a member of the Royal Medical Society of Edinburgh.

1120. Pete, Charles (fl.1675-1695). A Treatise on the Venereal Diseases. London, 1678; another ed. in 1694.

1121. Profily, John (fl.1745-1750). An Easy and Exact Method of Curing the Venereal Disease. London, 1748. 336pp.

1122. Renny, George (fl.1780-1795). A Treatise on the

Venereal Disease (contd.)

  Venereal Disease. London, 1782. 171pp.; another ed. in 1793.
1123. Robinson, Nicholas (1697?-1755). A Treatise of the Venereal Disease. London, 1736. See, also, #220.
1124. Rowley, William (1742-1806). An Essay on the Cure of the Gonorrhoea. London, 1771. 34pp. See, also, #222.
1125. Sawrey, Solomon (1765-1825). A Popular View of the Effects of the Venereal Disease upon the Constitution. Edinburgh, 1794. 205pp. The writer studied anatomy and surgery privately at London before gaining admittance to the Corporation of Surgeons (1796); he specialized in ophthalmic surgery; his published works include a tract on the membrane in the eye (1807) and an edition (with a biographical sketch) in 1814 of the posthumous works of Dr. Andrew Marshall (1742-1813), the Scottish anatomist who lectured at London.
1126. Simmons, Samuel Foart (1750-1813). A Treatise on the Gonorrhoea. London, 1780. See, also, #351.
1127. Sintelaer, John (fl.1705-1710). The Scourge of Venus and Mercury; or, Venereal Diseases. London, 1707; another ed., London, 1709.
1128. Spilsbury, Francis B. (fl.1785-1809). A Treatise on the Venereal Disease. London, 1789. The writer also published tracts on dentistry (1791) and ophthalmia (1802); see #250.
1129. Spinke, John (fl.1705-1720). Quackery Unmasked; or, [John] Martin on the Venereal Disease. London, 1709; another ed., London, 1711. Medical tracts by a John Martin (or Marten) reached publication at London between 1706 and 1740.
1130. _____. The Venereal Patient's Refuge. London, 1717. 124pp.
1131. Thomas, William (fl.1770-1808). An Essay on Gonorrhoea. London, 1780. The writer also published tracts on cancers (1805) and on the Egyptian ophthalmia (1808).
1132. The Tomb of Venus; or, A Plain and Certain Method by which all People that ever labour'd under any Venereal Distemper may infallibly know whether they are cured or not. London, 1710. 87pp.
1133. Turnbull, William (1729?-1796). An Inquiry into Lues Venerea. London, 1786. See, also #529.
1134. Wall, William (fl.1695-1700). A Description of a New System of the French Disease. London, 1696.
1135. Warren, George (fl.1725-1740). A New Method of Curing (without Internal Medicines) that Degree of Venereal Disease, call'd Gonorrhoea, or Clap. London, n.d.; a 3rd ed. at London, 1734. Perhaps the writer's most interesting publication concerned an essay on the dissection of an ostrich, which appeared in the Philosophical Transactions of the Royal Society (1726).
1136. Wastell, Henry (fl.1775-1800). Observations on the Efficacy of a New Mercurial Preparation for the

Venereal Disease (contd.)

Cure of the Venereal Disease. London, 1778. 104pp.
1137. Wathen, Jonathan (fl.1755-1785), ed. and trans. [Hermann] Boerhaave's Academical Lectures on the Lues Venerea; from the Latin. London, 1793. The writer practiced surgery in London.
1138. _____. Practical Observations on the Cure of Venereal Disease by Mercurials. London, 1765.
1139. Watson, John (fl.1740-1745). A Commentary upon Mr. [Francis] Hauksbee's Medicine for Venereal Disease. London, 1742; another ed., London, 1743. Hauksbee (1687-1763) held the office of curator of experiments to the Royal Society; his most important contributions to science focused upon his work in electricity and natural philosophy.
1140. Wynel, John (fl.1655-1665). An Essay on the Lues Veneres; wherein the Nature, Subject, Cause, and Cure are Handled. London, 1660.

VII

Cold, Sore Throat, Croup, Catarrh, Whooping Cough, Asthma, Consumption, Respiration, Lungs, Scrofula, Dropsy, Influenza

A. Cold

1141. Chandler, John (1700-1780). <u>A Treatise of the Disease Called a Cold</u>. London, 1761. 123pp. See, also, #988.
1142. Hayes, Thomas (fl.1765-1790). <u>A Serious and Friendly Address to the Public on the Dangerous Consequences of Neglecting Common Coughs and Colds</u>. London, 1783. 42pp.; 3rd ed., London, 1786; 4th ed., Dublin, 1786.
1143. Kelson, Thomas M. (fl.1795-1800). <u>A Treatise on the Nature of Colds</u>. London, 1797. The writer advances the thesis of a cold being a disease; as such, it needs to be placed in a class by itself.

B. Sore Throat

1144. Fothergill, John (1712-1780). <u>An Account of the Sore Throat Attended with Ulcers</u>. London, 1748. 72pp.; four eds. through 1754. See, also, #112.
1145. Huxham, John (1694-1768). <u>A Dissertation on the Malignant Ulcerous Sore-Throat</u>. London, 1757. Actually, this seventy-page tract represents a highly detailed account of diptheria; although Huxham failed (as did a number of his contemporaries) to differentiate that disease from scarlatina angina, he did emerge as the first physician to observe the paralysis of the soft palate; see, also, #334.
1146. Levison, George (fl.1775-1780). <u>An Essay on Epidemical Sore Throat</u>. London, 1778. The writer held the M.D. degree.
1147. Penrose, Francis (1718-1798). <u>A Dissertation on the Inflammatory, Gangrenous, and Putrid Sore Throat; also on the Putrid Fever, together with the Diagnostics and Method of Cure</u>. Oxford, 1766. 54pp. In this practical treatise, the writer

Sore Throat (contd.)

narrates cases from his own practice and observation; Penrose practiced surgery at Bicester, Oxford, before moving (1782) to Plymouth; he wrote largely upon electricity, magnetism, and physiology as they related to medicine; supposedly, he held a medical degree from "a German university."

1148. Perkins, William Lee (fl.1787-1798). <u>A Treatise on Putrid Sore Throat</u>. London, 1787; another ed., London, 1790. Perkins also published essays on hydrophobia (1786) and the angina pectoris (1798).

1149. Reeve, Thomas (d.1790; fl.1744-1789). <u>An Essay on the Erysipelatous Sore Throat</u>. London, 1789. Erysipelas, accompanied by diffused inflammation of the skin, also carried identifications as "St. Anthony's fire" and "the rose"; see, also, #700.

1150. Saunders, Robert (fl.1775-1780). <u>Observations on the Sore Throat and Fever that raged in the north of Scotland</u>. London, 1778. 50pp.

1151. Torrano, Nicholas (fl.1750-1755). <u>An Essay on Sore Throat, Translated from Chomel</u>. London, 1753. The translator, an M.D., practiced midwifery in London and published tracts on that subject.

C. Croup

1152. Alexander, David (fl.1790-1795). <u>A Treatise on the Croup</u>. Huddersfield, 1794. The writer, an M.D., practiced medicine at Huddersfield, Yorkshire.

1153. Home, Francis (1719-1813). <u>An Inquiry into the Nature, Cause, and Cure of the Croup</u>. Edinburgh, 1765. 60pp. See, also, #143.

D. Catarrh

1154. <u>Advice to the People, upon the Epidemic Catarrhal Fever</u>. Dublin, 1775. 48pp.

1155. Mudge, John (1721-1793). <u>A Radical and Expeditious Cure for Recent Catarrhous Cough</u>. London, 1778; further eds. in 1782, 1783. See, also, #1010. The work includes a drawing of a "remedial inhaler," a device that gained acceptance from Mudge's contemporaries.

E. Whooping Cough

1156. Butter, William (1726-1805). <u>A Treatise on the Kinkcough</u>. London, 1773. 206pp. See, also, #731. According to the <u>OED</u>, kinkcough has been dialectically synonymous with whooping cough since 1568.

1157. Jones, John Gale (1769-1838). <u>Observations on the Tussis Convulsiva, or Hooping Cough, as read at the Lyceum Medicum, Londonense</u>. London, 1794; 2nd ed., London, 1798. Although trained at Chelsea as a surgeon and apothecary, by 1795 Jones had turned his attention to politics; in fact, this tract

Cold, Sore Throat, Scrofula, Influenza 125

Whooping Cough (contd.)

reflects the obvious superficiality of his medical knowledge and qualifications.

F. Asthma

1158. Akenside, Mark (1721-1770). "Of the Use of Ipecacuanha in Asthma," Medical Transactions, 1 (1768):93. Far more recognized for his verse than for his medical practice and professional prose, Akenside received the M.D. from Leyden in 1744 and practiced for a time at Northampton; in 1759, he gained the appointment as principal physician to both Christ's Hospital and St. Thomas's Hospital, London; his interests in poetry, politics, and classical scholarship motivated his moves to Hampstead and then London; Samuel Johnson, in his "Life of Akenside" (Lives of the Most Eminent English Poets, ed. Peter Cunningham [London: John Murray, 1854] 3:379), provides us with a most interesting contemporary view of the eighteenth-century physician as seen through his subject: "At London, he [Akenside] was known as a poet, but was still to make his way as a physician; and would perhaps have been reduced to great exigencies, but that Mr. [Jeremiah] Dyson, with an ardour of friendship that had not many examples, allowed him three hundred pounds a-year. Thus supported, he advanced gradually in medical reputation, but never attained any great extent of practice, or eminence of popularity. A physician in a great city seems to be the mere plaything of Fortune; his degree of reputation is, for the most part, totally casual: they that employ him know not his excellence; they that reject him know not his deficience. By any acute observer, who had looked on the transactions of the medical world for half a century, a very curious book might be written on the 'Fortune of Physicians.'"
1159. Beddoes, Thomas (1760-1808), ed. Letters from Dr. [William] Withering [et al]. . .on Asthma, Consumption, Fever, and Other Diseases. Bristol, 1794. 48pp. See, also, #26 and #543.
1160. Floyer, Sir John (1649-1734). A Treatise on the Asthma. London, 1698; three eds. through 1745; a French ed., Paris, 1761. See, also, #106. This work has been praised by scholars for the detail of the writer's observations and for its being the first account (resulting from dissection) of the change in the lungs (emphysema) found in one of the forms of asthma; however, Floyer conducted his experiments not upon humans, but with "a broken winded mare."
1161. Lipscomb, George (1773-1846). Observations on the History and Cause of Asthma. Birmingham, 1800. 108pp. See, also, #943.
1162. Millar, John (1733-1805). Observations on the Asthma

Asthma (contd.)

and on the Whooping Cough. London, 1769. 207pp. The writer, a native of Scotland, received the M.D. from Edinburgh and began his medical practice at Kelso; in 1774, he gained an appointment as a physician to the Westminster General Dispensary, London, and became an active promoter of the Medical Society of London; although his practiced focused upon women and children, he wrote upon a variety of medical and professional issues.

1163. Ryan, Michael (1760?-1823). Observations on the History and Cure of the Asthma, in which the Propriety of Using the Cold Bath in that Disorder is fully considered. London, 1793. Ryan graduated M.D. in 1784 from Edinburgh, became a fellow of the Irish College of Surgeons, and then practiced at Kilkenny; apparently, he also practiced and lectured at Edinburgh, where he developed a large following.

1164. Withers, Thomas (fl.1772-1794). A Treatise on the Asthma. London, 1786. Withers received the M.D. from Edinburgh in 1772; he published tracts at London and Edinburgh on such topics as fevers, chronic weakness, abuses in medical practice, and medical education; see, also, #282 and #283.

G. Consumption

1165. Archer, John (fl.1660-1684). Secrets Disclosed: or, A Treatise of Consumptions, Their Various Causes and Cures. London, 1684; another ed., London, 1693. As was his usual practice, Archer provided nostrums of his own preparation to support the thesis of this volume; as usual, the majority of them proved useless; an Irishman of questionable medical qualifications, he managed to secure an appointment as a court physician to Charles II; see, also, #11.

1166. Barry, Sir Edward (1696-1776). A Treatise on a Consumption of the Lungs. Dublin, 1726. 227pp.; London, 1727. 276pp. An M.D. from Leyden in 1719 and a recipient of the same degree from Trinity College, Dublin, in 1740, Barry became a fellow of the Royal Society, a fellow of the King's and Queen's College of Physicians (Ireland), and a member of the Irish House of Commons; he practiced medicine in Dublin, then at London, where he achieved some degree of notice as the first person to undertake a "scientific" study of wines for medicinal purposes.

1167. Beddoes, Thomas (1760-1808). An Essay on the Causes, Early Signs, and Prevention of Pulmonary Consumption. Bristol, 1779. 274pp.; 2nd ed. under the title, A Popular Essay on Consumption. London, 1799. 340pp. A native of Shropshire, the writer received his education at London and Edinburgh, before taking the M.D. from Oxford; he worked with heat and light as they related to medical

Consumption (contd.)

and physical knowledge; see, also, #26.

1168. ____. A Letter to Erasmus Darwin, M.D., on a New Method of Treating Pulmonary Consumption. Bristol, 1793. 72pp. Erasmus Darwin (1731-1802), the grandfather of the nineteenth-century discoverer of natural selection, became a popular physician, known for his medical abilities, his radical and freethinking opinions, his verse, and his eight-acre botanical garden; a native of Elton, near Newark (Nottinghamshire), he studied at St. John's College, Cambridge, and at Edinburgh; he practiced medicine at Northampton, then moved to Lichfield, where he collected a large quantity of patients.

1169. Blackmore, Sir Richard (1650-1729). A Treatise on Consumptions. London, 1724. See, also, #839. Interestingly enough, Blackmore's professional tracts reached publication during the final productive period of his life (1720-1727), apparently after he had expended his poetic, philosophic, and political energies.

1170. Charles, Richard (fl.1785-1788). An Essay on the Treatment of Consumption. London, 1787. 30pp. See, also, #400.

1171. Godbold, Nathaniel (fl.1780-1790). An Essay on Consumption. London, 1784; another ed., London, 1787.

1172. Haworth, Samuel (fl.1680-1683). A Treatise on Curing Consumption. London, 1682. An M.D., the writer published tracts on anatomy and descriptions of the spas at Bath; see, also, #329.

1173. Marten, Benjamin (fl.1715-1725). A New Theory of Consumptions. London, 1720. 186pp.

1174. May, William (fl.1790-1795). An Essay on Pulmonary Consumptions. Plymouth, 1792. 107pp. See, also, #868.

1175. Neale, Henry St. John (fl.1795-1805). Practical Essays and Remarks on that Species of Consumption . . .commonly called Tabes Dorsalis. London, 1797; another ed., London, 1800. 223pp. The writer practiced surgery in London.

1176. Nevett, Thomas (fl.1695-1705). A Treatise on Consumption. London, 1697. See, also, #193.

1177. O'Ryan, Michael (fl.1790-1800). Advice in the Consumption of the Lungs. Dublin, 1798. 131pp. See, also, #482.

1178. Robinson, Nicholas (1697?-1775). A New Method of Treating Consumptions. London, 1727. See, also, #220.

1179. Ryan, Michael (1760?-1823). An Inquiry into the Nature, Causes, and Cure of Consumption of the Lungs. Dublin, 1787; another ed., Dublin, 1788. This volume represents a commentary upon William Cullen's First Lines of the Practice of Physick (see #80) and Thomas Reid's Essay on the Phthsis Pulmonalis (see #1195); see, also, #1163.

1180. Simmons, Samuel Foart (1750-1813). Observations on

Consumption (contd.)

the Treatment of Consumptions. London, 1780. See, also, #351.
1181. Smyth, James Carmichael (1741-1821). An Account of the Effects of Swinging Employed as a Remedy in the Pulmonary Consumption and Hectic Fever. London, 1787. 53pp. See, also, #686.
1182. Stephens, John (fl.1755-1765). An Essay on Consumptions. London, 1760.
1183. Stern, Philip (fl.1765-1770). Medical Advice to the Consumptive and Asthmatic People of England. London, 1767. 38pp.; twenty eds. through 1779. Although the writer held the M.D. degree, and despite the obvious popularity of his Advice, the volume has been dismissed as a piece of mere "quackery" (see Allibone 2:2242).
1184. Sutton, Thomas (1767?-1835). Considerations regarding Pulmonary Consumption. London, 1799. Sutton studied medicine at London, Edinburgh, and Leyden (M.D. 1787); after serving as a physician to the Royal Army, he settled at Greenwich and became consulting physician to the Kent Dispensary; he stands as the first modern British physician to advocate bleeding and an antiphlogistic treatment of fever; further, he identified the delerium tremens as being apart from those nervous diseases with which it had been traditionally associated.

H. Respiration

1185. Coleman, Edward (1765-1839). A Dissertation on Suspended Respiration from Drowning, Hanging, and Suffocation. London, 1791. 284pp.
1186. Dobson, Matthew (d.1784). A Medical Commentary on Fixed Air. Chester, 1779. 196pp.; 2nd ed., edited by William Falconer, Dublin, 1785. 230pp.; 3rd ed., London, 1787. 298pp. The writer held the M.D. degree and published various medical tracts between 1774 and 1781.
1187. Goodwyn, Edmund (1756-1829). The Connection of Life with Respiration. London, 1788. 274pp. The writer, an M.D., practiced medicine at London; ill-health forced his retirement to Framlingham, Suffolk; his published tracts focus upon submersion and respiration.
1188. Hoadley, Benjamin the younger (1706-1757). Three Lectures on the Organs of Respiration. London, 1746. Born in London, the son of the controversial Bishop of Bangor, Hereford, Salisbury, and Winchester, the younger Hoadley graduated M.B. and M.D. from Oxford; he then settled into medical practice at London, where he found the time to write for the stage (The Suspicious Husband, 1747, being one example); the three essays on respiration constitute the Gulstonian lectures delivered to the College of Physicians, London.
1189. Kite, Charles (1768-1811). An Essay on the Recovery

Cold, Sore Throat, Scrofula, Influenza 129

Respiration (contd.)

of the Apparently Dead. London, 1788. 274pp. See, also, #157.

1190. Mayow, John (1640-1679). Tractatus Quinque Medico-Physici quorum primus agit De Sal-Nitro, et Spiritu Nitro-Aero. Oxford, 1674. The writer identifies the function of breathing as merely to bring air in contact with the blood, to which it gives up oxygen and from which it carries off the vapors produced by the heating of the blood; further, according to the thesis of these tracts, the heart, as a muscle, drives the blood through the lungs and throughout the body; essentially a physiologist and a chemist, Mayow studied physic and natural philosophy before beginning his medical practice at Bath; although his work ranks high in the minds of those who now study the history of medicine, Mayow failed to impress or affect the work of his contemporaries, the majority of whom simply could not understand his theories; in 1790, however, Thomas Beddoes (see #26, #1167) published extracts from the Tractacus under the title Chemical Experiments and Opinions Extracted from a Work Published in the Last Century, ascribing to Mayow a number of significant discoveries concerning air.

1191. Menzies, Robert (fl.1785-1795). A Dissertation on Respiration. Edinburgh, 1796. This volume an obvious translation (a version of #1192?), since Menzies wrote the original in Latin.

1192. Sugrue, Charles (fl.1795-1800). A Dissertation on Respiration; from the Latin of Dr. [Robert] Menzies, with Notes. London, 1796. See #1191.

I. Lungs

1193. Davidson, William (fl.1790-1795). Observations, Anatomical, Physiological, and Pathological, on the Pulmonary System. London, 1795. 226pp. The writer contributed various essays to Medical Facts and Observations (see #2049) during 1792, 1793, and 1794.

1194. Packe, Christopher (1728-1800). An Explanation of that Part of Dr. [Hermann] Boerhaave's Aphorisms which treats the Phthisis Pulmonalis. London, 1754. 38pp. Boerhaave's Aphorismi de Cognoscendis et Curandis Morbis appeared initially in 1709, shortly after his appointment as professor of medicine and botany at Leyden.

1195. Reid, Thomas (1739-1802). An Essay on the Nature and Cure of the Phthisis Pulmonalis. London, 1782. 155pp.; another ed., London, 1785. See, also, #1179.

1196. White, William, of York (1744-1790). Observations on the Nature and Method of Cure of the Phthisis Pulmonalis. York, 1771; 2nd ed., York, 1793. The writer held the M.D. degree, practiced at York, and wrote tracts on diseases of the bile and on cures

Lungs (contd.)

for the fever; see, also, #537.

J. Scrofula

1197. Badger, John (fl.1745-1750). A Treatise on the Cures of the King's Evil by Royal Touch. London, 1748.
1198. Becket, William (1684-1738). An Inquiry into the Antiquity and Efficacy of Touching for the Cure of the King's Evil, with a Collection of Records. London, 1722. 24pp. Becket received assistance with this work from one John Anstis the elder (1669-1744), an antiquarian and writer on heraldry; see, also, #722. During the reign of Queen Anne, Anglican authorities revived the old belief (from the time of Edward the Confessor) that the English sovereign possessed the miraculous power to cure scrofulous tumors by his or her touch; the ceremony took place under scrutiny from the royal surgeons and the monarch's chaplains; "the tenacity with which it survived so many changes of civilisation and religion, is one of the most curious facts in ecclesiastical history" (for a thorough discussion of the tradition and the process of the royal touch --albeit from the view of a nineteenth-century Irish historical eye--see W.E.H. Lecky, A History of England in the Eighteenth Century, 3rd ed., rev. [London: Longmans, Green, and Company, 1883-1890] 1:67-73).
1199. Brown, Charles (fl.1795-1800). A Treatise on Scrofulous Diseases. London, 1798. 168pp.
1200. The Ceremonies for the Healing of Them That Be Diseased with the King's Evil. London, 1789. 8pp.
1201. Durant, Thomas (fl.1760-1765). A Treatise on the King's Evil. London, 1762. 52pp.
1202. Edmonstone, William (fl.1780-1785). A Dissertation on the Prevention of an Evil Injurious to Health. London, 1702. The work apparently came under attack by reviewers, which caused Edmonstone to publish, in 1785, a tract entitled The Reviewers Corrected.
1203. Fern, Thomas (fl.1705-1710). A Perfect Cure for the King's Evil. London, 1709. 58pp.
1204. Gibbs, John (fl.1710-1715). Cures of the King's Evil. London, 1712.
1205. Morley, John (d.1776?). An Essay on the Nature and Cure of Scrophulous Disorders. London, 1767; 31 eds. through 1797. As the principal "cure," the writer offers "a preparation of vervain root."
1206. Nisbet, William (1759-1822). An Inquiry into. . . Scrophula and Cancer. Edinburgh, 1795. 263pp. See, also, #478.
1207. Roberts, Daniel (fl.1790-1795). Remarks on the King's Evil. London, 1791. 44pp.; another ed. in 1792.
1208. Scott, William (fl.1759-1776). A Dissertation on the Scrofula. Edinburgh, 1759. 60pp. The writer held the M.D. degree.

Scrofula (contd.)

1209. Werenfels, Samuel (1657-1740). <u>A Dissertation upon Superstition in Natural Things. . .To which are added Occasional Thoughts on the Power of Curing the King's-Evil ascribed to the Kings of England</u>. London, n.d.; another ed., London, 1748. 75pp.
1210. White, Thomas (fl.1767-1801). <u>A Treatise on Struma, or Scrofula</u>. London, 1784. 110pp.; 2nd ed., London, 1787; 3rd ed., London, 1794. The writer served as a surgeon to the London Dispensary.
1211. Willan, Robert (fl.1746-1757). <u>A Treatise on the King's Evil</u>. London, 1746. 41pp.
1212. Withers, Philip (d.1790). <u>The History of the Royal Malady, with Variety of Entertaining Anecdotes</u>. London, 1789. 88pp. Withers had no association with the practice of medicine; rather, a doctor of divinity, he served (from 1783) as chaplain to the Lady Dowager Hereford; the publication of this <u>History</u> cost him dearly, for it contained attacks upon Mrs. Maria Fitzherbert, a devout Roman Catholic and the wife of George, Prince of Wales; sued for libel and found guilty, Withers received (on 21 November 1789) a sentence of one year in prison and a fine of fifty pounds; he died in Newgate Prison on 24 July 1790 (see Allibone 3: 2808; Jean Morris, <u>The Monarchs of England</u> [New York: Charterhouse, 1975] 339, 342, 347).

K. Dropsy

1213. Dease, William (1752?-1798). <u>Observations on the Different Methods Made Use for the Radical Cure of the Hydrocele</u>. Dublin, 1782. 149pp. See, also, #737.
1214. Dwight, Samuel (1669?-1737). <u>De Hydropibus: deque Medicamentis ad eos Utilibus Epellendas</u>. London, 1725. 48pp. See, also, #424.
1215. Earle, Sir James (1755-1817). <u>A Treatise on the Hydrocele</u>. London, 1791; expanded eds. in 1793 (with a forty-page appendix), 1796, 1805. See, also, #741.
1216. Lowther, William (fl.1770-1775). <u>A Treatise on Dropsy</u>. London, 1771. The writer, an M.D., practiced in London.
1217. Luxmore, William (fl.1790-1800). <u>Observations on Hydropic Patients</u>. London, 1792; another ed., London, 1796.
1218. Milman, Sir Francis (1746-1821). <u>Animadversiones de Natura Hydropis ejusque Curatione</u>. London, 1782. This tract initially published at Vienna in 1779; the writer developed this volume partially from his own observations during travels abroad; he does distinguish among dropsies from cirrhosis of the liver, from malignant growth of the peritoneum, or from renal disease; thus, he recommends purges and tonics and declares that the patient's fluid food need not be restricted; born in Devonshire, Milman

Dropsy (contd.)

received the M.D. from Oxford in 1776 and gained admission as a physician to the Middlesex Hospital and as a fellow of the College of Physicians of London; he practiced at London, lectured extensively there, but appears to have attained only a modest reputation.

1219. Patterson, William (fl.1793-1809). Letters to Dr. [Charles William] Quin on the Internal Dropsy of the Brain. Dublin, 1794. 93pp.; another ed., Dublin, 1795. See #1221. An M.D., the writer practiced medicine at Londonderry; he published (1804) some observations on the climate of Ireland and contributed various medical tracts to English and American periodicals.

1220. Pott, Percival (1714-1788). Practical Remarks upon the Hydrocele. London, 1762; 2nd ed., London, 1767; another ed. in 1771. Pott describes the cause of the problem, recommends a variety of treatments, and sets forth a rational process for cure; he also includes a dissertation upon the "sarocele," then an apparently unresolved affliction or condition; see, also #741 and #770-#771.

1221. Quin, Charles William (fl.1790-1795). A Treatise on Dropsy of the Brain. Dublin, 1790. 227pp.; 2nd ed., London, 1790. An M.D., the writer practiced in Dublin; see #1219.

1222. Whytt, Robert (1714-1766). Observations on the Dropsy of the Brain. Edinburgh, 1768. See, also, #538.

1223. Wilkes, Richard (1691-1760). A Treatise on Dropsy. London, 1730; reissued as An Historical Essay on Dropsy; with an Appendix by N.D. Falch, M.D. London, 1777. Born at Willenhall, Staffordshire, Wilkes studied for the ministry at Cambridge; after taking deacon's orders but failing to secure a preferment, he began to practice medicine at Wolverhampton; Dr. Nathaniel Falch (fl.1771-1779) published tracts on medicine and mechanics; see #1835.

L. Influenza

1224. Broughton, Arthur (d.1796). Observations on the Influenza. London, 1782. 31pp. An M.D. from Edinburgh in 1779, Broughton practiced medicine at Bristol and with the Bristol Infirmary; he spent the last thirteen years of his life at Kingston, Jamaica; his principal interest focused upon botany.

1225. Grant, William (d.1786). Observations on the Late Influenza. London, 1782. 40pp. An M.D., Grant published medical tracts on various topics between 1771 and 1782.

1226. Hamilton, Robert (1749-1830). A Description of the Influenza. London, 1782. 31pp. Born at Londonderry (or Derry) the writer studied medicine at

Influenza (contd.)

Edinburgh; he served with the army as a surgeon, then received (1780) the M.D. from Edinburgh; in 1784, he joined the College of Physicians and practiced at Ipswich (1785-1795); blindness brought an end to his medical career in 1795, following a rheumatic attack; in 1788, he wrote the first systematic treatise on the duties of regimental surgeons (see #1849).

1227. Leslie, Peter Dugud (d.1782). An Account of the Epidemical Catarrhal Fever, commonly called the Influenza. London, 1783. 100pp. Leslie, an M.D., practiced at Durham before moving on to London; he also published (1778) an essay on the causes of animal heat.

VIII

Gout, Rheumatism, Arthritis, Goiter, Back, Bones, Palsy

A. Gout

1228. Atkins, William (fl.1690-1695). <u>A Discourse on the Gout</u>. London, 1694.
1229. Barret, Onsow (fl.1780-1790). <u>A Treatise on the Gout</u>. London, 1785.
1230. Bennet, Thomas (fl.1730-1735). An Essay on the Gout. London, 1734. 134pp. The writer held the M.D. degree.
1231. Berdoe, Marmaduke (fl.1770-1775). <u>An Essay on the Nature and Causes of the Gout</u>. Bath, 1772. An M.D., the writer practiced at Bath, where he published various medical tracts there and at London between 1771 and 1773.
1232. Berkenhout, John (1730?-1791). <u>A Dissertation on the Gout, Examined and Refuted</u>. London, 1771. 38pp. This tract consists of a response to William Cadogan's <u>Dissertation</u> (see #1236); Berkenhout, a physician, naturalist, and miscellaneous prose writer, spent his childhood at Leeds; his father sent him to the Continent, where he joined the Prussian army; upon his return to Britain, he entered medical school at Edinburgh; after receiving the M.D., he moved on to England and settled in Middlesex; he traveled to America and wrote tracts on history, education, literature, and medicine.
1233. Blackmore, Sir Richard (1650-1729). <u>Discourses on the Gout, Rheumatism, and King's Evil</u>. London, 1726. See, also, #839, #896.
1234. Boulton, Richard (fl.1697-1724). <u>Physico-Chirurgical Treatises of the Gout, the King's Evil, and the Lues Venerea</u>. London, 1714. 32pp. See, also, #386.
1235. Buzaglo, Abraham (fl.1775?-1780?). <u>A Treatise on the Gout</u>. London, 1778. 55pp.; three eds. published in 1778.

Gout (contd.)

1236. Cadogan, William (1711-1797). A Dissertation on the Gout and on All Chronic Diseases. London, 1771. 88pp.; eleven eds. through 1785. Born at London, Cadogan studied medicine at Leyden (M.D. 1737), served as a physician to the Royal Army, practiced medicine at Bristol, and settled in London; elected a fellow of the Royal Society, he practiced in the London Foundling Hospital and later received M.A., M.B., and M.D. degrees from Oxford; in this Dissertation, Cadogan viewed gout as not being hereditary, but rather the results of indolence, intemperance, and vexations; the sufferer needed to restrict diet and partake of exercise; the popularity of the volume may be measured by it having reached no less than ten editions within two years of initial publication; for at least one detractor, see #1232.

1237. Cadwallader, Jonathan. The Physicians Out-done; or, the Gout Curable. London, n.d. 16pp. This title cited in the National Library of Medicine Short Title Catalogue.

1238. Carter, William (1711?-1799). A Free and Candid Examination of Dr. [William] Cadogan's Dissertation on the Gout. Canterbury, 1711(?). 46pp. See #1236. The writer, an M.D., practiced at London.

1239. Caverhill, John (d.1781). A Treatise on the Cause and Cure of the Gout. London, 1769. 187pp. Caverhill, a Scottish physician and a licentiate (1767) of the London College of Physicians, published tracts on the gout and the diseases of the bones; in 1777, he published a curious piece, An Explanation of the Seventy Weeks of Daniel.

1240. Cheshire, John (1695-1762). The Gouty Man's Companion. Nottingham, 1747. 97pp. An interestingly written but relatively unimportant tract by the Leicester physician: the writer advises temperance and strict diet (as did a number of his contemporaries), recommending tea in the afternoon, calomel and emetics during an attack of the gout, and mercury at intervals of calm; apparently, Cheshire himself suffered from gout and, in an egocentric sort of way, advanced the merits of his own recommendations.

1241. Cheyne, George (1671-1743). Observations concerning the Nature and Due Method of Treating the Gout. London, 1720; 3rd ed., London, 1721; 5th ed., enlarged, London, 1723; 7th ed., London, 1725; 8th ed., London, 1737; 10th ed., London, 1753. See, also, #55.

1242. Descherny, David (b.1730?-fl.1750-1765). An Essay on the Causes and Effects of the Gout. London, 1760. 47pp. See, also, #908.

1243. Douglas, John (d.1743). A Short Dissertation on the Gout. London, 1741. 24pp. See, also, #315.

1244. Drake, Richard (fl.1751-1771). A Candid and Partial Account of. . .a Specific for the Gout. London,

Gout, Rheumatism, Bones, Palsy 137

Gout (contd.)

1771. 70pp.
1245. ____. An Essay on the Nature and Manner of Treating the Gout. London, 1751. 72pp. This volume has been described as "A work of no merit, being little more than a quack advertisement" (see Allibone 1:519).
1246. ____. An Essay on the Nature and Manner of Treating the Gout. London, 1758. 185pp. This work a significant expansion of #1245.
1247. Dray, Thomas (fl.1770-1775). Reflections Serving to Illustrate the Doctrine Advanced by Dr. [William] Cadogan on the Gout. Canterbury, 1772. 33pp. See #1236, #92.
1248. An Essay on the Nature and Method of Treating the Gout. London, 1746. 22pp.
1249. Falconer, William (1744-1824). An Address to Dr. [William] Cadogan occasioned by his Dissertation on the Gout. London, 1771. 36pp. See #1236 and #100.
1250. Flower, Henry (fl.1760-1775). Incontestable Proofs of Curing the Gout. London, 1771. 26pp.
1251. ____. Observations on the Gout and Rheumatism. London, 1766. 31pp. This work described as "A mere quack advertisement" (see Allibone 1:608).
1252. Forbes, Murray (fl.1785-1795). A Treatise upon Gout. London, 1786. 180pp.
1253. Gardiner, John (fl.1771-1804). An Inquiry into the Nature, Cause, and Cure of the Gout. Edinburgh, 1792. 242pp.; another ed., Edinburgh, 1793. An M.D., the writer practiced medicine at Edinburgh.
1253a. Garlick, Thomas (fl.1719-1741). An Essay on the Gout. London, 1729. 64pp.
1254. Ghyles, Thomas (fl.1680-1690). A Treatise on Short Sickness, or Gout. London, 1685.
1255. Grant, William (d.1786). Some Observations on the . . .Atrabilious Temperament and Gout. 3 vols. London, 1779-1781. See, also, #854.
1256. Grey, Sir William de (1719-1781). A Treatise on the Gout. London, 1772. A parliamentarian and jurist, Lord Grey also suffered from the gout; although not a practitioner of medicine, he recorded, in this document, his own observations and thoughts relative to his affliction.
1257. Ingram, Dale (1710-1793). An Essay on the Cause and Seat of the Gout. Reading, 1743. 100pp. See, also, #454.
1258. James, Robert (1703-1776). A Treatise on the Gout and Rheumatism. London, 1745. See, also, #936.
1259. Jay, Sir James (1732-1815). Reflections and Observations on the Gout. London, 1772. 102pp. The writer, who died at New York, was the older brother of John Jay (1745-1729), the Chief Justice of the Supreme Court of the United States, held the M.D. degree; he published this tract initially in London.
1260. Jeans, Thomas (fl.1790-1795). A Treatise on the Gout.

Gout (contd.)

London, 1792. 108pp. The writer, held the M.D. degree and practiced medicine at London.

1261. Kentish, Richard (fl.1785-1790). Advice to Gouty Persons. London, 1789. 100pp. See, also, #689.

1262. Latham, John (1761-1843). A Dissertation on Gout and Rheumatism. Oxford, 1796. The writer matriculated from Brasenose College, Oxford; he then practiced medicine at that university town and published a variety of tracts, the most important being on diabetes.

1263. Marshall, Rev. Edmund (fl.1770-1799). A Candid and Impartial State of the Evidence of the Gout Medicine of Le Fevre. 2 vols. London, 1770-1771.

1264. Marten, John (fl.1706-1740). The Atilla of the Gout. London, 1713. 50pp.; 2nd ed., London, 1713. 101pp. See, also, #172.

1265. Martin, Charles (fl.1755-1760). A Treatise on Gout. London, 1759. 44pp. An M.D., the writer practiced medicine at London; see, also, #173.

1266. A Medical and Philosophical Essay on the Theory of the Gout. London, 1781. 38pp.

1267. "Misiastrus, Philander." The Honour of the Gout; or, a Rational Discourse. Demonstrating that the Gout is one of the Greatest Blessings which ever befell a Mortal Man. London, 1699; another ed., London, 1735. An obvious exercise in satire, as well as an attack upon contemporary cures and theories relative to the gout.

1268. Mooney, Matthew (fl.1755-1760). A Letter to a Physician concerning the Gout and Rheumatism. London, 1757. 28pp. The writer held the M.D. degree; see, also #1113.

1269. Nelson, Gilbert (fl.1725-1730). The Nature, Cause and Symptoms of the Gout. London, 1728. 32pp.

1270. Philips, George (fl.1685-1695). A Problem concerning the Gout. London, 1691. In 1689, the writer also published at London a political tract, The Interest of England in the Preservation of Ireland.

1271. Riollay, Francis (1748-1797). A Letter to Dr. [James] Hardy on the Hints he has given concerning the Origin of Gout. London, 1778. Riollay suggests that gout represents a disease of the nervous system; James Hardy, an London M.D., wrote a response to this letter in 1780; see, also, #958.

1272. Robinson, Nicholas (1697?-1775). An Essay on the Gout. London, 1755. See, also, #220.

1273. Rogers, John (fl.1730-1740). Dr. Rogers's Oleum Arthriticum, or Specifick Oil for the Gout. London, 1735. 22pp. An M.D., Rogers also translated Latin works by Hermann Boerhaave and published tracts on epidemic diseases.

1274. Rowley, William (1742-1806). A Treatise on the Regular, Irregular, Atonic, and Flying Gout. London, 1792. 90pp. See, also, #222.

1275. Scott, John (fl.1775-1785). An Enquiry into the Origin of the Gout. London, 1779. 176.pp; three

Gout (contd.)

eds. through 1783. The writer held the M.D. degree and practiced at London.

1276. _____. *A History of Gouty, Bilious, and Nervous Cases*. London, 1780. 24pp.

1277. Smith, Daniel (fl.1770-1780). *A Letter to Dr. [William] Cadogan on the Gout*. London, 1772. See #1236. An M.D., Smith practiced medicine at London.

1278. _____. *Observations on Dr. [John] Williams's Treatment of the Gout*. London, 1774. The substance of this tract derives, essentially, from the work of Thomas Sydenham; see #1286.

1279. Stephens, William (fl.1725-1735). *Dolaeus on the Cure of Gout by Milk Diet; with an Essay on Diet*. London, 1732. The writer, an M.D., practiced medicine at London.

1280. Stukeley, William (1687-1765). *A Treatise on the Cause and Cure of the Gout, with a New Rationale*. London, 1734. A native of Lincolnshire, Stukeley studied at Cambridge and then went to London to study medicine at St. Thomas's Hospital; returning to Lincolnshire, he began to practice medicine at Boston, but then departed once again for London; after receiving the M.D. from Cambridge, he gained admission to the College of Physicians and also helped to establish the Society of Antiquarians; shortly thereafter, Stukeley's studies of antiquity proved more attractive to him than the practice of medicine; his long suffering from gout resulted, in part, from the length and stress of various expeditions in search of ruins--to include coins, fossils, and pictures.

1281. Thompson, Thomas (fl.1735-1755). *A Treatise of the Gout*. London, 1740. See, also, #1015.

1282. Viviginis, Pierre de. (fl. 1770-1775). *A Description of the Four Situations of a Gouty Person*. London, 1774. The writer held the M.D. degree.

1283. Wallis, George (1740-1802). *An Essay on the Gout*. London, 1798. Wallis practiced medicine at York and wrote mock tragedy that achieved modest success upon the stages of York, Leeds, and Edinburgh; he moved to London in 1775, and there lectured on a practiced physic.

1284. Warner, Ferdinando (1703-1768). *A Full and Plain Account of the Gout. . . , with Some New and Important Instructions for Its Relief, which the Author's Experiences in the Gout above Thirty Years hath induced him to impart*. London, 1768; another ed., London, 1772. Unfortunately, following the publication of this piece, the writer died from the gout, an occurrence that did little to promote the cures advanced therein; a churchman and preacher, Warner's concerns about medicine appear to have been quite peripheral; instead, his published tracts tend to focus upon theology, history, and biography.

Gout (contd)

1285. Whyte, William Peter (fl.1700-1800). Observations on the Gout and Rheumatism. Stourbridge, 1800.
1286. Williams, John (fl.1770-1780). Advice to People Inflicted with the Gout. London, 1774. 86pp. See, also, #1278. An M.D., the writer practiced medicine at London.
1287. Wood, Samuel (fl.1770-1780). Strictures on the Gout. London, 1775. 66pp.

B. Rheumatism

1288. Cam, Joseph (fl.1715-1732). A Miscellaneous Essay on the Rheumatism, Gout, and Stone. London, 1722. 55 pp. See, also, #1088.
1289. Cheshire, John (1695-1762). A Treatise on the Rheumatism, as well Acute as Chronical. With Observations upon the Various Causes that may produce them. Leicester, 1723. 36pp.; enlarged ed., London, 1735. 202pp. Cheshire practiced medicine at Leicester and the surrounding area; this work never clearly distinguishes between acute and chronic rheumatism, thus seeming to demonstrate the writer's lack of depth in his subject and his reliance upon the works of others previously published; see, also, #1240.
1290. Dawson, Thomas (1725?-1782). Cases in the Acute Rheumatism and the Gout. London, 1774. 104pp.; five eds. through 1781. An M.D. from Glasgow in 1753, Dawson became a Presbyterian preacher, but abandoned that college for the practice of medicine, which he conducted at London in the wards of Guy's Hospital; he gained election as a physician to the Middlesex Hospital (1759) and admittance as a licentiate of the College of Physicians, London (1762); from 1764 to 1770, he served as a physician to the London Hospital; his efforts toward advancing treatment for rheumatism gained him only slight recognition.
1291. An Essay on the Nature, Causes, and Cure of the Rheumatism. London, 1776. 68pp.
1292. James, Robert (1703-1776). A Treatise on the Gout and Rheumatism. London, 1745. See, also, #1258 and #936.
1293. Jebb, John (1736-1786). Select Cases of the Disorder Commonly Termed the Paralysis of the Lower Extremities. London, 1782. 74pp; 2nd ed., London, 1783. 74pp. A native of London, Jebb studied at Trinity College, Dublin, and became a fellow of Peter House, Cambridge; he took Holy Orders and served as rector of Ovington, Norfolk; his embracing of Socinianism forced him to leave that office, and in 1775 he committed himself to the study of medicine; his publications on civil and religious liberty rise far above his medical tracts.
1294. Maillard, Nathaniel (fl.1760-1765). A Treatise on the

Rheumatism (contd).

Rheumatism. London, 1764.
1295. Sanden, Thomas (fl.1774-1801). An Essay on Acute Rheumatism. Edinburgh, 1782. An M.D., Sanden published at least four tracts on medicine, natural science, and bibliography between 1774 and 1801.

C. Arthritis

1296. Musgrave, William (1655?-1721). De Arthritide Anomala sive Interna. Exeter, 1707; 2nd ed., Amsterdam, 1710; a new ed., London, 1716. Musgrave studied medicine at Leyden and returned to England to distinguish himself in natural philosophy and physic; he served as secretary to the Royal Society and edited its Philosophical Transactions; in addition, he practiced medicine at Oxford and London and even devoted portions of his time to the pursuit of antiquarian studies.
1297. ____. De Arthritide Symptomatica Dissertatio. Exeter, 1703; a new ed., London, 1716.

D. Goiter

1298. Prosser, Thomas (fl.1769-1790). An Account and Method of Cure of the Bronchocele. London, 1769. 72pp.; 3rd ed., London, 1782. See, also, #209.

E. Back

1299. Earle, Sir James (1755-1817). Observations on the Cure of the Curved Spine. London, 1799. 81pp. See, also, #741.
1300. Sheldrake, Timothy the younger (fl.1780-1810). An Essay on the Various Causes and Effects of the Distorted Spine. London, 1783. 82pp. The writer, a London M.D., served as truss-maker to the East India Company and the Westminster Hospital.
1301. Worthington, Rev. Richard (fl.1785-1795). A Treatise on the Dorsal Spasm. London, 1792. An M.D., as well as a churchman, Worthington wrote on subjects relative to education and published his own sermons.

F. Bones

1302. Bell, John (1763-1820). Engravings to Illustrate the Structure of the Bones, Muscles, and Joints. London, 1790; further eds. between 1794 and 1804. See, also, #297.
1303. Cheselden, William (1688-1752). Osteographic, or Anatomy of the Bones; with Plates the Sizes of Life. London, 1728; 2nd ed., London, 1733. See, also, #301.
1304. Crowther, Bryan (1765-1840). Practical Observations of the Disease of the Joints, commonly called White Swelling. London, 1797. 122pp. A London surgeon,

Bones (contd.)

Crowther's medical publications appeared principally between 1797 and 1811.

1305. Ford, Edward (1746-1809). <u>Observations on the Disease of the Hip Joint, to which are added Some Remarks on White Swellings of the Knees</u>. London, 1794. 255pp.; revised eds. in 1810, 1818, ed. Thomas Copeland (fl.1810-1820). Born at Wells and trained for medicine at Bristol, Ford practiced surgery at London; he received an appointment as a surgeon to the Westminster General Dispensary.

1306. Fyfe, Andrew (1754-1824). <u>Views of the Bones, Muscles, Viscera, and Organs of the Senses</u>. Edinburgh, 1800. 50pp. See, also, #321.

1307. Havers, Clopton, (d.1702). <u>Osteologia Nova, or Some New Observations of the Bones, and the Parts belonging to Them</u>. London, 1691; Latin eds. at Frankfurt-am-Main (1692) and Amsterdam (1731). This work constitutes a series of papers presented to the Royal Society, in which the writer provides the first detailed account of the structure of the human bone; from this work, also, arose the term "Haversian canals" to describe the minute channels of bone in which run the blood vessels; Havers received the M.D. from Utrecht in 1685 and practiced medicine at London; he gained admittance to the College of Physicians and the Royal Society.

1308. Jackson, Alexander (1696-1767). <u>Osteology, a Treatise on the Anatomy of the Human Bones</u>. Edinburgh. 1726; six eds. through 1758. Contains accounts of the periosteum and the structures of bones and joints; includes detailed descriptions of the various bones; see, also, #1009.

1309. Jackson, William (fl.1780-1890). <u>A Treatise on the Ankle-Joints</u>. London, 1788.

1310. Nesbitt, Robert (d.1761). <u>An Essay on Human Osteogeny</u>. London, 1736. 170pp. The London-born writer studied medicine at Leyden (M.D. 1721) and Cambridge (M.D. 1728); practiced at London; be- to the College of Physicians and the Royal Society. College of Physicians and to the Royal Society.

1311. Park, Henry (1745-1831). <u>An Account of a New Method of Treating Diseases of the Joints of the Knee and Elbow</u>. London, 1783. 51pp. The writer served an apprenticeship to a surgeon at the infirmary in his native Liverpool, after which he studied in London with Percival Pott and then at Paris and Rouen; returning to Liverpool, he practiced surgery there and gained appointment as a surgeon to the infirmary (1766-1816); Park's colleagues hailed his methods for treating diseases of the joints as a significant surgical triumph.

1312. Russell, James (1754-1836). <u>A Practical Essay on a Certain Disease of the Bones termed Necrosis</u>. Edinburgh, 1794. 209pp. Educated at Edinburgh, Russell rose to become Regius Professor of clinical surgery at Edinburgh and the president of the Royal College of Surgeons of that city; beginning in

Gout, Rheumatism, Bones, Palsy 143

    Bones (contd.)

        1786, he presented clinical lectures in practical surgery, while at the same time demonstrating strong interests in art and literature.

1313. Sharp, William (fl. 1765-1770). <u>An Account of a New Method of Treating Fractured Legs</u>. London, 1767. 16pp. This work appeared initially in the <u>Philosophical Transactions</u> of the Royal Scoiety (1767).

1314. Sheldon, John (1752-1808). <u>An Essay on the Fracture of the Patella or Knee-Pan. . .with Observations on the Fracture of the Olecranon</u>. London, 1789. 79pp.; a new ed., London, 1819. Born in London, Sheldon studied anatomy under Henry Watson and lectured on that subject under the guidance of William Hunter; he then opened a private theatre in London, gained appointment as a surgeon to the General Medical Asylum, and served as a surgeon to the Westminster Hospital; Sheldon devoted considerable effort to studying the lymphatic system and to the art of embalming.

1315. Sheldrake, Timothy the younger (fl.1783-1806). <u>A Practical Essay on the Club-Foot</u>. London, 1798. 214pp. See, also, #1300.

1316. Sury, William (fl.1680-1690). <u>A Treatise on the Rickets</u>. Oxford, 1685.

1317. Wellis, Benjamin (fl.1660-1670). <u>A Treatise on the Joint-Evil</u>. London, 1669.

    G. Palsy

1318. Harwood, Edward (1729-1794). <u>The Case of the Rev. Dr. Harwood: An Obstinate Palsy. . .Relieved by Electricity</u>. London, 1784. 46pp. The writer, a Unitarian minister and schoolmaster, ministered to a congregation at Bristol from 1765 to 1760; he then moved on to London, where he wrote and tutored in the classics; he published volumes on the New Testament and criticisms of translations of Greek and Roman classics; this narrative appears to have been his only sojourn into medicine.

IX

Distemper, Epilepsy, Apoplexy, Lock Jaw, Rabies, Swelling, Suppuration, Poison, Infection

A. Distemper

1319. Arnold, Thomas (1742-1816). <u>A Case of Hydrophobia</u>. London, 1793. 245pp. Born at Leicester and educated at Edinburgh (M.D.), the writer became a fellow of the Royal College of Physicians and of the Royal Medical Society of Edinburgh; he practiced at Leicester, where he became the owner and director of a large lunatic asylum.
1320. _____. <u>Observations on. . .Inanity, Lunacy, or Madness</u>. 2 vols. Leicester, 1782-1786.
1321. Brookes, Richard (fl.1721-1763). <u>The History of the Most Remarkable Pestilential Distempers that have appeared in Europe for 300 Years last past; with the Method of Prevention and Cure of that Distemper</u>. London, 1721. 47pp.; 2nd ed., London, 1722. 72pp. The writer, a physician, traveler, and gazetteer, published translations and compilations of general medicine, surgery, natural history, and geography; he practiced medicine in Surrey and traveled to America and Africa; Brookes also wrote a volume on the art of angling.
1322. Cheyne, George (1671-1743). <u>The Natural Method of Cureing the Diseases of the Body, and the Disorders of the Mind Depending on the Body</u>. 3 parts. London, 1742.; five English eds. through 1753; a French ed., 2 vols., Paris, 1749. Cheyne dedicated this work to Philip Dormer Stanhope, fourth Earl of Chesterfield, one of his most ardent readers and admirers, as well as a friend; for his part, Chesterfield wrote to Cheyne in 1745: "I read with great pleasure your book [<u>Natural Method</u>], which your bookseller sent me according to your directions. The physical part is extremely good, and the metaphysical part may be so too, for what I know; and I believe it is; for, as I look upon all metaphysics to be guess-work of imagination, I know

Distemper (contd.)

> no imagination likelier to hit upon the right than yours; and I will take your guess against any other metaphysician's whatsoever. That part which is founded upon knowledge and experience, I look upon as a work of public utility; and for which the present age and their posterity may be obliged to you, if they will be pleased to follow it" (see Charles F. Mullett, ed., <u>The Letters of Doctor George Cheyne to Samuel Richardson (1733-1743)</u> [Columbia: The University of Missouri Studies, 18: 1], 10; this volume, with its wealth of biographical and bibliographical information, will prove most helpful to those interested in medicine and medical practice during the first half of the eighteenth century).

1323. Gilchrist, Ebenezer (1707-1774). <u>An Account of a Very Infectious Distemper</u>. Edinburgh, 1770. 26pp. See, also, #435.

B. Epilepsy

1324. Andree, John (1699?-1785). <u>Cases of Epilepsy, Hysteria, Fits, and St. Vitus Dance</u>. London, 1746. 298pp.; 2nd ed., London, 1753. 298pp. See, also, #366.

1325. Bland, Thomas (fl.1775-1780). <u>A Treatise upon Epilepsy</u>. London, 1780.

1326. Cole, William (1635-1716). <u>Consilium Aetiologicum de Casu quodam Epileptico; Annexa Disquisitione de Prespiratione Insensibili</u>. London, 1702. 151pp. See, also, #903. In this, his final prose tract, Cole responds to Dr. Thomas Hobart of Cambridge, who had written to him (also in Latin), seeking his advice relative to a specific case of epilepsy.

1327. Dick, Sir Alexander (1703-1785). <u>De Epilepsia</u>. Edinburgh, 1725. This work constitutes the writer's inaugural dissertation at Leyden (1725), where he had studied under Hermann Boerhaave prior to receiving the M.D. degree; Dick also received the M.D. from St. Andrews in 1727; from 1756 to 1763, he presided over the College of Physicians at Edinburgh.

1328. Smyth, James Carmichael (1741-1821). <u>A Description of the Jail Distemper</u>. London, 1795. 248pp. See, also, #686.

1329. Threlfal, William (fl.1765-1775). <u>An Essay on Epilepsy</u>. London, 1772. 33pp. The writer received the M.D. from Edinburgh in 1770.

C. Apoplexy

1330. Catherwood, John (fl.1710-1735). <u>Apoplexia</u>. London, 1715; 2nd ed., London, 1735; an English ed. under the title, <u>A New Method for Curing the Apoplexy</u>, London, 1715. 77pp. The writer held the M.D. degree.

Distemper, Epilepsy, Poison, Infection   147

        Apoplexy (contd.)

1331. Chandler, Benjamin (1737-1786). An Enquiry into the
      Various Theories and Methods of Cure in Apoplexies
      and Palsies. Canterbury, 1785. 148pp. See, also,
      #1032.
1332. Cole, William (1635-1716). A Physico-Medical Essay
      concerning the Late Frequency of Apoplexies.
      Oxford, 1689. See, also, #903. In this, the only
      medical tract written by Cole in English, the
      physician attributes the principal causes of
      apoplexy to cold temperatures, beginning with the
      severe winter of 1683. On 23 December 1683, John
      Evelyn noted that "The small-pox very prevalent and
      mortal; the Thames frozen." On 1 January 1684, the
      diarist observed, "The weather continuing
      intolerably severe, streets of booths were set upon
      the Thames; the air was so very cold and thick, as
      of many years there had not been the like. The
      small-pox was very mortal." Rain and thaw finally
      came to London on 9 February 1684; see The Diary of
      John Evelyn, ed. William Bray (London: Dent/Every-
      man's Library), 2:195-198.

     D. Lock Jaw

1333. Mackie, John (1748-1831). A Treatise on the Locked
      Jaw. London, 1795. Mackie began his medical
      studies at Edinburgh, then moved on to practice at
      Huntingdon, Southampton, and on the Continent;
      thus, his patients ranged from French immigrants at
      Southampton to royalty in Spain and Holland.
1334. Watson, Sir William (1715-1787). Observations on the
      Effects of Electricity applied to a Tetanus.
      London, 1763. 16pp. See, also, #532.

     E. Rabies

1335. Berkenhout, John (1730?-1791). An Essay on the Bite
      of a Mad Dog. London, 1783. 83pp. See, also,
      #379.
1336. Dalby, Joseph (fl.1760-1765). The Virtues of Cinnabar
      and Musk against the Bite of a Mad Dog.
      Birmingham, 1762. 55pp.; 2nd ed., Birmingham, 1764.
      55pp.
1337. Foot, Jesse (1744-1826). An Essay on the Bite of a
      Mad Dog. London, 1788. 86pp. See, also, #1104.
1338. ____. A Plan for Preventing the Fatal Effects from
      the Bite of a Mad Dog. London, 1793. 15pp.
1339. Fothergill, John (1712-1780). The Case of a
      Hydrophobia. London, 1778. 36pp. See, also, #112.
1340. Hamilton, Robert (1749-1830). Remarks on the Means of
      Obviating the Fatal Effects of the Bite of a Mad
      Dog. Ipswich, 1785. 265pp. See, also, #1226.
1341. James, Robert (1703-1776). A New Method of Preventing
      and Curing the Madness Caused by the Bite of a Mad
      Dog. London, 1741. See, also, #936. The writer
      recommends mercury in the treatment of hydrophobia;

Rabies (contd.)

the preface to this volume bears the date 4 December 1740, which means that James wrote the piece shortly after his arrival in London from Birmingham; interestingly, almost a quarter of a century later, Joseph Dalby, then residing at Birmingham, recommends (see #1336) cinnabar, a native red mercuric sulfide, for rabies treatment.

1342. ____. A Treatise on Canine Madness. London, 1760. This work essentially an expanded edition of the observations and opinions offered in #1341.

1343. Layard, Daniel Peter (fl.1750-1780). An Essay on the Bite of a Mad Dog. London, 1762. The writer, an M.D., practiced at London; see, also, #464.

1344. Mease, James (1771-1846). An Essay on the Disease Produced by the Bite of a Mad Dog. London, 1793. 179pp. The writer, an M.D., began his practice at London; he eventually moved to Philadelphia and gained prominence; his later American publications include tracts on the geology of the United States (1807), a description of Philadelphia (1811), and an essay on William Penn's treaty with the Indians (1836).

1345. Nugent, Christopher (d.1775). An Essay on the Hydrophobia. London, 1753. The writer clearly details his successful treatment, in 1751, of a female servant who had been bitten in two places by a mad "turnspit" dog (literally a dog kept to turn the roasting spit by running within a type of treadmill connected with the spit [see OED]; he treated her with "powders of musk and cinnabar" (see, also, #1336); the sixty-seven sections of the book that follow discuss the mental and physical characteristics of the hydrophobia, its parallels with hysteria, and the writer's proposed remedies; born in Ireland, Nugent studied medicine in France (M.D.), then practiced in southern Ireland, Bath, and London; he also counted himself one of the original members of the Literary Club that included Johnson, Boswell, Burke, and Goldsmith; Boswell described his attendance as "very constant" (see James Boswell, Life of Johnson, ed. R.W. Chapman, corrected by J.D. Fleeman [London: Oxford University Press, 1970] 363).

1346. Pearson, Richard (1765-1836). The Argument in Favour of an Inflammatory Disthesis in Hydrophobia Considered. Birmingham, 1798. 59pp. See, also, #424.

F. Swelling

1347. Akenside, Mark (1721-1770). "A Method of Treating White Swellings of the Joints," Medical Transactions, 1 (1768) 104. See, also, #1158.

1348. Burns, John (1774-1850). A Dissertation on Inflammation. 2 vols. Glasgow, 1800. Born at Glasgow, the writer studied medicine at the

Swelling (contd.)

University there; in 1792, he received an appointment as a surgeon's clerk at the Royal Infirmary, Glasgow; he lectured on anatomy, but eventually developed a special interest in midwifery and diseases of women and children; by 1815, he had risen to the professorship of surgery at Glasgow.

1349. Harrison, Thomas (fl.1780-1805). A Treatise on Inflammation. Dublin, 1785. 147pp. Harrison also published essays on botany.

1350. Magenise, Daniel (fl.1768-1778). A Treatise on the Doctrine of Inflammations. London, 1768. 168pp.; 2nd ed., London, 1776. An M.D. who practiced at London, Magenise also published tracts on the relationships among law, physic, and divinity.

1351. Rowley, William (1742-1806). A Treatise on the Causes and Cures of Swelled Legs. London, 1796. 132pp. See, also, #222.

1352. Russell, Richard (1687-1759). The Oeconomy of Nature in Acute and Chronical Diseases of the Glands. London, 1755. 253pp. See, also, #691.

G. Suppuration (Infectious Discharge)

1353. Barry, Sir Edward (d.1776). A Treatise on Three Different Digestions and Discharges of the Human Body. London, 1759. 434pp.; 2nd ed., London, 1763. 384pp. The writer studied medicine at Leyden under the direction of Hermann Boerhaave; he practiced at Dublin and London.

1354. Clare, Peter (1738-1786). An Essay on the Cure of Abscesses by Caustic. London, 1779. 154pp.; 2nd ed., London, 1779. 245pp. See, also, #401.

1355. _____. Observations on the Nature and Treatment of the Variolous Abscess. London, 1781. 61pp.

1356. Darwin, Charles (1758-1778). Experiments Establishing a Criterion between Mucaginous and Purulent Matter. Lichfield, 1780. 134pp. The writer the son of Erasmus Darwin (see #1168) by his first wife; his father published this volume after he had moved to Lichfield.

1357. Earle, Sir James (1755-1817). Observations on Haemorrhoid Excrescences. London, 1790. 18pp. See, also, #741.

1358. Fizes, Matthew (fl.1755-1760). An Essay on Suppuration. London, 1759.

1359. Home, Sir Everard (1756-1832). A Dissertation on the Properties of Pus. London, 1788. 63pp. The writer, a native of Greenlaw Castle, County Berwick, Scotland, studied medicine with John Hunter (his brother-in-law), after which he practiced in London for five years; he rose to become president of the Royal College of Surgeons; he also lectured and published on comparative anatomy.

H. Poisons

1360. Adams, Joseph (1756-1818). <u>Observations on Morbid Poisons, Phagedaena, and Cancer</u>. London, 1795.. 328pp. The writer studied medicine at Aberdeen (M.D. 1796), and later settled in Madeira to practice medicine; he also served a term as editor of the <u>Medical and Physical Journal</u> (see #2051).

1361. Baker, Sir George (1722-1809). <u>An Essay concerning the Cause of the Endemical Colic of Devonshire</u>. London, 1767. See, also, #17 and, particularly, #1445.

1362. Clutterbuck, Henry (1767-1856). <u>An Account of a New and Successful Method of Treating those Affections which arise from the Poison of Lead</u>. London, 1794. 69pp. See, also #1095.

1363. Coke, John (fl.1765-1775). <u>A Treatise on Poisons</u>. London, 1770. An M.D., the writer practiced in London. See, also, #1364; this entry cited in Allibone, 1:403.

1364. Cook, John (fl.1730-1770). <u>A Treatise of Poisons, Vegetable, Animal, and Mineral</u>. London, 1770. 81pp. See, also, #1363; this entry cited in National Library of Medicine <u>Short Title Catalogue</u>.

1365. Falconer, William (1744-1824). <u>Observations and Experiments on the Poison of Copper</u>. London, 1774. 116pp. See, also, #100.

1366. Fowler, Thomas (1736-1801). <u>Observations on the Effects of Arsenic</u>. London, 1786. A native of York, the writer (an M.D.) practiced at Stafford and York; he also published tracts on tobacco and on bleeding; at his death, Fowler left, in unpublished manuscripts, the records of more than six thousand cases that he had observed or treated during the years of his practice.

1367. _____. <u>Medical Reports of the Effects of Tobacco</u>. London, 1785.

1368. Houlston, Thomas (d.1787). <u>Observations on Poisons</u>. London, 1784. 72pp.; a new ed., Edinburgh, 1787. 95pp. The writer, an M.D., practiced at Liverpool; he published a variety of medical tracts at London between 1773 and 1787.

1369. Johnstone, John (1768-1836). <u>An Essay on Mineral Poisons</u>. Evesham, 1795. 168pp. See, also, #153.

1370. Mead, Richard (1673-1754). <u>A Mechanical Account of Poisons, in Several Essays</u>. London, 1702. By actually swallowing the venom extracted from the fangs of a viper, Mead, in this 176-page volume, confirms the necessity for puncture to produce the fatal effect; he concludes that hard particles in the poison interact mechanically with the blood, thus causing death; the essay also considers such subjects as opium and bites from mad dogs and tarantulas; see, also #176.

1371. Percival, Thomas (1740-1804). <u>A Treatise on the Poison of Lead</u>. London, 1774. See, also, #204.

1372. Prestwich, John (d.1795). <u>Dissertations on Mineral, Animal, and Vegetable Poisons</u>. London, 1775.

Poison (contd.)

Essentially an antiquarian writer rather than a medical practitioner, Prestwich published tracts on the English, Scottish, and Irish nobilities; he also produced histories of Liverpool and South Wales; he died at Dublin.

1373. Ramesay, William (b.1626?; fl.1651-1669). *De Venenis; or a Discourse of Poysons*. London, 1663. This work had been written in 1656 and dedicated (on 26 October 1660) to the restored Charles II; an edition of 1665 bears the title *Life's Security*; born at Westminster (London), Ramesay (or Ramsay) studied at Oxford and St. Andrews; he resided in Edinburgh before moving to London; after graduating M.D. from Montpellier in 1652, he remained in France and served as a physician-in-ordinary to Charles II during that monarch's period in exile; following the Restoration, Ramesay settled in Plymouth; his medical practices appear to have been guided by his deep interest in astrology.

1374. Robertson, Joseph (1726-1802). *An Essay on Culinary Poisons*. London, 1781. 45pp. The writer resides outside of the medical profession, he having taken Holy Orders in 1752; he eventually became rector of Sutton (Essex) and vicar of Horncastle, in Lincolnshire; his considerable published work focuses upon criticism of the "polite" literature of his day.

1375. Skinner, Joseph (fl.1787-1815). *A Treatise on the Venom of the Viper; from the French of Felix Fontana*. 2 vols. London, 1787; 2nd ed., London, 1795. The writer, a naval surgeon, also published tracts upon venereal diseases and the plague; Felice Fontana (1730-1805), a native of Tyrol, achieved a reputation as a practicing physician and anatomist, as well as for his work in the history of the natural sciences.

1376. Wilmer, Bradford (fl.1771-1802). *Observations on Poisonous Vegetables*. London, 1781. The writer practiced surgery at Stony-Stratford and then at Coventry; his publications include tracts on hernia and on surgery in general.

I. Infection

1377. Douglas, James (d. 1743). *A Short Account of Mortification*. London, 1742. 48pp. See, also, #312.

1378. O'Halloran, Sylvester (1728-1807). *A Complete Treatise on Gangrene and Sphacelus*. London, 1765. 288pp. Born at Limerick, the writer studied medicine and surgery at Paris and Leyden, with emphasis upon the diseases of the eye; beginning in 1750, he practiced at Limerick; his tract on glaucoma stands as the first work on that subject published by an Irish press; in 1760, he founded the Limerick Infirmary; in addition, he pursued an active study of Irish language and antiquity.

X

Stone, Urinary Diseases and Disorders, Liver, Jaundice

A. Stone

1379. Adams, William (fl.1770-1775). <u>A Disquisition on the Stone, Gravel, and the Diseases of the Bladder and Kidneys</u>. London, 1773. The writer practiced surgery in London.

1380. Austin, William (1754-1793). <u>A Treatise on the Origin and Component Parts of the Stone in the Urinary Bladder</u>. London, 1791. 123pp. The work describes a series of experiments that, erroneously, conclude that the stone owes its formation not from the urine secreted by the kidneys, but principally from the mucus produced from the sides of the different cavities through which the urine passes; that condition, according to Austin, could be relieved only through surgery; essentially, the writer had been misled by the imperfections of eighteenth-century chemical analysis; born at Wotton-under-Edge, in Gloucestershire, Austin studied Hebrew and botany at Oxford, then gravitated to medicine and an M.D. in 1783; he eventually practiced in London, where he became associated with the Radcliffe Infirmary and St. Bartholomew's Hospital.

1381. Awister, John (fl.1760-1770). <u>A Treatise on the Stone, Gravel, and Other Disorders</u>. London, 1767. 39pp. See, also, #368.

1382. Beddoes, Thomas (1760-1808). <u>Observations on the Nature and Cure of the Calculus, Sea Scurvy, Consumption, Catarrh, and Fever</u>. London, 1793. 278pp.; Philadelphia, 1797. 278pp. See, also, #26.

1383. Blackmore, Sir Richard (1650-1729). <u>A Dissertation on Dropsy and Stone</u>. London, 1727. See, also, #839.

1384. Blackrie, Alexander (d.1772). <u>A Disquisition on Medicines which Dissolve the Stone; in which Dr. Chittick's Secret is consider'd and discover'd</u>. London, 1766; 2nd ed., enlarged, London, 1771. A native of Scotland, Blackrie practiced at Bromley,

Stone (contd.)

Kent, as an apothecary; evidence suggests that he settled in that town as early as 1733; the identity of "Dr. Chittick" has proven as secretive as his medicine.

1385. Bracken, Henry (1697-1764). Lithiasis Anglicana; or, A Philosophical Enquiry into the Nature and Origin of the Stone. London, 1739. 55pp. A native of Lancaster, the writer studied medicine at St. Thomas's Hospital, London, then continued on to Paris and Leyden (M.D.); he practiced surgery at London and Lancaster, but encountered political problems; essentially, Bracken gained a reputation for his publications on farriery and midwifery.

1386. Butter, William (1726-1805). A Method of Cure for the Stone. Edinburgh, 1754. Butter, a native of the Orkney Islands, graduated M.D. from Edinburgh in 1761; he practiced at Derby, then moved on to London; in his several publications, he focused upon fevers, diseases, and the arteries.

1387. Cheselden, William (1688-1752). A Treatise on the High Operation for the Stone. London, 1723. See, also, #301. In this tract, Cheselden describes his own method for such an operation, as well as reprints accounts of procedures from among his predecessors at St. Thomas's Hospital, London; a rival lecturer on anatomy and a former pupil at St. Thomas's, John Douglas (see #1391), responded anonymously with a pamphlet attack upon Cheselden, Lithotomus Castratus (London, 1723); Douglas accused his former mentor of having plagiarized from him (specifically from #1391), but he did receive full credit and acknowledgement from Cheselden in this Treatise.

1388. Descherny, David (b.1730? fl.1750-1765). A Treatise of the Causes and Symptoms of the Stone. London, 1753. 146pp. An M.D., the writer also published tracts on the small pox and gout.

1389. The Distinct Symptoms of the Gravel and Stone, Explained to the Patient. London, 1759. 51pp.

1390. Douglas, James (1675-1742). An Appendix to the History of the Lateral Operation for the Stone. Containing Mr. [William] Cheselden's Present Method. London, 1731. 47pp. See #1387; also #312.

1391. Douglas, John (d.1743). Lithotomia Douglassiana; or, an Account of a New Method of Making the High Operation to extract the Stone. London, 1720. 28pp.; further eds. through 1724. A Scottish surgeon and brother of Dr. James Douglas (see #312 and #1390), Douglas practiced in London and lectured on anatomy at Fetter Lane; he became a surgeon-lithotomist at the Westminster Infirmary, and later gained election to the Royal Society; see, also, #1387 concerning his dispute with William Cheselden, his former tutor,

1392. Earle, Sir James (1755-1817). Practical Observations on the Operation for the Stone. London, 1793; 2nd

Stone (contd.)

ed., London, 1796. See, also, #741.
1393. Gem, Richard (fl. 1740-1745). An Account of the Remedy for the Stone, lately published in England . . . .Extracted from the Examination of this Remedy . . . .by M. [Sauveur Francois] Morand and M. [Etienne-Francois] Geoffroy. London, 1741. 54pp. Geoffroy (1672-1731), practiced chemistry and medicine at Paris.
1394. Houstoun, Robert (fl.1720-1725). Lithotomus Castratus; or, Mr. [William] Cheselden's Treatise on the High Operation for the Stone thoroughly Examin'd. London, 1723. 99pp. See, also, #819.
1395. Kirkpatrick, James (d.1743). An Account of the Success of Mrs. [Joanna] Stephens's Medicines for the Stone. Belfast, 1739. 61pp. See, also. #153 and #506.
1396. Perry, Charles (1698-1780). Disquisitions on the Stone and Gravel, with Other Diseases of the Kidneys. London, 1777. See, also, #624.
1397. Perry, Sampson (1747-1823). Farther Observations on the Stone, Gravel, and All Other Calculous Obstructions. London,1789. 68pp. Born at Birmingham, Perry eventually began his medical practice in surgery at London; he developed a solvent for the stone, known as "Adams' solvent"; in 1777, he gained appointment as a surgeon to the East Middlesex militia; his tracts on venereal diseases gained acceptance, but he suffered a reversal of fortune through involvement in several libel suits.
1398. Pitcairne, Omelius (fl. 1735-1740). The Truth Unveiled for the Public Good; or, A Treatise on the Stone. London, 1739.
1399. Robinson, Nicholas (1697?-1775). A Complete Treatise of the Gravel and Stone. London, 1721; 2nd ed., London, 1723; a second imprint of the 1723 ed., London, 1724; 3rd ed., London, 1734. The writer defends the theory of Charles Bernard (fl.1695-1700), who had advanced the notion of cutting into the kidney to remove renal calculus (or stone); Robinson also advances the notions of tinctura lithontriptica, pulvis lithontripticus, and elixir lithontripticum as principal remedies for the stone and the gravel; see, also, #220.
1400. Saunders, William (1743-1817). Observations and Experiments on the Power of the Mephytic Acid in Dissolving Stones of the Bladder. London, 1777. 32pp. See, also, #232.
1401. Shaw, William (fl.1730-1740). A Dissertation on the Stone in the Bladder. London, 1734; another ed., London, 1738. An M.D., the writer practiced at London.
1402. Sherley, Thomas (1638-1678). A Philosophical Essay declaring the Probable Cause whence Stones are produced in the Outer World. London, 1672. Born at Westminster, Sherley attended Oxford and studied

Stone (contd.)

> physic in France; returning to London, he practiced medicine there and secured an appointment as a physician-in-ordinary to Charles II; in addition to this Philosophical Essay, he published a number translations of European medical tracts; the Essay itself in German translations at Hamburg in 1675 and 1699.

1403. Touche, Henri Bernard de la (fl.1760-1765). An Essay on the Stone. London, 1764. A translation from the French.

B. Urinary Diseases and Disorders

1404. Bayford, Thomas (fl.1765-1775). The Effects of Injection into the Urethra. London, 1773. 100pp. The writer published various medical tracts at London between 1767 and 1772.
1405. Dufour, William (fl.1790-1810). Observations upon Diseases of the Urinary Passages. London, 1794; further eds. in 1801, 1808. The writer also published tracts on ruptures.
1406. Foot, Jesse (1744-1826). Cases of the Successful Practice of Vesicae Lotura in the Cure of Diseased Bladders. 2 vols. London, 1798-1803. See, also, #1104.
1407. _____. A Complete Treatise on the Lues Venerea and Obstructions in the Urethra. London, 1792. 675pp.
1408. _____. A Critical Enquiry into the Ancient and Modern Manner of Treating the Diseases of the Urethra. London, 1774. 65pp; four eds. through 1786.
1409. Forbes, Murray (fl.1785-1795). A Treatise upon Gravel and upon Gout. London, 1787. 184pp.; another ed., London, 1793. 258pp.
1410. Home, Sir Everard (1756-1832). Practical Observations on the Treatment of Strictures in the Urethra. London, 1795. 199pp.; 2nd ed., London, 1797. 528pp. See, also, #1359.
1411. Parsons, James (1705-1770). A Description of the Urinary Bladder. London, 1742. 283pp. An M.D., Parsons achieved a reputation for his publications in anatomy and antiquarian studies; he became the assistant foreign corresponding secretary of the Royal Society and published papers on natural history, obstetrics, hermaphrodites, seeds, human physiognomy, and the remains of Japhet.
1412. Reid, Alexander (fl.1765-1780). An Inquiry into the Merits of the Operation used in Obstinate Suppressions of Urine. London, 1778. 63pp. The writer also translated and edited works of Continental physicians.
1413. Rutty, William (1687-1730). A Treatise of the Urinary Passages. London, 1726. 54pp.; another ed., London, 1750. This volume constitutes the writer's Gulstonian lectures, delivered before the College of Physicians, London, in 1722; Rutty also published medical tracts in the Philosophical

Urinary Diseases and Disorders (contd.)

<u>Transactions</u> of the Royal Society between 1720 and 1730.

1414. Sherwin, John (1749-1826). <u>Observations on the Diseased and Contracted Urinary Bladder</u>. London, 1799. 56pp. Sherwen studied medicine at St. Thomas's Hospital, London, then journeyed to Sumatra and Calcutta in the service of the East India Company; upon his return to England, he practiced surgery in Middlesex, received the M.D. degree from Aberdeen (1798), visited France, and eventually settled at Bath; his interests extended beyond the practice of medicine to include the studies of English literature and antiquity.

1415. Tomkins, Thomas (fl.1745-1750). <u>Chirurgical Observations on the Disorders of the Urethra; from Davon and Others</u>. London, 1749.

1416. Trye, Charles Brandon (1757-1811). <u>Remarks on Morbid Retention of Urine</u>. Gloucester, 1784. 84pp. Born in Gloucestershire and later apprenticed to an apothecary at Worcester, Trye remained in that town to study surgery; he moved on to London to study with John Hunter, after which he received an appointment as a house surgeon to the Westminster Hospital; returning to Gloucester, he gained appointment as a house apothecary to the Gloucester Infirmary (1783) and election as a surgeon to the Gloucester Charity (1784-1810); with Rev. Thomas Stark, he established a lying-in charity hospital at Gloucester; Trye gained a considerable reputation for his surgical skills and for his having promoted inoculation.

1417. Wilson-Philip, Alexander Philip (1770?-1851?). <u>An Inquiry into the Remote Cause of Urinary Infection</u>. London, 1792. See, also, #542.

C. Liver

1418. Andree, John (fl.1779-1799). <u>Considerations on Bilious Diseases</u>. Hertford, 1788. 58pp.; 2nd ed., London, 1790. 61pp. See, also, #816.

1419. Bath, Robert (fl.1777-1805). <u>A Treatise on Diseases of the Liver and Biliary Ducts</u>. London, 1777. 65pp. A surgeon, Bath's medical tracts appeared at London between 1777 and 1805.

1420. Coe, Thomas (d.1761). <u>A Treatise on Biliary Concretions</u>. London, 1757. 345pp. The writer held the M.D. degree.

1421. Crawford, John (fl.1770-1795). <u>An Essay on the Nature, Cause, and Cure of a Disease Incident to the Liver</u>. London, 1772. 66pp. An M.D., Crawford also published a tract on the muscles (1772, 1786).

1422. Gibson, John (fl.1768-1800). <u>A Treatise upon Bilious Diseases</u>. London, 1799. 68pp. An M.D., the writer published a number of tracts upon midwifery, foreign substances in the body, fevers, and even fruit gardening.

Liver (contd.)

1423. McClurg, James (1746?-1823). Experiments upon the Human Bile. London, 1772. 217pp. A native of Hampton, Virginia, McClurg received his education at the College of William and Mary before removing to Edinburgh and Paris to study medicine; he then returned to America, practicing first at Williamsburg ((1772-1783) and then at Richmond (1783-1823); this piece, published at London, constitutes the writer's inaugural dissertation from Edinburgh; in Virginia, he also wrote a series of poetical character sketches of famous women.

1424. Monro, George (fl.1775-1780). A Practical Treatise upon Bilious Fevers. London, 1777. The writer held the M.D. degree.

1425. Pearson, George (1751-1828). Experiments and Observations tending to show the Composition and Properties of Urinary Concretions. London, 1798. 34pp. See, also, #623. This piece appeared initially in the Philosophical Transactions of the Royal Society.

1426. Pearson, Richard (1765-1836). Some Observations on the Bilious Fevers of 1797, 1798, and 1799. Birmingham, 1799. 30pp. See, also, #484.

1427. Powell, Richard (1767-1834). Observations on the Bile and Its Diseases, and on the Oeconomy of the Liver. London, 1800. 180pp. The writer notes, with detail, his own methods of clinical examination of the liver; the essays herein constitute the Gulstonian lectures delivered before the College of Physicians, London; Powell received the M.D. from Oxford, studied medicine at St. Bartholomew's Hospital, and eventually became a physician at that institution; he has been recognized as the first English medical writer to demonstrate that gall stones may remain fixed in the neck of the gall bladder (even to the extent of obliterating its cavity) without distinct symptoms or even injury to the patient.

1428. Priestley, Robert (fl.1795-1800). A Few Interesting Remarks on Bilious Disorders. Leeds, 1798. 102pp.

1429. Saunders, William (1743-1817). A Treatise on the Structure, Economy, and Diseases of the Liver. London, 1793. 292pp.; 2nd ed., London, 1803; 3rd ed., London, 1809. This work emerged from the Gulstonian lectures delivered by the writer to the College of Physicians, London, in 1792; Saunders may well have been the first English physician to observe that in certain forms of cirrhosis, the liver becomes enlarged and afterward contracted; see, also, #510.

1430. Wainewright, Jeremiah (fl.1705-1725). An Anatomical Treatise of the Liver, with the Diseases Incident to It. London, 1722. 100pp. An M.D., the writer practiced in London.

1431. White, William (fl.1744-1790). An Essay on the Diseases of the Bile, more particularly its

Liver (contd.)

Calculous Concretions called Gall-Stones. York, 1771. 66pp. See, also, #537.

D. Jaundice

1432. Corp. William (fl.1785-1795). *An Essay on the Jaundice, and Using the Bath Waters in that Disease.* Bath, 1785. 75pp.; 2nd ed., Bath, 1787. An M.D., the writer practiced medicine at Bath.
1433. Daniel, Samuel (fl.1775-1780). *Dissertatio de Ictero.* London, 1776. The writer held the M.D. degree.

XI

Stomach, Dysentery, Colic, Bowels

A. Stomach

1434. Jewel, Edward (fl.1675-1680). <u>A Practical Treatise on the Stomach</u>. London, 1678.
1435. Webster, Charles (1750-1795). <u>Facts tending to show the Connection of the Stomach with Life, Disease, and Recovery</u>. Edinburgh, 1793. A native of Dundee, Webster went, in 1760, to Edinburgh, where he practiced physic; eventually, he became a minister of the nonjurors' Scottish Episcopal Church at Carrubber's Close, Edinburgh, moving later to St. Peter's Chapel in Roxburgh Place, a structure built under his own direction; he died in the West Indies; in addition to medical tracts and sermons, Webster wrote a biography of Dr. Archibald Pitcairne (see #55).

B. Dysentery

1436. Akenside, Mark (1721-1770). <u>De Dysenteria Commentarius</u>. London, 1764. 81pp.; an English ed., London, 1767. 96pp. See, also, #1158.
1437. Baker, Sir George (1722-1809). <u>De Catarrho et de Dysenteria Londonensi Epidemicus Utrisque</u>. London, 1761. This tract constitutes an Harverian oration by the Devonshire physician; see, also, #17.
1438. Boag, William (fl.1790-1795). "An Essay on Fevers and Dysentery of Hot Climates." <u>Medical Facts and Observations</u>, 3 (1793).
1439. Geach, Francis (1724-1798). <u>Some Observations on the Present Epidemic Dysentery</u>. London, 1781. 41pp. See, also, #121.
1440. Hopson, Charles Rivington (1744-1796). <u>A Treatise on Dysentery, from the German of J.G. Zimmermann</u>. London, 1771. Hopson graduated M.D. in 1767 from Leyden, practiced medicine at London, and served as a physician to the Finnsbury Dispensary; he also

Dysentery (contd.)

translated, from the German, several volumes of travel narrative; Johann Georg Zimmermann (1728-1795), a Swiss physician and miscellaneous writer, studied medicine under Albrecht von Haller at Gottingen; after practicing at Berne, he received (1768) an appointment as a physician to George III at Hanover, as well as to Frederick of Prussia; he died from "a hypochondriac disease."

1441. Moseley, Benjamin (1742-1819). Observations on the Dysentery of the West Indies, with a New and Successful Method of Treating It. Jamaica, 1781; London, 1781. In this, the writer's first publication, Moseley suggests administering (Robert) James's powder (see #446) or another diaphoretic and wrapping the patient in blankets to induce profuse sweating; born in Essex, Moseley studied medicine at London, Paris, and Leyden, then settled (1768) in Jamaica; he became surgeon-general there, traveled throughout the West Indies, visited Newfoundland, and eventually returned to England; after receiving the M.D. from St. Andrews, Moseley toured hospitals at Stroursbourg, Dijon, Montpellier, Aix, Lausanne, Venice, and Rome; from 1788 until his death, he served as a physician to the Royal Hospital at Chelsea.

1442. Rollo, John (d.1809). Observations on the Acute Dysentery. London, 1786. Born in Scotland and educated at Edinburgh, Rollo joined the army as an artillery surgeon; he spent time at Barbados, St. Lucia, Woolwich, and Deptford; in 1794, Rollo received appointment as surgeon-general to the military.

1443. Wilson, Andrew (1718-1792). An Essay on the Autumnal Dysentery. London, 1760; 2nd ed., London, 1777. See, also, #683.

C. Colic

1444. Alcock, Thomas (1709-1798). The Endemical Colic of Devon, not caused by a Solution of Lead in the Cider. Plymouth, 1768(?). 141pp. This piece constitutes an response to George Baker's Essay of the previous year (see #1445); Alcock, a miscellaneous writer, received his education from Oxford; he entered the Church and spent most of his time at Cheshire before moving on to Plymouth; he also published his sermons and an essay on the poor laws.

1445. Baker, Sir George (1722-1809). An Essay concerning the Cause of the Endemical Colic of Devonshire. London, 1767. This tract stands as an important addition to medical knowledge by the Devonshire physician; he discovered "the Devonshire colic" and the colica Pictonum to have been forms of lead poisoning and existed because of the large pieces of lead in Devonshire cider presses and vats (as

Stomach, Dysentery, Colic, Bowels

Colic (contd.)

opposed to those counties that utilized presses and vats of stone, wood, or iron); after he extracted the lead from Devonshire cider, the citizens of that region attacked him because of his supposed "faithlessness" toward his native county; Baker finally convinced people of his theory and findings, and thus colic ceased to exist as a serious health problem in Devon; see, also, #1444 and #17.

1446. Purcell, John (1674-1730). A Treatise on the Colick. Dublin, 1702; London, 1714. 188pp.; 2nd ed., London, 1715. The work contains the description of an autopsy witnessed by the writer at Montpellier; he provides the earliest record of an observation in any book in English of the irritation produced by the exudation in peritonitis on the hands of a morbid anatomist; born in Shropshire, Purcell studied medicine at Montpellier (M.D. 1699); upon his return to England, he practiced and wrote at London.

D. Bowels

1447. Cockburn, William (1669-1734). An Account of the Nature, Causes, Symptoms, and Cure of Looseness. London, 1710. 262pp. See, also, #65.
1448. ____. The Nature and Cures of Fluxes. London, 1724. 344pp.
1449. ____. Profluvia Ventris; or, the Nature and Causes of Looseness. London, 1701. 178pp.
1450. ____. Some Observations of the Power and Efficacy of a Medicine against Looseness. London, 1757. 72pp. This tract published posthumously.
1451. Lettsome, John Coakley (1744-1815). The History of an Extraordinary Introsusception. London, 1786. 8pp. See, also, #160.
1452. Wilson, Andrew (1718-1792). Short Remarks upon Autumnal Disorders of the Bowels. London, 1760; Newcastle-upon-Tyne, 1765; 2nd ed., London, 1777. See, also, #683.

XII

Cancer, Ulcers, Tumors

A. Cancer

1453. Akenside, Mark (1721-1770). "Observations on Cancers," <u>Medical Transactions</u>, 1 (1768), 64. See, also, #1158.
1454. Andree, John (fl.1779-1799). <u>Some Few Cases and Observations on the Treatment of Fistula in Ano.</u> London, 1799. 47pp. See, also, #816.
1455. Becket, William (1684-1738). <u>New Discoveries relating to the Cure of Cancers.</u> London, 1711; 2nd ed., London, 1712. See, also, #722 and #1198.
1456. Bell, George (fl.1785-1805). <u>Thoughts on the Cancer of the Breast.</u> Birmingham, 1788. 34pp.
1457. Burrows, John (fl.1760-1775). <u>A New Practical Essay on Cancers.</u> London, 1767. 76pp. The writer held the M.D. degree.
1458. Ewart, John (fl.1790-1795). <u>The History of Two Cases of Ulcerated Cancer of the Mamma.</u> Bath, 1794. 62 pp. The writer, a Bath physician, held the M.D. degree.
1459. Fearon, Henry Bradshaw (fl.1784-1825). <u>Observations on Cancers . . .</u> [and] <u>Memoirs on Medicine.</u> London, 1784. 77pp.; three eds. through 1790. The writer practiced surgery in London; however, his literary recognition came from a narrative of a five thousand miles journey through the eastern and western United States.
1460. Guy, Melmoth (1775-1780). <u>Observations upon Cancerous Cases.</u> London, 1777.
1461. Guy, Richard (fl. 1755-1765). <u>The Answer to Certain Inuendious Falsehoods and Reflections upon His Method of Curing Cancers.</u> London, 1754. 60pp.; further eds to 1765.
1462. ____. <u>An Essay on Schirrhous Tumours and Cancers.</u> London, 1759. 96pp.
1463. ____. <u>Practical Observations on Cancers and Disorders of the Breast.</u> London, 1762. 173pp.

Cancer (contd.)

1464. Howard, John (d.1811). *The Plan Adopted by the Governors of the Middlesex Hospital for the Relief of Persons Afflicted with Cancer.* London, 1792. 81pp. See, also, #453.
1465. Justamond, John Obadiah (d.1786). *An Account of the Methods Pursued in the Treatment of Cancerous and Schirrhous Disorders.* London, 1780. 176pp. See, also, #748.
1466. Norford, William (1715-1793). *An Essay on the General Method of Treating Cancerous Tumours.* London, 1753. 171pp. In this piece, the writer attempts to establish rules for the treatment of cancer based upon previous cases; thus, he advances "sulphur electuary" and an ointment of his own preparation as the principal remedies; Norford, himself, began to practice medicine at Halesworth, Suffolk, principally as a surgeon and midwife; he then moved his practice to Bury St. Edmunds, Suffolk.
1467. Pearson, John (1758-1826). *Practical Observations on Cancerous Complaints.* London, 1793. 122pp. See, also, #766.

B. Ulcers

1468. Baynton, Thomas (1761-1820). *A Descriptive Account of a New Method of Treating Old Ulcers of the Legs.* Bristol, 1797. 115pp. 2nd ed., Bristol, 1799. 151pp. The writer served as a surgeon at Bristol; he achieved a reputation resulting from his treatments of ulcers and wounds; those medical tracts appeared, essentially, between 1795 and 1813.
1469. Bell, Benjamin (1749-1806). *A Treatise on the Theory and Management of Ulcers: with a Dissertation on White Swellings of the Joints.* London, 1778; Edinburgh, 1778; 7th ed., Edinburgh, 1801; an American ed. at Boston, 1797. The writer provides a clear classification of the various types of ulcers; a native of Dumfriesshire and the recipient of an M.D. from Edinburgh, Bell began his practice in the Scottish capital; then, he became a surgeon of the Royal Infirmary and of Watson's Hospital (both Edinburgh), achieving recognition for having been the first English speaking physician to distinguish between gonorrhoea and syphilis; in addition, Bell engaged in and wrote about agriculture; this *Treatise* extends to 264 pages in length.
1470. *An Essay on the Most Efficacious Means of Treating Ulcerated Legs.* London, 1783. 31pp.
1471. Home, Sir Everard (1756-1832). *Practical Observations on the Treatment of Ulcers of the Legs.* London, 1797. 295pp.; an American ed., Philadelphia, 1811. A pupil, colleague, and close friend of John Hunter, Home gained recognition not so much for his medical achievements but for his burning of

Cancer, Ulcers, Tumors 167

Ulcers (contd.)

Hunter's manuscripts and papers in 1823; a native of Greenlaw Castle, Berwick (Scotland), Home established a profitable London practice and contributed significantly, between 1797 and 1828, to the annals of medical literature.

1472. Rowley, William (1742-1806). An Essay on the Cure of Ulcerated Legs. London, 1770. 46pp. See, also, #222.

C. Tumors

1473. Dowman, George (fl.1745-1750). A Treatise on the Schirrhous Tumours. London, 1748. An M.D., the writer practiced at London.
1474. Ogle, William (fl.1750-1755). A Practical Essay on the Cure of Tumours. London, 1754.
1475. Saffray, Henry (fl.1773-1787). A Treatise on the Causes and Effects of Schirrhous Tumours and Cancers. London, 1787. 55pp; another ed., London, 1789. As with the largest portion of Saffray's published work, this piece has been attacked as the work of a quack; see, also, #509.

XIII

Nutrition and Exercise, Scurvy, Indigestion, Spirits, Diabetes, Worms

A. Nutrition and Exercise

1476. Eales, Mary (fl.1740-1745). The Complete Confectioner. London, n.d. 103pp.; three eds. through 1742. This volume includes recipes, instructions for pickling, and "receipts in. . . family physick."
1477. Ferris, Samuel (1760-1831). A Dissertation on Milk. London, 1785. 206pp. A London M.D., Ferris belonged to the College of Physicians.
1478. Forster, William (fl.1735-1745). A Treatise on the Various Kinds and Qualities of Foods. Newcastle-upon-Tyne, 1738. 108pp. See, also, #110.
1479. Fuller, Francis (1670-1706). Medicina Gymnastica; or, a Treatise concerning the Power of Exercise. London, 1705. 283pp.; seven eds. through 1740. The writer graduated B.A. (1691) from Cambridge and received the M.A. (1704) from the same university; however, he had little or no training in or knowledge of medicine; nonetheless, he advocated strenuous exercise and emetics as principal cures of distempers and diseases.
1480. Manning, James (fl.1755-1760). The Nature of Bread, Honestly and Dishonestly Made, and Its Effects. London, 1757. The writer, a London physician, held the M.D. degree.
1481. Markham, Peter (fl. 1755-1760). Syhoroc, or Considerations on the Ten Ingredients used in the Adulteration of Bread Flower and Bread; to which is added a Plan of Address. London, 1758; reprinted, London, 1758, as A Dissertation on Adulterated Bread. The writer attempts to expose the abuses in the manufacture of bread during the scarcity of 1757; as a result, Parliament approved an act setting forth specific processes for and ingredients of the manufacture of bread.
1482. Mason, Simon (fl.1745-1756). The Good and Bad Effects

Nutrition and Exercise (contd.)

of Tea Considered. London, 1745. Mason published tracts on fevers and agues, as well as memoirs and autobiographical pieces.

1483. Moseley, Benjamin (1739-1819). A Treatise concerning the Properties and Effects of Coffee. London, 1755; 3rd ed., London, 1785; 5th ed., London, 1792. See, also, #1441. The writer cites particulars relative to the drinking of coffee in the West Indies and suggests that the drink had not yet become common practice in England. Taxation more than taste may have contributed to restricting the popularity of coffee during the middle of the eighteenth century.

1484. ____. A Treatise on Sugar. London, 1799; 2nd ed., London, 1800. This tract contains little of scientific or medical value; However, Moseley does relate the event of the death of one "Three-Fingered Jack," a known Black outlaw slain by three Maroons; the latter had, in 1781, described their experiences to the writer.

1485. Robinson, Bryan (1680-1754). A Dissertation on Food and Discharges of Human Bodies. London, 1748. 120pp. See, also, #499.

1486. Short, Thomas (1690?-1772). Discourses on Tea, Sugar, Milk, Made Wines, Spirits, Punch, and Tobacco. London, 1750. See, also, #514.

1487. ____. A Dissertation upon Tea. London, 1750; 2nd ed., London, 1754.

1488. Valangin, Francis de (fl.1765-1770). A Treatise on Diet, or, Management of Human Life. London, 1768. The writer has been identified (Allibone 3:2504) as an M.D. who practiced physic at London.

1489. Willich, Anthony Florian Madinger (fl.1790-1804). Lectures on Diet and Regimen. London, 1798; 2nd ed., London, 1799; further eds. at Boston, 1800, and New York, 1801; 4th ed., London, 1809. An M.D., the writer published on such subjects as hot-well water in Bristol and physical exercise for school children.

B. Scurvy

1490. Case, Henry (fl.1675-1680). Treatises on the Scurvy and Dropsy. London, 1676.

1491. Crosfield, Robert James (fl.1795-1800). A Treatise on the Scurvy. London, 1797. An M.D., the writer practiced in London.

1492. Edwards, John (b.1742; fl.1775-1790). A Short Treatise on the Plant Called Goose Grass, or Clivers, for Scurvy. London, 1784. 15pp. The writer promotes what had been termed "silver-weed" (Potentilla anserina) as a potential remedy.

1493. Hayman, John (fl.1790-1795). A Treatise on the Scurvy. London, 1791. 80pp.

1494. Jervey, William (fl.1765-1770). Practical Thoughts on the Prevention and Cure of the Scurvy. London,

Nutrition, Scurvy, Diabetes, Worms   171

Scurvy (contd.)

1769. 83pp. An M.D., the writer practiced medicine at London.
1495. Lind, James (1716-1794). <u>A Treatise of the Scurvy</u>. Edinburgh, 1753. 456pp.; three eds. through 1772. See, also, #942.
1496. Lubbock, Richard (1759-1808). <u>De Principio Scorbili</u>. London, 1784. An M.D., the writer resided and practiced medicine at Norwich.
1497. MacBride, David (1726-1778). <u>An Historical Account of a New Method of Treating the Scurvy at Sea</u>. London, 1767. 62pp. See, also, #167.
1498. Mead, Richard (1673-1754). <u>A Discourse on Scurvy</u>. London, 1749. The writer promotes the notion of ventilating the holds of ships to prevent disease, supporting his argument with evidence in the form of observations of the scurvy as it occurred during George Anson's voyage around the world, September 1740 to June 1744. See, also, #176.
1499. Milman, Sir Francis (1746-1821). <u>An Enquiry into the Source from whence the Symptoms of the Scurvy and Putrid Fevers Arise</u>. London, 1782. 231pp. This work has been described as a compendium of others' observations and experiments, evidencing little of the writer's own knowledge of the subject. See, also, #1218.
1500. Paterson, David (fl.1790-1800). <u>A Treatise upon the Scurvy</u>. Edinburgh, 1795. 87pp.
1501. Sherwen, John (1749-1826). <u>Cursory Remarks on the Marine Scurvy</u>. London, 1782 The writer published this work anonymously; see, also, #1414.
1502. Spilsbury, Francis (fl.1775-1809). <u>Free Observations on the Scurvy, Gout, Diet, and Remedy</u>. London, 1780. 19pp.; seven eds. through 1792. See, also, #250, #1128.
1503.   . <u>Physical Dissertations; in which the Various Causes, Qualities, and Symptoms Incident to the Scurvy and Gout are comprehensively Treated</u>. London, 1778. 20pp.
1504. Thomson, Frederick (fl.1785-1795). <u>An Essay on the Scurvy</u>. London, 1790. 206pp.
1505. Trotter, Thomas (1760-1832). <u>Observations on the Nature and Cause of the Marine Scurvy</u>. Edinburgh, 1786. 83pp.; 2nd ed., enlarged, Edinburgh, 1792. This volume emerged from the writer's notes during his service with the Channel Fleet in the West Indies; a native of Roxburghshire, Trotter studied medicine at Edinburgh (M.D. 1788) and then served as a surgeon with the Channel Fleet, as well as in the same capacity on board several slave ships; he rose to become Surgeon of the Fleet and then physician to the Royal Hospital at Haslar, near Portsmouth; upon his retirement, Trotter practiced medicine at Newcastle-upon-Tyne and published extensively on medicine, social problems, and health conditions in the military services.

C. Indigestion

1506. Fordyce, George (1736-1802). A Treatise on the Digestion of Food. London, 1791. 204pp.; 2nd ed., London, 1791. 204pp. See, also, #109.
1507. Squirrel, Robert (fl.1790-1806). An Essay on Indigestion and Its Consequences; and on Bathing. London, 1795. This essay as been described as totally "empirical" (see Allibone 2:2216); an M.D., Squirrel published tracts upon the cow pox and on general health; however, his works tended to receive negative reviews from the literary periodicals of the day: thus, "Never was any thing [his Observations on the Cow-Pox (London, 1805)] so ill written, or so vulgar and absurd, produced by a person entitling himself a Doctor of Medicine" (Edinburgh Review [October 1806] 49).
1508. Wilson-Philip, Alexander Philip (1770?-1851?). Disputatio Inauguralis de Dyspepsia. Edinburgh, 1792. As the title would indicate, this piece constituted part of the writer's academic degree requirements; see, also, #542.

D. Spirits (including wine)

1509. Landford, William (fl.1785-1795). Reports of Observations on the Medical Effects of Wines and Spirits. London, 1790.
1510. MacBeth, William (fl.1790-1800). A Treatise upon Wines. London, 1794.
1511. Observations concerning the Medical Virtues of Wine. London, 1786. 16pp.
1512. Sandford, William (fl.1795-1800). A Few Practical Remarks on the Medicinal Effects of Wine and Spirits. Worcester, 1799. 152pp.; an ed. at London also in 1799.
1513. Sedgwick, James (fl.1720-1730). A New Treatise on Liquors. London, 1725. 407pp.
1514. _____. Vinum Britannicum: or, an Essay on the Properties and Effects of Malt Liquors. London, 1727. 52pp.
1515. Wright, John (fl.1790-1800). An Essay on Wines, especially on Port Wines. London, 1795. 68pp. The writer held the M.D. degree.

E. Diabetes

1516. Girdleston, Thomas (1758-1822). A Case of Diabetes, with an Historical Sketch of that Disease. Yarmouth, 1799. 112pp. Born at Norfolk, the writer served as an army physician, then settled and practiced at Great Yarmouth for thirty-six years; he possessed an extensive medical library and contributed regularly (and often under an assortment of assumed names) to the medical periodicals and transactions of the day; he also translated the odes of Anacreon into English verse.
1517. A Mechanical Enquiry into the Nature, Causes, Seat,

Diabetes (contd.)

and Cure of the Diabetes. Oxford, 1745. 34pp.
1518. Pearson, George (1751-1828). <u>Communications to Dr. [John] Rollo's Work on Diabetes</u>. London, 1798. 28pp. See #1519; also, #623.
1519. Rollo, John (d.1809). <u>Diabetes Mellitus: Notes of a Diabetic Case</u>. Deptford, 1797; further eds. in 1798, 1806. In the first edition of this tract, the writer described the improvement of officers with diabetes after they had been placed on meat diets; the editions of 1798 and 1806 contain observations of additional cases; all instances occurred at military stations in the West Indies; see, also, #1442 and #1518.

F. Worms

1520. <u>An Account of the Tenia, and Method of Treating It</u>. London, n.d.; 2nd ed., London, 1778. 77pp.
1521. <u>An Inquiry into the Original Production of Insects in Human Bodies, especially of the Seminal Animacula</u>. London, 1727. 40pp.
1522. Ramesay, William (b.1626?; fl.1651-1669). <u>Some Physical Considerations of Worms in Mens Bodies</u>. London, 1668. 125pp. See, also, #1373.
1523. <u>A Short Historical Account of the Several Kinds of Worms residing in Human Bodies</u>. London, 1716. 63pp.
1524. Simmons, Samuel Foart (1750-1813). <u>A Treatise on Taenia, or Tape Worm</u>. London, 1778. This piece representative of the writer's "elegant and unaffected style" (see Allibone 2:2104); see, also, ##351.

XIV

Heart, Spleen, Pulse, Blood, Bleeding, Sweating, Weakness

A. Heart

1525. Barclay, John (1758-1826). <u>Remarks on Mr. John Bell's Anatomy of the Heart and Arteries. By Jonathan Dawplucker, Esq.</u> London, 1799. 68pp. Born in Perthshire, Barclay served as an assistant to the anatomist John Bell (see #297. #298); he received the M.D. from Edinburgh in 1796, studied further at London, then returned to Edinburgh as a lecturer in anatomy; he achieved a reputation from his development of a nomenclature of human anatomy based upon scientific principles.
1526. Butter, William (1726-1805). <u>A Treatise on the Disease Commonly Called Angina Pectoris</u>. London, 1791. 62pp. See, also, #731.
1527. Mason, Henrich (fl.1750-1765). <u>Lectures upon the Heart</u>. Reading, 1763. See, also, #754.
1528. Morland, Joseph (fl.1700-1720). <u>Disquisitions concerning the Force of the Heart</u>. London, 1713. 88pp. Morland published a variety of medical tracts at London between 1703 and 1720.
1529. Walker, John (1759-1830). <u>On the Necessity for Contracting Cavities between the Venous Trunks and the Ventricles of the Heart</u>. Edinburgh, 1799. 34pp. A native of Cockermouth, Cumberland, Walker went to Dublin in 1779 to learn the craft of engraving, then removed to London to study medicine at Guy's Hospital; he visited Paris, then entered the University of Leyden, where in 1799 he received the M.D. degree; eventually, he became an advocate of and a specialist in vaccination, claiming that he had vaccinated in excess of one hundred thousand persons.
1530. Wilson, James (1765-1821). <u>A Description of a Very Unusual Formation of the Human Heart</u>. London, 1798. 13pp. An M.D., Wilson practiced as a surgeon and apothecary, as well as lectured on anatomy.

Heart (contd.)

1531. Wood, William (b.1688?; fl.1715-1730). <u>A Mechanical Essay upon the Heart</u>. London, 1729. 42pp.

B. Spleen

1532. Blackmore, Sir Richard (1650-1729). <u>A Treatise on the Spleen and Vapours</u>. London, 1725. See, also, #839.
1533. Robinson, Nicholas (1697?-1775). <u>A New System of the Spleen, Vapours. and Hypochondriak Melancholy</u>. London, 1729. This work, dedicated to Sir Hans Sloan, describes (from reports by secondary sources) the symptoms of the last illness of John Churchill, Duke of Marlborough (1650-1722), who had suffered three major strokes between 1716 and 1722, the last one being the direct cause of his death; the writer also relates examples of the occasional disease identified then as "vapours" (actually depression or melancholia); see, also, #220.
1534. Stukeley, William (1687-1765). <u>An Essay of the Spleen</u>. London, 1723. The writer initially read this tract as the Gulstonian lecture for March 1722; see, also, #1280.

C. Pulse

1535. Cox, Daniel (d.1759?). <u>Observations on the Intermitting Pulse</u>. London, 1758. 144pp. See, also, #1033.
1536. Falconer, William (1744-1824). <u>Observations respecting the Pulse</u>. London, 1796. 158pp. See, also, #100.
1537. Floyer, Sir John (1649-1734). <u>The Physician's Pulse Watch</u>. 2 vols. London, 1707-1710. See, also, #106.
1538. Nihill, James (fl.1740-1750). <u>New and Extraordinary Observations concerning the Predictions of Various Crises by the Pulse</u>. London, 1741. 153pp; another London ed. in 1750; a Latin ed. at Amsterdam in 1746. The writer held the M.D. degree.
1539. Rumball, John (fl.1795-1800). <u>The Pulse in a State of Health</u>. London, 1797.

D. Blood

1540. Averell, John (1711?-1771). <u>The Question about Eating of Blood Stated and Examin'd</u>. London, 1732. 40pp.
1541. Beale, Barton (fl.1695-1710). <u>A Treatise upon Diseases from Vicious Blood</u>. London, 1700.
1542. Betts, John (d.1695). <u>De Ortu et Natura Sanguinis</u>. London, 1669. Betts, born at Winchester, received the M.B. and M.D. degrees from Oxford in 1654 and later practiced among the Roman Catholics in London; he received an appointment as a physician-in-ordinary to Charles II, became a fellow of the College of Physicians, and eventually gained a

Blood (contd.)

seat in the House of Lords; he wrote and published almost entirely in Latin.

1543. Blizard, Sir William (1743-1835). A Popular Lecture on the Situation of the Large Blood Vessels of the Extremities and the Methods of Making Effectual Pressure on Them. London, 1786; 3rd ed., London, 1798. This volume recognized as the most lucid of the writer's works; see, also, #35.

1544. Boyle, Robert (1627-1691). Memoirs of the Natural History of Humane Blood, especially the Spirit of that Liquor. London, 1684. In this, his most important medical publication, Boyle summarized the contemporary knowledge of blood chemistry; he had intended to write a natural history of urine and to compare its properties with those of blood; however, he never actually published the written accounts of his experiments on that subject; born at Munster, Ireland, Boyle attended Eton College, studied at Geneva and Oxford, and then established residences at both London and Oxford; he became one of the first members of the so-called "invisible college," an association of Oxford intellectuals opposed to the prevalent doctrines of scholasticism; surprisingly an alchemist, Boyle's form of alchemy emerged as a logical outcome of his atomism, in which he declared that every substance exists as a rearrangement of the same basic elements; thus, transmutations should be possible; in the end, modern physics proved him correct.

1545. Brown, Joseph (fl.1700-1721). A Lecture of Anatomy, against the Circulation of the Blood. London, 1701. 30pp. See, also, #44.

1546. A Complete System of the Blood Vessels and Nerves, taken from Albinus's edition of Eustachius, also from Ruysch. London, 1758. 35pp. Bernard Siegfried Albinus (1696-1770), born at Frankfurt am-Main, became one of the most recognized anatomists of his day; he studied at Leyden under Hermann Boerhaave and eventually gained an appointment as professor of anatomy there and edited the work of Bartholomew Eustachius (d.1570); the latter, an eminent Italian physician, practiced and studied at Rome, where he formed his anatomical tables and reached such important conclusions as the discovery of the passage from the throat to the internal ear (thus, the Eustachian tube); in 1707, Boerhaave published his Opuscula Anatomica; finally, Frederick Ruysch (1638-1731), born at the Hague, rose to become one of the most eminent among the Continental anatomists.

1547. Corrie, James (fl.1790-1795). An Essay on the Vitality of the Blood. London, 1791. 100pp. An M.D., the writer practiced medicine at London.

1548. Davies, Richard (d.1762). A Proposal To Promote the Experimental Analysis of the Human Blood. Bath, 1760. 55pp. See, also, #847.

Blood (contd.)

1549. Falconer, Magnus (1754-1778). Experimental Inquiries on Blood. London, 1776. This work actually constitutes four chapters of William Hewson's Experimental Inquiry (see #1551), which the latter had never committed to a formal published volume before he died; see, also, #319.

1550. Gardiner, John ((fl.1700-1705). An Essay on the Circulation of the Blood. London, 1700; 2nd ed., London, 1702.

1551. Hewson, William (1739-1774). An Experimental Inquiry into the Properties of the Blood, in Three Parts. London, 1771; 2nd ed., London, 1772; 3rd ed., London, 1780. This work helped to establish the essential character of the process of coagulation and the forms of the red corpuscles in different animals; essentially an anatomist and physiologist, Hewson, born in Northumberland, studied at St. Thomas's and Guy's hospitals, London, with John and William Hunter; he practiced surgery, lectured, performed anatomical demonstrations, and published widely and variously.

1552. Hey, William (1736-1819). Observations on the Blood. London, 1779. 81pp. Hey lost the sight of his right eye at age four; after an apprenticeship to a surgeon at Leeds, he studied (1757-1759) surgery at St. George's Hospital, London; he began his surgical practice at Leeds and rose to become senior surgeon at the Leeds Infirmary (1773-1812); after he had formed a close relationship with Joseph Priestley, the latter sponsored him for a fellowship in the Royal Society.

1553. Hill, Oliver (fl.1695-1705). An Essay against the Circulation of the Blood. London, 1700. The writer also published, in 1702, a tract with the interesting title, A Rod for the Back of Fools.

1554. Home, Sir Everard (1756-1832). Experiments and Observations on the Blood when mixed with Urine. London, 1796. 8pp. See, also, #1359.

1555. Hunter, John (1728-1793). A Treatise on the Blood, Inflammation, and Gunshot Wounds. London, 1794; four eds. through 1828. This volume constitutes the writer's most important work, one in which he merged the studies of physiology, pathology, and surgery; in general, the writer managed in this essay to contribute significantly to furthering the practice of surgery in England; see, also, #1110.

1556. Knight, Thomas (fl.1725-1750). An Essay on the Transmutation of Blood, containing the Aetology . . . of Putrid Fevers. London, 1725. 52 pp. See, also, #462, #1557.

1557. _____. A Vindication of a Late Essay on the Transmutation of Blood. London, 1731. 240pp. See #1556.

1558. Levison, George (fl.1775-1785). An Essay on the Blood. London, 1776. See, also, #1146.

1559. Sharp, Thomas (1693-1758). A Defense of the Inquiry

Blood (contd.)

about the Lawfulness of Eating Blood. London, 1734. 32pp. See #1560. Educated at Trinity College, Cambridge, and later a fellow there, Sharp took Holy Orders; he received appointments as rector of Rothbury (1720) and archdeacon of Northumberland (1722); he published works on the Book of Common Prayer, the canons of the Church of England, textual analyses of various Holy Scriptures; he neither studied nor practiced medicine, and thus this work (as well as #1560) concern theological issues as well as matters related to general health.

1560. ____. An Enquiry about the Lawfulness of Eating Blood. London, 1733. 72pp. See, also, #1559.

1561. Wilson, Andrew (1718-1792). An Enquiry into the Moving Powers Employed in the Circulation of the Blood. London, 1774; an Italian translation at Milan, 1779. See, also, #683.

E. Bleeding

1562. Butler, Richard (fl.1730-1735). An Essay concerning Blood-letting. London, 1734. 148pp. An M.D., the writer practiced in London.

1563. Dickson, Thomas (1726?-1784). A Treatise on Blood-letting. 2 parts. London, 1765. The writer, an M.D., served as a physician to the London Hospital.

1564. Farr, Samuel (1741-1795). An Enquiry into the Propriety of Blood-Letting in Consumptions. London, 1775. 42pp. The writer argues against the practice indicated in the title of his tract; born at Taunton, Somersetshire, Farr received the M.D. degree from Leyden in 1765, served the Bristol Infirmary (1767-1780), practiced medicine at Bristol, and then returned to Taunton; he published, between 1769 and 1789, no less than eight major tracts on medicine.

1565. Fowler, Thomas (1736-1801). The Effects of Blood-Letting. London, 1795. A native of York, Fowler practiced medicine at Stafford and at York.

1566. Griffith, Richard (1635?-1691). A-la-Mode Phlebotomy No Good Fashion; or, the Copy of a Letter to Dr. [Francis] Hungerford, complaining. . .of the phantistick Behaviour and unfair Dealing of Some London Physitians. . .whereupon a fit Occasion is taken to Discourse of the profuse way of Blood-Letting. London, 1681. The writer complains, essentially, of unnecessary bleeding that accelerated the deaths of patients; Griffith received his M.D. from the University of Caen, Normandy, in 1664; he then returned to England and practiced medicine at Richmond, Surrey; Francis Hungerford practiced medicine at Reading.

1567. Horn, George (fl.1795-1800). An Entire New Treatise on Leeches. London, 1798. 29pp.

1568. Kellie, George (fl.1795-1805). Observations on the

Bleeding (contd.)

Medical Effects of Compression by the Tourniquet. Edinburgh, 1797. 114pp. The writer, an M.D., published various medical treatises between 1797 and 1803.

1569. Neale, George (also Neal; fl.1755-1760). Some Observations on the Use of the Agaric and Its Insufficiency in Stopping Haemorrhages. London, 1757. 50pp. See, also, #763.

1570. Ruspini, Bartholomew (fl.1768-1805). Observations of the Styptic. London, 1786. Works on the teeth and on surgical instruments under this writer's name also bear London imprints.

1571. Smith, Hugh (d.1790). Essays Psychological and Practical on the Nature and Circulation of the Blood, with Reflections on Blood-Letting. London, 1761. 132pp. Smith studied medicine at Edinburgh (M.D. 1755) and practiced first at Essex before removing to London; in 1760, he initiated a series of lectures on the theory and practice of physic; he gained election to the Middlesex Hospital as a surgeon, and, around 1772, began the practice of medicine in his own home; for two days of each week, he devoted his labors to treating the poor, from whom he would demand nor take no fees.

F. Sweating

1572. Cruikshank, William (1745-1800). Experiments on the Invisible Perspiration of the Human Body. London, 1795. 104pp. See, also, #309.

G. Weakness

1573. Withers, Thomas (fl.1772-1794). Observations on Chronic Weakness. York, 1776. The writer held the M.D. degree from Edinburgh (1771) and practiced medicine at York and London.

XV

Muscles, Nerves

A. Muscles

1574. Blane, Sir Gilbert (1749-1834). <u>A Lecture on Muscular Motion</u>. London, 1790. 57pp. This work comprises the Scottish physician's Croonian Lecture, read before the Royal Society on 18 and 20 November 1788; a native of Ayrshire, Blane studied medicine at Edinburgh and Glasgow (M.D. 1778); he then served as a physician to Admiral Sir George Brydges Rodney (1719-1792) on an expedition to the West Indies (1779) and became the principal medical officer for the West Indian fleet; thus, Blane contributed, through his practice and publications, to discoveries and investigations relative to disease and sickness among seamen; see, also, #1833.

1575. Browne, John (1642-1700?). <u>Myographia Nova, or a Complete Treatise of the Muscles, as they appear in the Human Body, and arise in Dissection</u>. London, 1671; further eds. in 1681, 1691, 1705. A native of Norwich, Browne studied medicine at St. Thomas's Hospital, London, then served as a naval surgeon; eventually, he received an appointment as a surgeon in ordinary to Charles II; he wrote no less than five major tracts on surgery and tumors.

1576. ____. <u>Myographia Nova sive Musculorum Omnium (in Corpore Humano hactenus repertorum) Accuratissima Descriptio</u>. London, 1684. This work a Latin version of #1575.

1577. Cowper, William (1666-1709). <u>Myotamia Reformata; or, a New Administration of all the Muscles of the Human Body, wherein the true uses of the Muscles are explained, the Errors of former Anatomists concerning them confuted, and several Muscles not hitherto taken notice of described; to which are subjoined a graphical Description of the Bones and other Anatomical Observations</u>. London, 1694. A

Muscles (contd.)

new edition, edited by Richard Mead and three of his colleagues, came forth in 1724; the initial edition included Cowper's original manuscripts (with additions and corrections), a short historical preface, and a lengthy introduction on muscular mechanics; see, also, #301.

1578. Croone, William (1633-1684). De Ratione Motus Musculorum. London, 1664; Amsterdam, 1667. Born at London, Croone held the the professorship of rhetoric at Gresham College, London; a royal mandate in 1662 created him doctor of medicine from Cambridge, after which he received an appointment as one of the first fellows of the Royal Society; the Company of Surgeons installed him as a lecturer in anatomy, and he also gained admission as a fellow of the College of Physicians; he founded a course of algebraic lectures in seven colleges at Cambridge; the first of the Croonian lectures in anatomy before the Royal Society came in 1738.

1579. Douglas, James (1675-1742). Mygraphiae Comparatae Specimen, or a Comparative Description of all the Muscles in a Man and in a Quadruped; added is an Account of the Muscles Peculiar to a Woman. London, 1707. 216pp.; six eds. through 1777. Douglas, born in Scotland, received the M.D. from Rheims; he settled in London and established a reputation as a skilled practitioner in anatomy and midwifery; in 1726, he participated in the exposure of one Mary Tofts, a Guildford woman who professed to have given birth to rabbits.

1580. Home, Sir Everard (1756-1832). Observations on the Structure of Muscles. London, 1795. 19pp. See, also, #1359.

1581. Innes, John (1739-1777). A Short Description of the Human Muscles, arranged as they appear in Dissection. Edinburgh, 1776; revised ed., by Alexander Monro, Edinburgh, 1778; seven eds. published at London; two American eds. through 1818. A Scottish anatomist, Innes served as Alexander Monro's dissector during the latter's term as professor of anatomy at Edinburgh (see, also, #339); the Short Description survived as the standard text at Edinburgh for at least half a century beyond the writer's death.

1582. Langrish, Browne (d.1759). The Croonian Lectures on Muscular Motion. London, 1748. 66pp. See, also, #159.

1583. ____. A New Essay on Muscular Motion. London, 1733. 103pp.

1584. Lawrence, Thomas (1711-1783). De Natura Musculorum Praelectiones Tres. London, 1759. Born at Westminster and schooled in Dublin, Lawrence studied anatomy with Dr. Frank Nichols (see #340) and practiced medicine at St. Thomas's Hospital, London, before receiving the M.D. from Oxford in 1740; he lectured extensively in anatomy, but his

Muscles (contd.)

reputation appears to have grown from his association with Samuel Johnson (his patient) and Hester Lynch Thrale Piozzi; he wrote exclusively in Latin, regarding that language as the only one fit for medical tracts; interestingly enough, when Dr. Johnson wrote to his friend and physician concerning medical matters, he did so only in Latin.

1585. Parsons, James (1705-1770). The Croonian Lectures on Muscular Motion for the Years MDCCXLIV [1744] and MDCCXLV [1745]. London, 1745. 86pp. See, also, #1411.

1586. Pugh, John (fl.179-1795). A Treatise on Muscular Motion for Restoring the Power of the Limbs. London, 1794. 106pp. See, also, #346.

1587. Stuart, Alexander (1673-1742). Dissertatio de Structura et Mortu Musculari. London, 1711; another ed., Bordeaux, 1738. An M.D., the writer published, between 1702 and 1738, numerous papers on medicine and antiquarian studies in the Philosophical Transactions of the Royal Society.

1588. _____. Three Croonian Lectures on Muscular Motion, before the Royal Society. London, 1739.

1589. Wright, Thomas (1758?-1812). A Concise History of the Human Muscles. Dublin, 1793. 224pp. The writer practiced surgery at Dublin.

1590. Ypey, Adolphus (fl.1775-1785). Observationes Phsyiologicae de Mortu Musculorum Voluntaria et Vitalia. London, 1776. The writer identified as an M.D.; this tract may have been published initially in France.

B. Nerves

1591. Cruikshank, William (1745-1800). Experiments on the Nerves, Particularly on Their Reproduction. London, 1751. 12pp. This essay originally appeared in the Philosophical Transactions of the Royal Society; see, also, #309.

1592. Johnstone, James (1730-1802). An Essay on the Use of the Ganglions of the Nerves. Shrewsbury, 1771. 96pp. See, also, #861.

1593. Kinneir, David (fl.1735-1740). A New Essay on the Nerves. . .shewing the great Benefit and true Use of. . .the Bath Waters. London, 1738. 167pp.; 2nd ed., London, 1739. 200pp.

1594. Musgrave, Samuel (1732-1780). Speculations and Conjectures on the Qualities of the Nerves. London, 1776. 146pp. See, also, #870.

1595. Neale, Henry St. John (fl.1795-1805). Practical Dissertations on Nervous Complaints. London, 1788. 68pp.; three eds. through 1796. See, also #1175.

1596. Smith, Hugh (1736?-1789). An Essay on the Nerves. London, 1780. 80pp. See, also, #242.

1597. Walker, Sayer (1748-1826). A Treatise on Nervous Diseases. London, 1796. 224pp. Born at London,

Nerves (contd.)

> the writer became a Presbyterian minister at Enfield, Middlesex; he went on to study medicine at London, Edinburgh, and Aberdeen (M.D. 1791); in 1792, he gained admittance as a licentiate of the College of Physicians of London, after which he stood successfully for election to the London Lying-in Hospital; his practice focused upon midwifery.

XVI

Head, Hair, Skin

A. Head

1598. Dease, William (1752?-1798). <u>Observations on Wounds of the Head</u>. Dublin, 1776. 131pp.; London, 1776, 175pp.; 3rd ed., Dublin, 1778, 302pp. See, also, #737.
1599. Mynors, Robert (1739-1806). <u>A History of the Practice of Trepanning the Skull</u>. Birmingham, 1785. 152pp. See, also, #762. The process of trepanning involved cutting out small pieces of bone from the skull with a trepan, a surgical instrument in the form of a crown-saw (see <u>OED</u>).
1600. O'Holloran, Sylvester (1728-1807). <u>A New Treatise on the Different Disorders arising from External Injuries of the Head</u>. London, 1793. 335pp. See, also, #1378.
1601. Parry, Caleb Hillier (1755-1822). <u>An Inquiry into the Symptoms and Causes of the Syncope Anginosa</u>. Bath, 1799. 167pp. See, also, #1048.
1602. Pott, Percival (1713-1788). <u>Observations on the Nature and Consequences of Those Injuries to which the Head is Liable from External Violence</u>. London, 1760; three eds. through 1773. The writer's systematized treatment of head injuries includes the first description of what came to be known as "Pott's tumour"; see, also, #741.
1603. Simson, Thomas (1696-1764). <u>An Enquiry on the Vital and Animal Actions: Five Essays</u>. Edinburgh, 1752. A native of Ayrshire, Simson held the first medical professorship at St. Andrews (1722-1764), a chair established in 1721 by James Brydgers, Duke of Chandos.
1604. Stevens, J.N. (fl.1755-1760). <u>A Treatise on Diseases of the Head and Neck</u>. London, 1758. An M.D., the writer practiced at Bath and London; see, also, #649.
1605. Young, James (fl.1679-1713). <u>Wounds of the Brain</u>

Head (contd.)

> Proved Curable. London, 1682. The writer practiced surgery at Plymouth; he wrote tracts on surgery and anatomy and, between 1702 and 1713, contributed numerous essays to the Philosophical Transactions of the Royal Society.

B. Hair

1606. Mather, John (fl.1790-1795). A Treatise upon Preservation of the Hair. London, 1794.
1607. Ritchie, David (fl.1765-1775). A Treatise on the Hair. London, 1770.
1608. Stewart, Alexander (fl.1785-1795). The Natural Production of Hair, or Its Growth and Decay. London, 1795.

C. Skin

1609. Chamberlaine, William (fl.1780-1815). A Practical Treatise on the Efficacy of Stizolobium, or Cowhage. London, 1783. 77pp.; five eds. through 1792. A London surgeon, the writer published medical tracts between 1784 and 1813; cowhage has been defined as the "stinging hairs" of the pod of the tropical plant macuna pruriens (see OED).
1610. Dickinson, Robert (fl. 1795-1800). An Essay on Cutaneous Diseases. London, 1800. 72pp.
1611. Jackson, Seguin Henry (1752?-1816). Deromo-Pathologica; or, Practical Observations... on the Pathology and Proximate Causes of Diseases of the True Skin. London, 1792. The writer held the M.D. degree.
1612. Kentish, Edward (fl.1795-1815). An Essay on Burns. London, 1797. 176pp. The writer held the M.D. degree.
1613. ____. A Second Essay on Burns. Newcastle-upon-Tyne, 1800. 117pp.
1614. Willan, Robert (1757-1812). The Description and Treatment of Cutaneous Diseases. 5 vols. London, 1798-1808. The writer concerns himself with papulous eruptions, scaly diseases, rashes, and bullae (blisters); the entire work republished in 1809 and again in 1849; according to the Edinburgh Review (October 1809, p.64), Willan "is the oracle of the metropolis [London] in all cutaneous disorders, and has more practice in that department than all the rest of his brethren put together"; see, also, #657.

XVII

Eyes, Ears

A. Eyes

1615. Adams, George (1750-1795). <u>An Essay on Vision</u>. London, 1789. 153pp.; 2nd ed., London, 1792. 157pp. See, also, #361.
1616. Ayscough, James (d.1762?). <u>A Short Account of the Eye and Nature of Vision</u>. London, 1754. 26pp.; six eds. through 1763.
1617. Bischoff, Frederick (fl.1790-1795). <u>A Treatise on the Extraction of the Cataract</u>. London, 1793. 80pp. The writer has been identified as a London oculist (see Allibone 1:194).
1618. Borthwick, George (fl.1772-1796). <u>A Treatise upon the Extraction of the Crystalline Lens</u>. Edinburgh, 1775. 30pp. See, also, #840.
1619. Briggs, William (1642-1704). <u>Ophthalmographia</u>. Cambridge, 1676; 2nd ed., Cambridge, 1687. The writer dedicated this work, an anatomical description of the eye, to Ralph Montagu, then British ambassador to France; the latter had sponsored Briggs' journey to France, where he had attended lectures in ophthalmology at Montpellier; Briggs, himself, practiced at St. Thomas's Hospital, London; in this tract, he recognized the retina as an expansion in which the fibers of the optic nerve are spread out; he also emphasized the hypothesis of vibrations as an explanation of the phenomenon of nervous action.
1620. _____. <u>A Theory of Vision</u>. London, 1682; 2nd ed., London, 1683; a Latin translation, London, 1685. Sir Isaac Newton wrote a laudatory preface to the Latin edition of 1685, noting that he had benefitted from Briggs' anatomical skills and knowledge.
1621. Chandler, George (fl.1775-1780). <u>A Treatise of a Cataract</u>. London, 1755. 116pp. The writer practiced surgery at London.

Eyes (contd.)

1622. ____. A Treatise on the Diseases of the Eye. London, 1780. 191pp.
1623. Coward, William (1657?-1725). Ophthalmiatria. London, 1706. 188pp. The writer practiced medicine at Northampton, then settled in London; he achieved recognition for his attempts to destroy the Cartesian notion of "an immaterial soul" residing in the pineal gland.
1624. Crisp, John (fl.1795-1800). Observations on the Nature and Theory of Vision. London, 1796. 178pp.
1625. Crosse, William (fl.1705-1710). A Brief Treatise of the Eyes. London, 1708.
1626. Dawson, Thomas (1725?-1782). An Account of a Safe and Efficacious Medicine in Sore-Eyes and Eye-Lids. London, 1782. 15pp. See, also, #1290.
1627. Elliott, Sir John (1736-1786). Philosophical Observations on the Senses of Vision and Hearing. London, 1780. 222pp. See, also, #96.
1628. Emerson, William (1701-1782). The Elements of Optics. 2 parts. London, 1768. Emerson's intellectual and academic reputations arose from his work in mathematics; a native of Hurworth, near Darlington, he published treatises upon such problems as natural philosophy, astronomy, and the branches of mathematics.
1629. Gataker, Thomas (d.1769). An Account of the Structure of the Eye. London, 1761. 86pp. See, also, #120.
1630. Grant, Roger (d.1724). An Account of a Miraculous Cure of a Young Man in Newington Born Blind. London, 1709. The writer described himself as a Baptist preacher, a cobbler, and an illiterate; after having lost an eye while in the service of the German army, he established an oculist's shop in London; without even the barest of academic or professional credentials, Grant managed to obtain appointments as oculist to Queen Anne and, later, to George I.
1631. Home, Sir Everard (1756-1832). An Account of the Orifice in the Retina of the Human Eye. London, 1798. 16pp. See, also, #1359.
1632. Kennedy, Peter (fl.1710-1738). Ophthalmographia; or, A Treatise on the Eye. London, 1713. 109pp.; a supplement published at London in 1739, 166pp. See, also, #459.
1633. Mauclerc, John Henry (fl.17740-1770). Nomenclatura Critica Morborum Ocularum; or, A Critical Index to the Distempers of the Eye. London, 1768. 32pp.
1634. Monro, Alexander secundus (1737-1817). Three Treatises on the Brain, the Eye and the Ear. Edinburgh, 1787. This piece represents the final bound volume published by the Edinburgh anatomist; see, also, #339.
1635. Noble, Edward Moore (fl.1790-1805). A Treatise on Ophthalmy. 2 vols. Birmingham, 1800-1801.
1636. Observations on the Use of Spectacles. London, 1753. 31pp.

Eyes (contd.)

1637. O'Halloran, Sylvester (1728-1807). A New Treatise on the Glaucoma, or Cataract. Dublin, 1750. 115pp. See, also, #1378.
1638. Peacock, Henry Barry (fl.1790-1795). Observations on Blindness by Cataracts. London, 1792. 36pp. The writer also published tracts on theology.
1639. Phipps, Jonathan W. (fl.1790-1795). A Dissertation on the Treatment after the Operation for the Cataract. London, 1792.
1640. Porterfield, William (1696-1771). A Treatise on the Eye. 2 vols. Edinburgh, 1759.
1641. Pott, Percival (1714-1788). Remarks on the Cataract. London, 1775. The writer argues for the operation of "couching" (or displacing the lens of the eye into the vitreous humor), as opposed to the more common practice of extracting the opaque lens; see, also, #741.
1642. Read, Sir William (d.1715). A Short but Exact Account of all the Diseases Incidental to the Eye. London, 1706. The writer presents his remedy, known as "styptic water," which he advanced as a substitute for the "barbarous" cauterizations then in fashion; originally a tailor, Read began to practice his own form of healing in and around Northampton, Yorkshire, Oxford, Devonshire, Wiltshire, Somerset, Bath, and Windsor; through some miraculous reason (or pure fortune), he managed to "cure" a number of soldiers and seamen of their blindness, and for those exercises he received knighthood; he also managed to gain an appointment as an oculist-in-ordinary to Queen Anne.
1643. Rowley, William (1742-1806). An Essay on the Ophthalmia, or Inflammation of the Eyes. London, 1771. 47pp. See, also, #222.
1644. ____. A Treatise on the Hundred and Eighteen Principal Diseases of the Eyes and Eyelids. London, 1790. 360pp.
1645. ____. A Treatise on the Principal Diseases of the Eyes. London, 1773. 159pp. This work stands as an earlier and less ambitious version of #1644.
1646. Sloane, Sir Hans (1660-1753). An Account of a Medicine for Soreness, Weakness, and Other Distempers of the Eyes. London, 1743; reprinted 1745; 2nd ed., London, 1750; French translation, Paris, 1746. The only medical volume published by the noted Irish physician, surgeon, and bibliophile; born in County Down, Sloane studied medicine at Paris and Montpellier; at the latter institution, he learned botany; after receiving the M.D. from Orange in 1683 and then spending more than a year in the West Indies, he settled at London and devoted his time to cataloguing plants and writing travel narratives; from 1727 to 1741, he presided over the Royal Society, having succeeded Sir Isaac Newton at that position; other of his appointments included first physician to

Eyes (contd.)

George II and physician in charge of Christ's Hospital, London; his extensive library and collections (which he sold to the government) formed the nucleus of what would eventually become the British Museum.

1647. Stockton, John (fl.1740-1745). St. Yves's Diseases of the Eyes; from the French. London, 1741; 2nd ed., London, 1744. The translator did hold the M.D. degree.

1648. Taylor, John the elder (1703-1772). An Account of the Mechanism of the Globe of the Eye. Norwich, 1727. A native of Norwich, Taylor initially served as an apothecary's assistant in London; afterward, he studied medicine at St. Thomas's Hospital, London, with emphasis upon diseases of the eye; he practiced at Norwich as a general surgeon and oculist, but soon determined to travel throughout Britain, France, and Holland; after receiving M.D. degrees from Basle, Liege, and Cologne, Taylor returned to England to continue his itinerant medical practice; because of his questionable methods and claims in advertisements, he came under attack by the periodical satirists of the day; indeed, on one occasion, Samuel Johnson termed Taylor "the most ignorant man I ever knew; but sprightly"; on another instance, the London sage described the physician as proving "how far impudence could carry ignorance" (see James Boswell, Life of Johnson, ed. R.W. Chapman, rev. ed. J.D. Fleeman [London: Oxford University Press, 1970] 1022); Horace Walpole viewed the Norwich physician in a more poetic light:

Why Taylor the quack calls himself Chevalier
  'Tis not easy a reason to render;
Unless blinding eyes, that he thinks to make clear,
Demonstrates he's but a Pretender!

1649. ____. An Exact Account of 243 Different Diseases to which the Eye and Its Coverings are Exposed. Edinburgh, 1759.

1650. ____. An Impartial Inquiry into the Seat of the Immediate Organ of Sight. London, 1743; a German ed. in 1750.

1651. ____. A New Treatise on the Crystalline Humour of a Human Eye; or, Of the Cataract and Glaucoma. London, 1735; 2nd ed., London, 1736; another ed. at Edinburgh, 1736. This tract proved extremely popular and underwent editions and translations throughout the Continent.

1652. ____. A Practice on the Diseases of the Immediate Organ of Sight. London, 1735.

1653. Ware, James (1755-1815). Chirurgical Observations relative to the Epiphora, or Watery Eye, the Scrophulous and Intermittent Ophthalmy, the Extraction of the Cataract, and the Introduction of the Male Catheter. 2 vols. London, 1792; 2nd ed.,

Eyes (contd.)

London, 1800. Born at Portsmouth, Ware served as an apprentice at the Halsar (Portsmouth) Naval Hospital, then entered as a student at St. Thomas's Hospital, London; in 1788, he became one of the founders of the Society for the Relief of the Widows and Orphans of Medical Men, London; professionally, he helped to elevate ophthalmic surgery from its low state and to remove it from the hands of quacks and incompetents.

1654. ____. Chirurgical Observations relative to the Eye; Observations on the Cataract. 2 vols. London, 1798; 2nd ed., London, 1805-1812; a German translation at Gottingen in 1809.

1655. ____. An Enquiry into the Causes which have prevented Success in the Operation of Extracting the Cataract. London, 1795.

1656. ____. Remarks on the Fistula Lachrymalis, to which are added Observations on Haemorrhoids and additional Remarks on Ophthalmy. London, 1798.

1657. ____. Remarks on the Ophthalmy, Psororophthalmy, and Purulent Eye. London, 1780; 2nd ed., London, 1785; reprinted, London, 1787; 3rd ed., London, 1795; five English eds. through 1814; a Spanish translation at Madrid in 1796.

1658. ____. A Treatise on the Cataract; from the French of M. de Wenzel, jun.; with Additional Remarks. London, 1793.

1659. Warner, Joseph (1717-1801). A Description of the Human Eye and Its Adjacent Parts, together with their Principal Diseases. London, 1773; 2nd ed., London, 1775. See, also, #791.

1660. Wathen, Jonathan (fl.1763-1792). A Dissertation on the Cataract. London, 1785. The writer practiced surgery at London; in addition to his tracts on practical medicine, he published an edition and translation of Herman Boerhaave's academic lectures on venereal diseases (1763).

1661. ____. Observations on the Tube for the Fistula Lachrymalis. London, 1781; 2nd ed., London, 1782.

1662. Wells, William Charles (1757-1817). An Essay on Single Vision with Two Eyes. London, 1792. 144pp. Born at Charlestown, South Carolina, and educated at Edinburgh, Wells returned to his native Charlestown to serve as apprentice to a physician there (1771-1775); he continued his medical studies at Edinburgh (1775-1778), then moved on to London as a student of St. Bartholomew's Hospital; after serving in Holland as a surgeon to a Scottish regiment, he pursued further medical studies at Leyden and again at Edinburgh (M.D. 1780); he spent time in Charlestown and St. Augustine, Florida, journeyed to Paris, and finally settled at London to practice medicine; his various appointments included physician to the Finsbury Dispensary (1789-1799) and to St. Thomas's Hospital (1800-1817).

Eyes (contd.)

1663. Wemyss, William (fl.1770-1775). <u>Dissertatio Medica Inauguralis de Ophthalmia</u>. Edinburgh, 1773. This tract constitutes the writer's principal exercise for the M.D. degree at Edinburgh.

B. Ears

1664. Cooper, Sir Astley Paston (1768-1841). <u>Observations on the Effects which take place from the Destruction of the Membrana Tympani of the Ear</u>. London, 1800. 12pp. This tract originally appeared in the <u>Philosophical Transactions</u> of the Royal Society; Cooper studied at St. Thomas's Hospital, London, and at the Edinburgh Medical School; he devoted his attention to the separation of surgery from anatomy and rose to the positions (in 1822) of examiner for the College of Surgeons and consulting surgeon at Guy's Hospital, London; in 1827, he succeeded to the presidency of the College of Surgeons and, a year later, received an appointment as physician to George IV; the extent of his medical practice may be appreciated from the knowledge that in 1822, he earned £22,000--then the largest income received by a medical practitioner (see <u>DNB</u> and Allibone 1:424).

1665. Home, Sir Everard (1756-1832). <u>On the Structure and Uses of the Membrana Tympani of the Ear</u>. London, 1800. 22.pp. See, also #1359.

XVIII

Teeth, Gums, Salivating

A. Teeth, Gums

1666. Allen, Charles (fl.1685-1690). <u>A Treatise on an Operator for the Teeth</u>. York, 1685; another ed. at Dublin, 1687.
1667. Bennet, William (fl.1775-1780). <u>An Essay on the Teeth and Gums</u>. London, 1778. 58pp.
1668. Berdmore, Thomas (1740-1785). <u>A Treatise on Disorders and Deformities of the the Teeth and Gums</u>. London, 1768. 267pp.; 2nd ed., London, 1770. 279pp.
1669. Curtis, Richard (fl.1765-1770). <u>A Treatise on the Structure and Formation of the Teeth</u>. Oxford, 1769. 82pp.; a German ed. at Altenburg, 1770. 79pp.
1670. De Chemant, Daniel (fl. 1785-1790). <u>Observations upon Artificial Teeth</u>. London, 1798.
1671. Hunter, John (1728-1793). <u>The Natural History of the Human Teeth: explaining their Structure, Use, Formation, Growth, and Diseases</u>. London, 1771; an ed. bound with #1672, London, 1778. Hunter proved to have been the first English medical practitioner and theorist to have conducted a truly scientific study of the human teeth, as well as being the first to recommend complete removal of the pulp in filling them; he also introduced the classification of the teeth (cuspids, bicuspids, molars, incisors), enlarged upon the topic of dental malocclusion (abnormal spacing of the teeth), and devised an apparatus for correcting spatial abnormalities; see, also, #1048.
1672. _____. <u>A Practical Treatise on the Diseases of the Teeth; intended as a Supplement to the Natural History of Those Parts</u>. London, 1778. Bound with #1671.
1673. Hurlock, Joseph (fl.1740-1745). <u>A Practical Treatise upon Dentition; or, The Breeding of Teeth in Children</u>. London, 1742. 285pp.
1674. Lewis, Merer (fl.1770-1775). <u>An Essay on the Teeth</u>.

Teeth, Gums (cont.d)

London, 1772.
1675. Ruspini, Bartholomew (fl.1768-1805). *A Treatise on the Teeth*. London, 1768; further eds. in 1778, 1797. See, also, #1570.
1676. Spilsbury, Francis B. (fl.1789-1802). *Every Lady and Gentleman Their Own Dentist*. London, 1791. 56pp. See, also, #250.
1677. Tolver, Alexander (fl.1750-1770). *A Treatise on the Teeth*. London, 1750; 2nd ed., London, 1752. The writer also published a discussion on the state of midwifery at Paris (1770).
1678. Wooffendale, Robert (1742-1828). *Practical Observations on the Human Teeth*. London, 1783. 158pp.

B. Salivating

1679. Cam, Joseph (fl.1715-1732). *The Practice of Salivating Vindicated*. London, 1724. See, also, #1088, #1089. The writer held the M.D. degree.

XIX

Pregnancy, Birth, Midwifery, Infants and Children, Women

A. Pregnancy and Childbirth

1680. Bland, Robert the elder (1730-1816). <u>Observations on Human and Comparative Parturition</u>. London, 1794. 223pp. An M.D. from St. Andrews, Bland practiced midwifery at London and hired out to write all of the articles on midwifery for Rev. Abraham Rees's <u>New Cyclopaedia</u> (1781-1786); he also published a collection of proverbs.

1681. Blunt, John (fl.1790-1795). <u>The Obstetric Family Instructor</u>. London, 1793.

1682. Butter, William (1726-1805). <u>An Account of Puerperal Fevers</u>. London, 1775. 124pp. See, also, #731.

1683. Clarke, John (1761-1815). <u>An Essay on the Epidemic Disease of Lying-in Women</u>. London, 1788. 43pp. A native of Wellingborough, Northamptonshire, Clarke attended St. Paul's School and studied medicine at St. George's Hospital, London; he practiced medicine in London and lectured on midwifery in the school founded by William Hunter; after rising to status of the principal London practitioner of midwifery, he shifted his attention to those diseases peculiar to women and children.

1684. _____. <u>Practical Essays on the Management of Pregnancy and Labour</u>. London, 1793. 170pp.

1685. Couper, Robert (1750-1818). <u>Speculations on the Mode and Appearances of Impregnation in the Human Female</u>. Edinburgh, 1789. 149pp.; 2nd ed., Edinburgh, 1797. 194pp. The writer studied medicine at Glasgow, practiced at Wigtonshire, and then went to Fochabers as a physician to the Duke of Gordon; he also published a collection of his own <u>Poetry, Chiefly in the Scottish Language</u> (Edinburgh, 1802) and a <u>History of the British Isles</u> (Edinburgh, 1807).

1686. Denman, Thomas (1733-1815). <u>An Essay on Difficult Labours</u>. 3 vols. London, 1787-1791. See, also,

Pregnancy and Childbirth (contd.)

#684.
1687. ____. An Essay on Natural Labours. London, 1786. 52pp.
1688. ____. An Essay on Preternatural Labours. London, 1786. 56pp.
1689. ____. An Essay on the Puerperal Fever, and on Puerperal Convulsions. London, 1768. 74pp.; three eds. through 1785.
1690. ____. On the Separation of the Symphysis of the Pubes in Labour. London(?), 1780. 15pp.
1691. Dickson, David (fl.1710-1715). An Essay on the Possibility and Probability of a Child's Being Born Alive, and Live, in the Latter End of the Fifth Solar. . .Month. Edinburgh, 1712. 120pp. The writer held the M.D. degree.
1692. Douglas, G. Archibald (fl.1758-1784). The Nature and Causes of Impotence. London, 1758. 54pp.; six eds. through 1772. The writer held the M.D. degree.
1693. Douglas, William (1712-?). A Letter to Dr. [William] Smellie: Shewing the Impropriety of his newly invented Wooden Forceps. London, 1748. 25pp. A second letter on the same subject came from Douglas to Smellie in the same year. See, also #51, #1721, #1768-#1772.
1694. Fleming, James (fl.1765-1770). A Treatise on the Formulation of the Human Species. London, 1768. The writer practiced surgery and midwifery at London.
1695. Garthshore, Maxwell (1732-1812). A Remarkable Case of a Numerous Birth. London, 1787. 22pp. This essay appeared initially in the Philosophical Transactions of the Royal Society. After serving an apprenticeship to an Edinburgh physician, the writer attended classes at Edinburgh, and then entered the army as a surgeon's mate; he practiced medicine at Uppingham (1756-1764), moved to London, and received the M.D. degree from Edinburgh in 1764; Garthshore gained admittance as a licentiate of the London College of Physicians (1764), received an appointment as a physician to the British Lying-in Hospital, and eventually became a fellow of the Royal Antiquarian Society.
1696. Gordon, Alexander (1752-1799). A Treatise on the Epidemic Puerperal Fever of Aberdeen. London, 1795. 124pp. The writer also published tracts on botany.
1697. Harvie, John (fl.1765-1770). Practical Directions, Showing a Method of Preserving the Perinaeum in Birth. London, 1767. 48pp.
1698. Hull, John (1761-1843). A Defence of the Caesarean Operation. Manchester, 1799. 229pp. The writer held the M.D. degree, practiced medicine in Manchester and published (between 1792 and 1809) a number of tracts on botany; see, also, #1709.
1699. Krohn, Henry (d.1816). Foetus Extra Uterium Historia. London, 1791. The writer held the M.D. degree.

Pregnancy, Midwifery, Infants, Children, Women   197

          Pregnancy and Childbirth (contd.)

1700. Leake, John (1728-1792). <u>Practical Observations on the Child-Bed Fever</u>. London, 1773; further eds. in 1774, 1784. This volume comprises a series of lectures delivered at the Westminster Lying-in Hospital; the writer, an M.D. from Rheims, specialized in midwifery.
1701. Mauclerc, John Henry (fl.1740-1770). <u>Dr. [James] Blondel Confuted; or, The Ladies Vindicated with Regard to the Power of Imagination in Pregnant Women</u>. London, 1747. 56pp. See #1702; also, #1633.
1702. _____. <u>The Power of Imagination in Pregnant Women Discussed</u>. London, 1740. 56pp. In this, a slight variant of #1701, the writer reacts to a dispute between James Blondel (d.1734?), an M.D. who practiced at London, and another London physician, Daniel Tower.
1703. <u>The Nurse's Guide; or, Short and Safer Rules for the Management of Women. . .in Child-Bed</u>. London, 1744. 52pp.
1704. Osborne, William (1736-1808). <u>An Essay on Laborious Parturition, in which the Division of the Symphysis Pubis is particularly Considered</u>. London, 1783. 255pp. Osborne argued against the Frenchman Jean Sigault and Dr. William Hunter, believing the operation he describes herein to have been useless and dangerous; born in London, Osborne received his medical education at St. George's Hospital, London, then practiced in that city as a surgeon and midwife at the lying-in hospital, Store Street; he received the M.D. in 1777 from St. Andrews and lectured in London on midwifery, claiming to have educated at least 1200 practitioners in that process.
1705. Parsons, James (1705-1770). <u>Pralecturi. . .J.P. . . . Elenchus Gyniacopathologicus Obstetricarius</u>. London, 1741. 56pp. This work focuses upon the diseases of women at childbirth; educated at Dublin, Parsons studied medicine at Rheims (M.D. 1736), then came to London to learn anatomy; after an appointment to the public infirmary at St. Giles, he embarked upon an extensive practice of obstetrics; Parsons published tracts on medicine, natural history, and antiquity (principally as pertained to Wales and Ireland).
1706. Pearson, George (1751-1828). <u>Observations on the Effects of Variolous Infection on Pregnant Women</u>. London, 1794. 48pp. See, also, #623.
1707. Rawlins, Richard (fl.1790-1795). <u>A Dissertation on the Structure of the Obstetric Forceps</u>. London, 1793. 125pp.
1708. Sibly, Ebenezer (1751-1800). <u>The Medical Mirror; or, a Treatise on the Impregnation of the Human Female</u>. London, 1794. 180pp.; four eds. through 1800. The writer studied surgery at London and eventually (1792) received the M.D. degree from King's

Pregnancy and Childbirth (contd.)

College, Aberdeen; he resided at Ipswich, there practicing medicine and studying astrology; his later publications evidence an attempt to relate medicine with the celestial and occult sciences.

1709. Simmons, William (fl.1795-1810). A Treatise on Dr. [John] Hull's Defense of the Caesarean Operation. London, 1798; another ed., London, 1799. John Hull (1761-1843), a Manchester physician and holder of the M.D., published principally on matters relating to botany (see #1698); Simmons published tracts on the Caesarean operation and on lithotomy.

1710. _____. A Treatise on the Caesarean Operation. London, 1798. This essay brought a response from George Tomlinson (see #1711).

1711. Tomlinson, George (fl.1795-1800). A Letter [to William Simmons] on the Caesarean Operation. London, 1798. This piece a reaction to #1710.

1712. Trye, Charles Brandon (1757-1811). An Essay on the Swelling of the Lower Extremities incident to Lying-in Women. London, 1792. 80pp. See, also, #1416.

1713. Walsh, Philip Pitt (d.1788). Practical Observations on the Puerperal Fever. London, 1787. 59pp. An M.D., the writer practiced surgery and midwifery at London.

1714. Watts, Giles (fl.1754-1767). Reflections on Slow Labours. London, 1755. The writer also published tracts on inoculation; see, also, #1053.

1715. Whitehead, John (1740?-1804). A Report of a Memoir containing a New Method of Treating Puerperal Fever; from the French [of Denis Claude Boulcet]. London, 1783. Although he had received the M.D. degree from Leyden in 1779, served as a physician to the London Dispensary and the London Hospital, and gained admittance as a licentiate of the College of Physicians, Whitehead's literary reputation resides in an arena removed from medicine; a former member of the Society of Friends, he attended to the medical needs of John and Charles Wesley and eventually joined the ranks of the Methodists; he, alone, attended John Wesley during his final days, preached his funeral sermon in March 1791, served as his literary executor, and published (1793) a biography of the Methodist founder and leader; in Marshall Claxton's painting of The Death-Bed of Wesley (1844), Whitehead stands most prominently at the extreme left (see Nehemiah Curnock, ed., The Journal of the Rev. John Wesley, A.M. [London: Charles H. Kelly, 1909-1916] 8:141).

1716. Woollcombe, William (fl.1795-1810). Dissertatio Inauguralis de Peritonitide Puerperarum. Edinburgh, 1796. This piece represents the writer's principal dissertation for the M.D. degree from Edinburgh; he then served as a physician to the Plymouth Dispensary.

B. Midwifery

1717. Aitken, John (d.1790). Principles of Midwifery, or Puerperal Medicine. Edinburgh, 1784. 95pp.; 2nd ed., Edinburgh, 1785. 216pp.; 3rd ed., London, 1786. 210pp. See, also, #288.
1718. Bracken, Henry (1697-1764). The Midwife's Companion. London, 1737. 321pp. See, also, #1385.
1719. Brudenell, Exton (fl.1750-1755). A Treatise on the System of Midwifery. London, 1751.
1720. Burton, John (1710-1771). An Essay toward a Complete New System of Midwifery, Theoretical as well as Practical. London, 1751. 391pp.; 2nd ed., London, 1753. An antiquary, physician, and classical scholar, Burton earned a reputation for skill in midwifery; the Yorkshire novelist Laurence Sterne, in his Tristram Shandy (1759-1767), unfairly satirized Burton in the character of "Dr. Slop"; the political differences between the two Yorkshire men had, prior to the publication of Tristram Shandy, manifested themselves into a climate of total animosity; Burton, born at Rippon, Yorkshire, studied at Leyden and received the M.D. from Rheims; he then settled in York.
1721. _____. A Letter to William Smellie, M.D., containing Critical and Practical Remarks upon his Treatise on the Theory and Practice of Midwifery. London, 1753. 250pp. See #1772. In this polemic tract, Burton attacks Smellie, concluding that the latter came forward only as a pure theorist and a poor practitioner; Burton appears to have been the first English physician to suggest that puerperal fever may well be contagious.
1722. Chamberlen, Hugh (1664-1728). Mauricenus's Midwifery. London, 1683. Educated at Trinity College, Cambridge, the writer achieved recognition as the inventor of an obstetric forceps, an instrument eventually approved by William Smellie the elder; Chamberlen developed a large practice, which also yielded him a considerable fortune; see, also, #51-#52.
1723. _____. A Treatise on Midwife's Practice. London, 1685.
1724. Chapman, Edmund (1680?-1756). An Essay on the Improvement of Midwifery, chiefly with regard to the Operation. London, 1733. 119pp.; 2nd ed., London, 1735. 186pp.; 3rd ed., London, 1759. 164pp. The writer practiced surgery at London.
1725. _____. A Reply to Mr. [John] Douglas's Short Account of the State of Midwifery. London, 1737. 68pp. See, also, #1738.
1726. Clark, William (1698-1780?). Observations upon the Province Midwifery. London, 1751. A native of Wiltshire, the writer received the M.D. degree from Leyden in 1727; he then settled at Bradford, Wiltshire.
1727. Clubbe, John (fl.1775-1790). A Treatise upon the Inflammation of the Breasts, Peculiar to Lying-in

Midwifery (contd.)

Women. Ipswich, 1779. 66pp. See, also, #1093.
1728. Cooper, Thomas (fl.1765-1770). A Compendium of Midwifery. London(?), 1766. 300pp.
1729. ____. Proposals for Teaching the Art of Midwifery. London, 1766(?). 15pp.
1730. Counsell, George (fl.1750-1760). The Art of Midwifery. London, 1752. 195pp.
1731. ____. The New London Art of Midwifery. London, 1758. 195pp.
1732. Culpeper, Nicholas (1616-1664). A Directory for Midwives. London, 1724. 374pp. This work published posthumously. See, also, #18.
1733. The Danger and Immodesty of...Employing Men Midwives. London, 1772. 64pp.; 2nd ed., London, 1772. 73pp.
1734. Daventer, Henry (fl.1715-1720). Midwifery Improved. London, 1716.
1735. Dawkes, Thomas (fl.1735-1750). The Midwife Rightly Instructed. London, 1736. 90pp.
1736. Dease, William (1752?-1798). Observations in Midwifery. Dublin, 1783. 212pp. See, also, #737.
1737. Denman, Thomas (1733-1815). Introduction to the Practice of Midwifery. London, 1782. 148pp.; 2 vols. London, 1794-1795; 2nd ed., 2 vols., London, 1798. See, also, #684.
1738. Douglas, John (d.1743). A Short Account of the State of Midwifery in London. London, 1736. 75pp. See, also, #315.
1739. Douglas, William (d.1752). A Treatise on Midwifery. London, 1736. A native of Scotland, Douglas settled in Boston, Massachusetts, in 1748, where he managed to achieve a considerable professional reputation.
1740. Fores, S.W. (fl.1790-1795). Men-Midwifery Dissected; or, the Obstetric Family Instructor. By John Blunt. London, 1793. 236pp.
1741. Foster, Edward (d.1780). The Principles and Practices of Midwifery, completed and corrected by James Sims, M.D. London, 1781. 316pp. A native of Canterbury and holder of the M.D. degree, Sims (d.1831) also published prose tracts on epidemics.
1742. Giffard, William (d.1731). Three Hundred and Twenty-Five Cases in Midwifery; Revised and Published by Edward Hody, M.D. London, 1734. 520pp. Edward Hody (1698-1759) published, in 1735, several of Gifford's medical essays in the Philosophical Transactions of the Royal Society.
1743. Hamilton, James (d.1839). A Collection of Engravings Designed to Facilitate the Study of Midwifery. London, 1796. 59pp. The writer received his medical training from his father and rose to the professorship of midwifery at Edinburgh; he published tracts on midwifery and on professional standards and practices in medicine.
1744. ____. Select Cases in Midwifery. Edinburgh, 1795. 159pp.

Midwifery (contd.)

1745. Harvie, John (fl.1765-1770). <u>An Essay on Midwifery</u>. London, 1767. See, also, #1697.
1746. Heath, John (FL.1785-1800). <u>Bondeloque's System of Midwifery. Translated from the French</u>. 3 vols. London, 1790.
1747. Henly, Thomas (fl.1710-1720). <u>Observations and Commentary upon a Case in Midwifery</u>. Oxford, 1715.
1748. Hunter, William (1718-1783). <u>The Anatomy of the Gravid Uterus Exhibited in Figures</u>. Birmingham, 1774. See, also, #332.
1749. Johnson, Robert Wallace (fl.1768-1786). <u>A New System of Midwifery, in Four Parts</u>. London, 1769. 440pp. The writer held the M.D. degree.
1750. Leake, John (1729-1792). <u>An Introduction to the Theory and Practice of Midwifery</u>. London, 1777. See, also, #1700.
1751. Manningham, Sir Richard (1690-1759). <u>An Abstract of Midwifery for the Use of the Lying-in Infirmary</u>. London, 1744. 32pp. See, also, #866.
1752. Mawbray, John (d.1732). <u>Midwifery brought to Perfection, by Manual Operation</u>. London, 1725. 46pp. The writer appears to have been one of the first teachers of obstetrics in London; he has been identified as lecturing in London in 1725; shortly thereafter, he established a lying-in hospital in that city, to which he admitted patients and instructed students.
1753. Mears, Martha (fl.1795-1800). <u>A Treatise upon Midwifery</u>. London, 1797.
1754. Memis, John (fl.1760-1767). <u>A Midwife's Pocket Companion</u>. London, 1764; further London eds. in 1765, 1766; another ed., Aberdeen, 1786. The writer held the M.D. degree and practiced in London.
1755. Moore, William (fl.1775-1780). <u>A Treatise on the Elements of Midwifery</u>. London, 1777. 234pp. An M.D., the writer practiced in London.
1756. Nihell, Elizabeth (1723-?). <u>A Treatise on the Art of Midwifery</u>. London, 1760. 471pp. The writer denounces all male midwives, particularly William Smellie the elder; the editors of the <u>Critical Review</u> attempted to discredit both the writer and her book, but she responded directly to them in 1760; see, also, #1768.
1757. Nisbet, William (1759-1822). <u>The Clinical Guide; or, A Concise View of. . .Midwifery</u>. London, 1800. 348pp. See, also, #478.
1758. Osborne, William (1736-1808). <u>Essays on the Practice of Midwifery in Natural and Difficult Labours</u>. London, 1792. 415pp.; another ed., London, 1795. This work stands, essentially, as an expanded version of #1704; Osborne opposed birth by Caesarian section, and thus he sets forth arguments to that effect in this tract--supported, interestingly enough, by Biblical quotation and inference.

Midwifery (contd.)

1759. Ould, Sir Fielding (1710-1789). A Treatise on Midwifery, in Three Parts. Dublin, 1742. 203pp. The writer dedicated this volume to the Dublin College of Physicians: the first part focuses upon normal labor, the second on various instances of abnormal labor, and the third upon obstetric operations; after studying medicine at Paris, Ould returned to Dublin in 1736 to begin his practice in midwifery; in 1759, he received the appointment as master of the lying-in hospital, Dublin.

1760. Perfect, William (1737-1809). Observations of Cases of Midwifery. 2 vols. Rochester, 1781; three eds. through 1789. An M.D., Perfect practiced medicine at Kent and also wrote tracts on insanity.

1761. Pole, Thomas (1753-1829). Lectures on Midwifery. London, 1797. A Quaker, Pole studied medicine at Maidenhead, Reading, and Falmouth--most likely under practicing physicians in those towns; in 1781, he settled in London, concentrating his practice upon obstetrics and diseases of women and children; he also lectured upon midwifery at London and Bath.

1762. Portal, Paul (1630-1703). The Compleat Practice of Men and Women Midwives. London, 1705. 345pp.; further eds. in 1753, 1763.

1763. Pugh, Benjamin (fl.1748-1785). A Treatise of Midwifery. London, 1748; another ed., London, 1754. 152pp. See, also, #629.

1764. Ritson, John ((fl.1770-1775). The Danger and Immodesty of. . .Unnecessarily Employing Men Midwives. London, 1772. This seventy-page tract has proven an extremely rare and unrecorded volume in the history of midwifery.

1765. Ryley, Samuel (fl.1765-1770). Elements of Midwifery; from the French of J[ean] Astruc. London, 1766. An anonymous translation of this piece appeared in London in 1867; the French physician, Astruc (1684-1766), treated Louis XV and taught medicine; however, his literary reputation rests upon his scholarly investigations of Moses and his establishing the foundation for modern criticism of the Pentateuch.

1766. Sharp, Jane (fl.1671-1725). A Complete Midwife's Companion. London, 1725.

1767. ____. A Midwife's Book. London, 1671. This piece an obvious companion to or revision of #1766.

1768. Smellie, William the elder (1697-1763). A Collection of Cases and Observations in Midwifery. London, 1754. A conscientious and brilliant physician, Smellie had once been attacked by a London female midwife as "a great horse godmother of a he-wife"; however, in the face of such ignorance and unfounded criticism, he advanced obstetrics into the "modern" age and transformed it into a genuine science; more than any other medical writer of the eighteenth century, Smellie described exactly the

Pregnancy, Midwifery, Infants, Children, Women   203

Midwifery (contd.)

mechanism of parturition and the curves followed by the infant during birth; he taught William Hunter and served the novelist (and physician) Tobias George Smollett as both teacher and friend.

1769. ____. A Collection of Preternatural Cases and Observations in Midwifery. London, 1764. In this piece, Smellie describes in more detail (even more than in #1768) than any previous writer in English the mechanism of parturition and the curves followed by the infant during birth; further, the writer demonstrates the importance of exact measurement of the pelvis.

1770. ____. A Sett [sic] of Anatomical Tables, with Explanations and an Abridgement, of the Practice of Midwifery, with a View To Illustrate a Treatise on That Subject, and a Collection of Cases. London, 1754; further eds., London and Edinburgh, 1761, 1786, 1787.

1771. ____. A Treatise on the Theory and Practices of Midwifery. London, 1752. In this tract, Smellie became the first practitioner to set forth "safe" rules for the employment of the forceps, as well as to differentiate the contracted pelvis from the normal pelvis by actual measurement; the illustrations provided herein proved extremely accurate and even "faultless"; see, also, #1721 and #1773.

1772. ____. A Treatise on the Theory and Practice of Midwifery; Illustrated by a Collection of Cases and Observations. 3 vols. Dublin, 1764; 3 vols., Edinburgh, 1784; 5th ed., 3 vols., London, 1766; a later ed. and revision (by others) of #1771 above. This piece essentially a digest of all of the writer's works on midwifery.

1773. Southwell, Thomas (fl.1740-1760). Remarks on Some of the Errors, Both in Anatomy and Practice, Contained in a Late Treatise on Midwifery. Dublin, 1742. This work essentially an attack upon Sir Fielding Ould's Treatise on Midwifery (1742); see #1759.

1774. Spence, David (fl.1767-1785; d. 1786). A System of Midwifery. Edinburgh, 1784. 589pp. The writer received the M.D. degree from Edinburgh in 1766.

1775. Stone, Sarah (1735-1740). A Complete Practice of Midwifery. London, 1737. 163pp.

1776. Thicknesse, Philip (1719-1792). Midwifery Analysed. London, 1764; another ed., London, 1768. The writer underwent, at an early age, a term as an apprentice to an apothecary; however, that experience proved to have been his only real contact with the medical profession; he spent some time as a soldier and administrator in Georgia, Jamaica, and on the European Continent; his piece on midwifery appears as only one of a host of his miscellaneous, political, historical, and social tracts.

1777. Thompson, Thomas (fl.1740-1773). A Vindication of

Midwifery (contd.)

Man-Midwifery. London, 1752. The writer held the M.D. degree and practiced at London.
1778. Torrano, Nicholas (fl.1750-1755). A Tract upon Midwifery. London, 1753. See, also, #1151.
1779. Wallace, Johnson Robert (fl.1765-1770). Observations on a New System of Midwifery. In Four Parts. London, 1769.
1780. White, Charles (1728-1813). A Treatise on the Management of Pregnant and Lying-in Women. London, 1773; five eds. through 1791; American ed., Worcester, Massachusetts, 1793; German ed., Leipzig, 1775. See, also, #795.
1781. Wolveridge, James (fl.1665-1675). An Irish Midwife's Handmaid. London, 1670. The writer held the M.D. degree.

C. Infants and Children

1782. Armstrong, George (1719-1789). An Account of the Diseases Most Incident to Children. London, 1777. 216pp.; a new ed., London, 1783. 200pp. Armstrong practiced as an apothecary at Hampstead, then moved directly to London and established (1769) a dispensary in Red Lion Square for the relief of poor children; that institution continued until 1781 and reportedly served more than 35,000 patients; indeed, within the first eight years of its existence, Armstrong's hospital treated 20,962 children, 699 of whom actually died there (see M. Dorothy George, London Life in the Eighteenth Century [New York: Alfred A. Knopf, 1926] 51, 336).
1783. _____. An Essay on the Diseases Most Fatal to Infants. London, 1767. 148pp.; 2nd ed., London, 1771; 3rd ed. (dedicated to Queen Charlotte), London, 1777; 4th ed., London, 1788.
1784. Armstrong, John (1709-1779). A Full View of All the Diseases Incident to Children. Containing Dr. [Walter] Harris's Book. London, 1742. 263pp. See, also, #12, #1793.
1785. Butter, William (1726-1805). A Treatise on the Infantile Remittent Fever. London, 1782. 50pp. through 1770. Butter, born on the Orkney Islands, studied medicine at Edinburgh (M.D. 1761), practiced at Derby, and finally settled and practiced in London.
1786. Cadogan, William (1711-1797). An Essay on the Nursing and Management of Children. London, 1748. 38pp.; 2nd ed., London, 1750; nine eds. through 1770. According to the writer--a physician at the London Foundling Hospital--children enjoyed too many clothes and too much food, the combination of which caused most of their medical problems; see, also, #1232.
1787. Clarke, Matthew (1701-1778). The Management of Children, from the Time of Birth to the Age of Seven Years. London, 1773. The writer, born at

Infants and Children (contd.)

London, received the M.D. from Leyden in 1726 and gained admission as M.D. to Cambridge in 1728; from 1732 to 1754, he served as a physician to Guy's Hospital, London.

1788. Clough, James (fl.1795-1800). An Essay on the Diseases of Children. London, 1796.

1789. Conyers, Richard (1707?-1764?). De Morbis Infantum Dissertatio. London, 1748. 48pp. The writer published both medical tracts and sermons.

1790. Cook, John (fl.1730-1770). A Plain Account of the Diseases Incident to Children. London, 1769. 66pp. See, also, #307.

1791. Farrer, William (fl.1765-1775). Observations on the Rickets for Children. London, 1773. The writer, an M.D., practiced medicine at London.

1792. Gower, Richard (fl.1680-1685). Observations on Children's Diseases. London, 1682.

1793. Harris, Walter (1647-1732). De Morbis Acutis Infantum. London, 1689. This volume served as a standard work on the treatment of children's diseases and illnesses until 1784, when Michael Underwood (see #1801) published his treatise on the Diseases of Children; born at Gloucester, Harris received appointment as a physician to William III; an M.D., he published consistently on matters related to medicine and surgery; see, also, #1784.

1794. Jones, Philip (fl.1785-1790). An Essay on Crookedness or Distortions of the Spines of Children. London, 1788. 149pp.

1795. Lettsome, John Coakley (1744-1815). Hints respecting the Chlorosis of Boarding Schools. London, 1795. 31pp. See, also, #160.

1796. Mantell, Sir Thomas (1751-1831). Short Directions for the Management of Infants. London, 1787. 62pp.; another ed., London, 1792.

1797. Moss, William (fl.1780-1800). An Essay on the Management, Nursing, and Diseases of Children and Women. Liverpool, 1782; other eds. at Liverpool, 1794; at Egham, 1794. See, also, #192.

1798. Nisbet, William (1759-1822). The Clinical Guide; or, A Concise View of. . .Infancy and Childhood. London, 1800. 407pp. See, also, #478.

1799. Observations upon the Proper Nursing of Children. London, 1761. 24pp.

1800. Tytler, Henry William (1752-1808). Paedotrophia; or, the Art of Nursing and Rearing Children, a Poem in Three Books; translated from the Latin of Scevele de Ste. Marthe, with Medical and Historical Notes. London, 1797. Born at Forfarshire, Tytler received the M.D. degree in 1797; his publications reveal a deep interest in translation from the Greek and Latin, as well as in travel narrative.

1801. Underwood, Michael (1736-1820). A Treatise on the Diseases of Children. 2 vols. London, 1784; further eds. at London in 1789, 1795, 1797 (3

Infants and Children (contd.)

vols.). A male midwife at London, the writer has received credit for first having described sclerema neonatorum ("Underwood's disease"); this Treatise has been described as the best treatment of the subject that had yet appeared in English; see, also, #789, #1793.

1802. ____. A Treatise on the Disorders of Childhood. 3 vols. London, 1797. A variant title for #1801.
1803. Wilson, Andrew (1718-1792). Aphorisms on Diseases of Children. London, 1783. See, also, #278.

D. Women

1804. Berdoe, Marmaduke (fl.1770-1775). An Essay on the Pudendagra. Bath, 1771. 80pp.
1805. Brown, Sarah (fl.1775-1780). A Medical Letter to a Lady on the Mode of Conducting Herself during Pregnancy. London, 1777. 32pp.
1806. Burns, John (1774-1850). The Anatomy of the Gravid Uterus. Glasgow, 1799. 248pp. See, also, #1348.
1807. The Complete Gentlewoman and Chamber-maid's Closet Newly Opened: Richly Stored with Many Choice Receipts in Physick and Chirurgury. London, n.d. 24pp. This work published at some time between 1701 and 1709.
1808. Denman, Thomas (1733-1815). An Essay on Uterine Haemorrhages. London, 1786. 76pp. See, also, #684.
1809. Douglas, Andrew (1736-1806). Observations on an Extraordinary Case of Ruptured Uterus. London, 1785. 74pp. Educated at Edinburgh, Douglas joined the navy as a surgeon in 1756, and eventually received the M.D. degree from Edinburgh in 1775; he settled in London, where he practiced midwifery and published treatises on women's diseases; in 1776, he gained admittance as a licentiate of the College of Physicians.
1810. ____. Observations on the Rupture of the Gravid Uterus. London, 1789. 135pp.
1811. Every Lady Her Own Physician; or, the Closet Companion. London, 1788. 124pp.
1812. Goldson, William (fl.1785-1805). An Extraordinary Case of Lacerated Vagina. London, 1787. 77pp. The writer published medical tracts at London between 1787 and 1805; in addition, he wrote a narrative of the Passage between the Atlantic and Pacific (Portsmouth, 1793).
1813. Grigg, John (fl.1785-1795). Medical Advice to the Female Sex in General, Particularly those in a State of Pregnancy. Bath, 1789. 319pp. another ed., Bath, 1793.
1814. Hull, John (1761-1843). An Essay on Phlegmatic Dolens. Manchester, 1800. 369pp. See, also, #1698.
1815. Jones, Thomas (fl.1735-1745). An Essay on the Diseases of Women. London, 1740.

Women (contd.)

1816. Leake, John (1729-1792). Medical Instructions toward the Prevention and Cure of Chronic or Slow Diseases Peculiar to Women. 2 vols. London, 1771. This work addressed to women in general and thus not directed to medical "professionals"; it also contains extraneous narrative and verse; an M.D., Leake practiced physic and midwifery in London; see, also, #1700.

1817. Manning, Henry (fl.1771-1780). A Treatise on Female Diseases. London, 1771. 431pp.; 2nd ed., London, 1775. 430pp. See, also, #168.

1818. Mawbray, John (d.1730). The Female Physician, containing all the Diseases Incident to that Sex. London, 1724. 420pp.; 2nd ed., London, 1730. See, also, #1752.

1819. Pole, Thomas (1753-1829). An Anatomical Description of a Double Uterus and Vagina. London, 1792. 6pp. See, also, #345.

1820. Rigby, Edward the elder (1747-1821). An Essay on the Uterine Heamorrhage which precedes the Delivery of the full-grown Foetus. London, 1775; six eds. through 1824; French and German translations. This work placed the writer among the first rank of his profession; a native of Chowbent, Lancashire, Rigby studied medicine at Norwich and London, eventually settling into practice at Norwich; in 1786, he led the effort to establish the Norfolk Benevolent Society for the relief of widows and orphans of medical practitioners; he toured Europe and later involved himself in the study of agriculture.

1821. Rowley, William (1742-1806). A Practical Treatise on Diseases of the Breasts. London, 1772. 55pp.; 2nd ed., London, 1777. See, also, #222.

1822. _____. A Treatise on Female, Nervous, Hysterical, Hypochondriacal, Bilious, Convulsive Diseases; Apoplexy and Palsy; with Thoughts on Madness and Suicide. London, 1788. 521pp.

1823. Simson, Thomas (1696-1764). A Treatise on the System of the Womb. Edinburgh, 1729. See, also, #1603.

1824. Smith, Hugh (1736?-1789). Letters to Married Women on Nursing. London, 1767. 246pp.; 3rd ed., London, 1774; another ed. edited by Dr. John Vaughan (fl.1775-1795), London, 1792; further eds. at Wilmington, Delaware, 1801, and New York, 1827. Smith received the M.D. degree from Leyden in 1755 and practiced at London.

1825. Tryer, Mary (fl.1670-1680). Medicatrix; or, The Woman's Physician. London, 1675. The writer identified as the daughter of one "M.O. Doude" (see Allibone 3:2462).

1826. Turner, Robert (fl.1654-1686). The Feminine Physician: The Enlarged Women's Counsellor. London, 1686. A graduate of Cambridge, the writer appears not to have studied medicine (at least formally); his published works reflect his interests in botany and astrology.

Women (contd.)

1827. Wallis, George (1740-1802). *An Essay on the Evil Consequences attending Injudicious Bleeding in Pregnancy.* London, 1778; 2nd ed., London, 1781. See, also, #1283.

XX

Seamen, Soldiers and Sailors, Farmers

A. Seamen (principally nonmilitary)

1828. Addington, Anthony (1713-1790). An Essay on the Sea-Scurvy, wherein is proposed an Easy Method of Curing that Distemper at Sea, and of preserving Water sweet for any Cruise or Voyage. Reading, 1753. 47pp. This piece dedicated to the lords of the British Admiralty; it proved popular and interesting to read, but the writer failed to transmit significant or practical information; Addington proposed, for example, the addition of muriatic acid (later known as hydrochloric acid) as the sole method of preserving the freshness of water at sea; an Oxfordshire man by birth, Addington graduated M.D. from Oxford in 1744, practiced physic at Reading, and later specialized in the treatment of mental disorders and diseases; in 1754, he moved to London.

1829. Arbuthnot, John (1667-1735). An Essay concerning the Effects of Air upon Human Bodies. London, 1733. 242pp.; another ed. London, 1751. 224pp. The writer received the M.D. degree from St. Andrews, then went to London, and initially supported himself by teaching mathematics; eventually, he gained entrance into the prominent literary and intellectual circles of the Augustan age; he became a member of the Royal Society and helped to establish the celebrated Scriblerius Club that included Alexander Pope, Jonathan Swift, John Gay, Robert Harley, Bishop Francis Atterbury, and William Congreve; he served as physician extraordinary to Queen Anne, wrote history and satire, and authored a significant quantity of political and satirical pamphlets (as well as medical and scientific tracts).

1830. Arthy, Elliott (fl.1795-1800). The Seamen's Medical Advocate. London, 1798. 248pp.

Seamen (contd.)

1831. Aubrey, Thomas (fl.1725-1730). The Sea-Surgeon; or, The Guinea Man's Vade Macum. London, 1729. 135pp.
1832. Bates, Thomas (fl.1704-1719). Enchiridion of Fevers Common to Seamen in the Mediterranean. London, 1709. Bates, a surgeon, served in that capacity with the Royal Navy in the Mediterranean, after which he practiced physic in London; he achieved recognition for his efforts in helping to alleviate the cattle plague of 1714 that affected the cowyards at Islington; in January 1719, he gained admission to the Royal Society.
1833. Blane, Sir Gilbert (1749-1834). Observations on the Diseases Incident to Seamen. London, 1785. 502pp.; 2nd ed., London, 1790; 3rd ed., London, 1803. The 1803 edition includes a "Pharmacopoeia" for the naval service. See, also, #1574.
1834. Cockburn, William (1669-1739). Sea Diseases. London, 1706. 272pp.; three eds. through 1736. See, also, #65.
1835. Falch, Nathaniel (fl.1771-1779). The Seamen's Medical Instructor. London, 1774. See, also, #1223.
1836. Fletcher, Charles (fl.1786-1800). An Essay on the Maritime State Considered, as to the Health of Seamen. Dublin, 1786. 342pp. The writer also penned a satiric piece of verse on cock-fighting in Dublin (1787).
1837. Hales, Stephen (1677-1671). A Description of Ventilators: whereby great Quantities of Air may with ease be conveyed into Mines, Gaols, Hospitals, Workhouses, and Ships, in Exchange for their Noxious Air. 2 vols. London, 1743; another ed., London, 1758. A plant physiologist and inventor, Hales also contributed to the study of animal physiology and to experiments on the distillation of fresh water from salt water; see, also, #689, #701.
1838. Northcote, William (d.1783). The Marine Practice of Physic and Surgery. 2 vols. London, 1770. See, also, #480. As the writer's principal published work, this piece abounds with descriptions of his own experiments; in an appendix entitled "Some Brief Descriptions to be Observed by the Sea Surgeon previous to and in an [military] Engagement," Northcote graphically relates the difficulties confronted by the surgeon during combat at sea.
1839. Sutton, Samuel (fl.1740-1750). An Historical Account of a New Method for Extracting the Foul Air out of Ships. London, 1745. 48pp.; 2nd ed., London, 1749.
1840. Trotter, Thomas (1760-1832). Medica Nautica; or, an Essay on the Diseases of Seamen. 3 vols. London, 1797-1803; 2nd ed., 3 vols., London, 1804. See, also, #1505.
1841. Wilkinson, John (fl.1755-1765). Tutamen Nauticum: or, Seamen's Preservations in Shipwreck. London, 1759. 91pp.; another ed., London, 1764. The writer held

Seamen (contd.)

the M.D. degree.

B. Soldiers and Sailors (military)

1842. Atkins, John (1685-1757). <u>The Navy Surgeon; or, a Practical System of Surgery</u>. London, 1732; 2nd ed., London, 1734; another ed. at London, 1742. This work exists as a general treatise on surgery, with discussions on such subjects as mineral springs, empirics, amulets, and infirmaries; the writer describes, however, specific cases relative to the naval service and cites a number an variety of medical sources; a naval surgeon, Atkins sailed with various military expeditions between 1707 and 1723.

1843. Bell, John (d.1801). <u>An Inquiry into the Causes which Produce Diseases among British Soldiers in the East Indies</u>. London, 1791. 180pp. The writer held the M.D. degree.

1844. Bisset. Charles (1717-1791). <u>The Medical Constitution of Great Britain. . .with an Account of the Throat Distemper and Military Fever which were Epidemic in 1760</u>. London, 1760. See #31 for full title.

1845. Blair, William (1766-1822). <u>The Soldier's Friend; or, The Means of Preserving the Health of Military Men; containing Familiar Instructions to the Loyal Volunteers, Yeomanry Corps, and Military Men in General, on the Preservation and Recovery of Their Health</u>. London, 1798. 158pp.; 2nd ed., London, 1803; 3rd ed., London, 1804. Born at Lavenham, Suffolk, Blair trained for medical practice in London; there he associated himself with the Lock Hospital, London Asylum, Finsbury Dispensary, Bloomsbury Dispensary, Female Penitentiary, and the New Rupture Society; he also edited the <u>London Medical Review and Magazine</u> (see #2047).

1846. <u>The Cure of the Military Fever. To which is annex'd, Advice to the Apothecaries</u>. London, 1751. 92pp.

1847. Curtis, Sir Roger (1746-1816). <u>The Means used to eradicate a Malignant Fever. . .on. . .His Majesty's Ship Brunswick</u>. London(?), 1791. 24pp. <u>H.M.S. Brunswick</u> will be remembered by some as the vessel upon which, on 29 October 1792, in Portsmouth harbor, three of the <u>H.M.S. Bounty</u> mutineers (Thomas Ellison, Thomas Burkitt, and John Millward) were hanged for their actions; Curtis, himself, sat on the court martial board that tried the <u>Bounty</u> mutineers from 12 to 18 September 1792 (see Sir John Barrow, <u>The Mutiny of the Bounty</u> [1831], ed. Gavin Kennedy [Boston: David R. Godine, Publisher, Inc., 1980] 124-127, 146, 162).

1848. Hamilton, Sir David (1633-1721). <u>Tractatus Duplex: prior de Praxeos Regulis, alter de Febre Miliari</u>. London, 1710. 247pp.; Ulm, 1711; English translation, London, 1737. A native of Scotland, Hamilton received the M.D. from Rheims in 1686 and

Soldiers and Sailors (contd.)

rose to become one of the leading practitioners of midwifery in England; he served Queen Anne and Charlotte, Princess of Wales.

1849. Hamilton, Robert (1749-1830). The Duties of a Regimental Surgeon. 2 vols. London, 1787; 2nd ed., 2 vols. London, 1794. See, also, #1226.

1850. Hunter, John (d.1809). Observations of the Diseases of the Army in Jamaica. London, 1788. 328pp.; 2nd ed., London, 1796. 342pp. Born in Perthshire and educated at Edinburgh (M.D. 1775), Hunter, in 1777, gained admittance as a licentiate of the College of Physicians in London; his various appointments include physician to the army and (1781-1783) superintendent of the military hospitals in Jamaica; he returned to London to practice medicine; his various contributions include published papers on typhus fever and tropical diseases and Gulstonian and Croonian lectures.

1851. Lempriere, William (fl.1790-1812). Observations upon Diseases of the Army in Jamaica, 1792-1797. 2 vols. London, 1799. Prior to receiving the M.D. degree, the writer served as an apothecary to the Royal Army; he also wrote, in 1791, a narrative of a military tour to Gibraltar and Morocco.

1852. Lind, James (1716-1794). An Essay on the Most Effectual Means of Preserving the Health of Seamen in the Royal Navy. London, 1757. 119pp.; three eds. through 1779. See, also, #942.

1853. Maclean, Hector (fl.1785-1800). An Inquiry into the Nature of the Causes of the Great Mortality among the Troops at St. Domingo. London, 1797. 358pp. The writer held the M.D. degree; this tract focuses upon the terrible effects of malaria among British troops during the campaign of 1795.

1854. Monro, Donald (1727-1802). An Account of the Diseases which were Most Frequent in the British Military Hospitals in Germany, from January 1761...to March 1763. London, 1764. This work also includes an essay on the means for preserving the health of soldiers and the procedures for maintaining military hospitals. See, also, #473, #1855.

1855. _____. Observations on the Means of Preserving the Health of Soldiers and of Conducting Military Hospitals, and on the Diseases Incident to Soldiers. 2 vols. London, 1780. This work constitutes a significant expansion of the essay appended to Monro's Account of the Diseases (see #1854).

1856. Pringle, Sir John (1707-1782). Observations on the Diseases of the Army in Camp and in Garrison. London, 1752; seven eds. through 1775. See, also, #872.

1857. Ranby, John (1703-1773). The Method of Treating Gunshot Wounds. London, 1744; 2nd ed., London, 1760; 3rd ed., London, 1781. This volume represents an account of surgical cases that came

Soldiers and Sailors (contd.)

under Ranby's care during the German campaign of 1743-1745, including those of the Battle of Dettingen (17 June 1743); the writer alludes to the need for an army medical corps; advances the the application of Peruvian bark for suppuration following gunshot wounds; anticipates quinine and its applications; provides details of a leg wound to William, Duke of Cumberland (and son to King George); and relates cases of death from tetanus following gunshot wounds; see, also, #775.

1858. Reide, Thomas Dickson (fl.1790-1800). A View of Diseases of the Army in Great Britain, America, and the West Indies. London, 1793. 396pp. The writer also published, in 1798, a tract on the duties of infantry officers.

1859. Renwick, William (1740?-1814). An Address to Parliament on the Situation of Naval Surgeons. London, 1785. Renwick, born at Berwick-on-Tweed, went to sea as a surgeon's mate as early as 1760; after a temporary loss of sight and period of poverty (1766-1773), he managed to return to naval service as surgeon on board several ships of the line; he also found time to write verse, drama, and highly autobiographical romantic tales.

1860. ____. A Treatise on the Medical Service of the Royal Navy. London, 1783.

1861. Rollo, John (d.1809). Observations on the Diseases in the Army on St. Lucia. London, 1781. The writer concerns himself with those problems (principally malaria) brought about by the climate in that part of the world; see, also, #1442.

1862. Rowley, William (1742-1806). Medical Advice for the Use of the Army and Navy in the Present American Expedition. London, 1776. 47pp. See, also, #222.

1863. Rymer, James (fl.1775-1822). An Essay on Medical Education, with Advice to Young Gentlemen who go into the Navy as Mates. London, 1776. See, also, #692.

1864. ____. Observations and Remarks respecting the more effectual Means of Preservation of Wounded Seamen and Mariners on board H.M.'s Ships in Time of Action. London, 1780; 2nd ed., London, 1782.

1865. Wade, John Peter (fl.1790-1795; d.1802). A Treatise on the Disorders of Seamen and Soldiers in Bengal. London, 1793. The writer, an M.D., published extensively on diseases peculiar to the European residents of Bengal; see, also, #2002, #2003.

1866. White, Charles (1728-1813). Observations on Gangrenes and Mortifications during War. Warrington, 1790; an Italian translation in 1791. See, also, #795.

1867. Williams, William Henry (1771-1841). Hints on the Ventilation of Army Hospitals and on Regimental Practice. London, 1798. Williams studied medicine at the Bristol Infirmary and in London at St. Thomas's Hospital and Guy's Hospital; he became associated with a number of military regiments

Soldiers and Sailors (contd.)

> prior to his appointment as Physician-General to the army; in 1797, he designed a simple but efficient tourniquet that came to bear his name and achieved for him a niche in military medical history: thus, "Williams's Field Tourniquet."

C. Farmers

1868. Falconer, William (1744-1824). <u>An Essay on the Preservation of the Health of Persons Engaged in Agriculture, and on the Cure of the Diseases Incident to that Way of Life</u>. Bath, 1789. 88p. This work first appeared in Volume IV of <u>The Letters and Papers</u> of the Bath and West of England Agricultural Society, later to be reprinted in Dr. Alexander Hunter's (see #598) <u>Georgical Essays</u>, 4 (1803-1804), 503-529; an Italian translation came forth in London (n.d.), while a third English edition appeared at London in 1794; born at Cheshire, Falconer studied medicine at Edinburgh (M.D. 1766), then received the M.D. from Leyden in 1767; he practiced medicine both at Cheshire and at Bath; essentially, the writer, in this work, discusses the employment of rural laborers, their diets, their living accommodations, and the medical treatment afforded them; see, also, #100.

XXI

History, Biography, Hospitals, Institutions and Organizations, Dictionaries, Glossaries, General References

A. History

1869. Antes, John (fl.1795-1805). <u>Observations on the Manners and Customs of the Egyptians. . . with Remarks on the Plague</u>. London, 1800; Bohn's 1841 Catalogue (2:1181, #13981-#13982) lists another ed. in 1800: the first sold for four shillings, the second for six; both contain a large map of Egypt.

1870. Black, William (1749-1829). <u>An Historical Sketch of Medicine and Surgery, from Their Origin to the Present Time</u>. London, 1792; a French translation published at Paris. Black studied medicine at Leyden (M.D. 1772) and practiced in London; his principal contributions appear to have been the application of statistical methods to medical research, he having been the first writer in Britain to to do so: see his <u>A Comparative View of the Mortality of the Human Species at All Ages, and of Diseases and Casualties, with Charts and Tables</u> (London, 1788); according to the critical commentator for the London <u>Monthly Review</u> (35:1783), the <u>Historical Sketch</u> represents an endeavor whereby "the execution of it is more to be commended than the plan" (see Allibone 1:195).

1871. Bradley, Henry (fl.1730-1735). <u>Remarks on the Ancient Physicians' Legacy</u>. London, 1733. These <u>Remarks</u> actually written by Thomas Dover (1662-1742; see #420) in 1732; see #1878.

1872. Bryant, Jacob (1715-1804). <u>Observations upon the Plagues inflicted upon the Egyptians</u>. London, 1794. 441pp. Born at Plymouth, Devonshire, Bryant received his education at Eton and King's College, Cambridge; he had no formal medical education or training, but devoted himself to literary, Biblical, and antiquarian studies; he served as tutor to the sons of the Duke of Marlborough and as

History (contd.)

the Duke's secretary during the latter's military campaigns; his employer ceded to him a lifetime annuity, as well as two rooms at Blenheim Palace and keys to the library there--a gift that yielded most unfortunate results: in stepping on a chair to reach a book in the library, Bryant slipped, seriously cut his leg, and died (14 November 1804, age eighty-nine) from infection; his Observations upon the Plague examines the miracles of the Old Testament with the intent of supporting the divine mission of Moses.

1873. Carter, Francis (fl.1785-1790). An Account of the Various Systems of Medicine, from the Days of Hippocrates to the Present Time. 2 vols. London, 1788. An M.D., Carter practiced medicine at London; according to the London Monthly Review (41: 1789), "So far is the author from giving an account of the various systems. . .that he wholly omits several, touches but slightly on a few, and fully explains only one system, viz., that of Dr. [John] Brown [1735-1788; see #42]. Dr. Carter seems no less inclined to abuse, than was his late friend Dr. B. [see #43]; but he abuses with less art and less keenness. We shall conclude with an humble hint to the defenders of the Bruonian doctrine: a weak cause requires a strong advocate; but we have not observed that any very powerful champion hath not yet entered the lists in favour of the opinions maintained by the late Dr. Brown" (see Allibone 1: 348).

1874. Clinch, William (fl.1720-1750). Historiae Medicae. London, 1733. 63pp. An M.D., the writer published various medical tracts between 1724 and 1750.

1875. _____. An Historical Essay on the Rise and Progress of the Small-Pox. London, 1725. 20pp.

1876. Davidson, Samuel (fl.1790-1800). The History of Medicine; and a Review of. . .Prevailing Theories on Fevers. Newcastle-upon-Tyne, 1791. 150pp. See, also, #569.

1877. Davis, Richard (fl.1785-1795). An Important Narrative of Facts. . .on the History of the Royal Malady. London, 1789. 56pp. The writer also published, in 1794, a survey of agricultural activity throughout Oxfordshire.

1878. Dover, Thomas (1662-1742). The Ancient Physician's Legacy to His Country. London, 1732. 155pp.; eight eds. through 1771 (see #1871). See, also, #420.

1879. Farr, Samuel (1741-1795). The History of Epidemics, by Hippocrates, in seven books; translated from the Greek, with Notes and Observations. London, 1781. See, also, #1564. One needs to keep in mind, obviously, that in all likelihood none of the books preserved under the name of Hippocrates can be labeled as genuine; rather, those works came to Alexandria as the remnants of medical literature which had circulated in the fifth and fourth

History, Biography, Institutions, References 217

History (contd.)

centuries and had been attributed to Hippocrates on the basis of accepted Hippocratic doctrine from the previous historical periods; for concise discussion of this issue and bibliographic guides, see (as but one source) N.G.L Hammond and H.H. Scullard (eds.), The Oxford Classical Dictionary, 2nd ed. (Oxford: At the Clarendon Press, 1970) 518-519, 660-664.

1880. Ferrier, John (1761-1815). Medical Histories and Reflections. 3 vols. Warrington, 1792-1798. See, also, #428.

1881. Fothergill, John (1712-1780). An Essay on the Character of the Late Alexander Russell. London, 1770. 19pp. See, also, #112, #224. Actually, this short piece contains as much medical history as it does biography.

1882. Freeman, Samuel (fl.1780-1785). An Address relative to the Universal Medicine of the Ancient Magi. London, 1781. An M.D., the writer practiced medicine and lectured at London.

1883. Freind, John (1675-1728). The History of Physick, from the Time of Galen to the Beginning of the Sixteenth Century. Parts 1-2. London, 1725-1726; 2 vols., London, 1727; 2 vols., London, 1758; Latin translation by Dr. John Wigan (1696-1739; see, also, #974, #116), under the title Historia Medicinae a Galeni Tempore usque ad Initium Saeculi Decimi Sexti (London, 1733); Latin eds. at Venice, 1733, and again at Venice, 1735. Scholars continued to believe, well into the twentieth century, that Freind's History stood as a classic example of extensive learning and as the best treatment of the subject for the period covered by the writer; see, also, #115-#116, #1903.

1884. Glass, Thomas (d.1786). An Account of the Antient Baths; and their Use in Physick. London, 1752. 42pp. See, also, #923.

1885. Good, John Mason (1764-1827). The History of Medicine as far as it relates to the Profession of an Apothecary. London, 1795. 239pp.; 2nd ed., London, 1796. The writer produced this piece at the request of certain members of the Pharmaceutic Association, the intent being to improve the education of illiterate and mistake-prone apothecaries; born at Epping, Good studied medicine at London and associated himself with the Physical Society of Guy's Hospital; he wrote frequently on miscellaneous and medical subjects, in addition to lecturing and practicing medicine; he received the M.D. degree in 1820 from Marischal College, Aberdeen.

1886. Goodall, Charles (1642-1712). The Royal College of Physicians of London founded and established by Law. London, 1684. The writer presents an account of all of the acts of Parliament, royal charters, and judicial decisions that established the College of Physicians; born at Suffolk, Goodall studied

History (contd.)

medicine at Leyden and received the M.D. degree from Cambridge in 1670; his association with the College of Physicians dated from 1676; from 1691 until his death, he served as a physician to the Charterhouse, London.

1887. Harle, Jonathan (fl.1725-1730). An Historical Essay on the State of Physick in the Old and New Testaments and the Apocryphal Interval. London, 1729. 179pp. An M.D., the writer practiced physic in London.

1888. James, Robert (1703-1776). A Medical Dictionary; including Physic, Surgery, Anatomy, Chymistry, and Botany, in all the Branches relative to Medicine. Together with a History of Drugs; an Account of their various Preparations, Combinations, and Uses; and an Introductory Preface, Tracing the Progress of Physic, and Explaining the Theories which have principally prevail'd in all Ages of the World. 3 vols. London, 1743-1745. Samuel Johnson assisted James in writing the proposals for this work; he also provided a number of entries and may even have written the dedication to Dr. Richard Mead. See, also, #936.

1889. Lettsom, John Coakley (1744-1815). A History of the Origin of Medicine, an Oration at the Medical Society. London, 1778; a French translation at Paris, 1787. See, also, #160.

1890. Mackenzie, James (1680?-1761). The History of Health and the Art of Preserving It. Edinburgh, 1758. 436pp.; three eds. through 1760; a French translation, The Hague, 1759. This work begins with an account of human beings' food before the fall from Eden, then follows with summaries for general health, as set forth by prominent physicians (beginning with Moses!); the writer also includes biographical, anecdotal, and professional notes on a variety of Continental and British medical practitioners; Mackenzie studied at Edinburgh and Leyden and later practiced at Worcester; he served as an attending physician at the Worcester Infirmary.

1891. Mead, Richard (1673-1754). Medicina Sacra, deu de Morbis Insignioribus qui in Biblis Memorantur. London, 1749. The writer explains various diseases mentioned in Holy Scriptures: Job's disease being elephantiasis, Saul suffering from melancholia, Jehoram from dysentery, Hezekiah from an abscess, Nebuchadnezzar from hypochondriasis; further, various Biblical personages demonstrated effects from leprosy, palsy, and Demoniacal possession; see, also, #176.

1892. ____. Oratio Anniversaria Harveiana. . .1723. . . Dissertatio de Nummis quibusdam a Smyrnaeis in Medicorum honorem Percussis. London, 1724. 56pp. This volume includes three pages of engravings of coins; Mead initially explicates a tract on coins

History, Biography, Institutions, References   219

History (contd.)

by Edmund Chishull (d.1733)--chaplain of the English factory at Smyrna (1698-1705), vicar of Walthamstow (1711), and rector of South Church, Essex (1731-1733)--within the context of the controversies over the status of physicians in the ancient world; further, Mead defends the position of physicians in Greece and Rome, arguing that they stood as honored and (often) wealthy members of ancient society; the argument receives support from the writer's reliance upon passages from the classics and from representations of physicians on coins and medals.

1893. Middleton, Conyers (1683-1750). A Dissertation on the State of Physicians among the Old Romans. London, 1734. 41pp. An native of York, educated at Trinity College, Cambridge, and appointed (1706) a fellow of that College, Middleton became the principal librarian of the University library at Cambridge; toward the end of his life, he received the living at Hascomb, Surrey; he appears to have spent his entire mature life embroiled in literary controversy; his most noteworthy pieces include a Letter from Rome (1729), a life of Cicero (1741), and his Free Inquiry into the Miraculous Powers which are supposed to have subsisted in the Christian Church (1749); in the last title, he attacked the authenticity of post-apostolic miracles, bringing about considerable debate.

1894. Northcote, William (d.1783). A Concise History of Anatomy. London, 1772. See, also, #342, #480.

1895. Quincy, John (d.1722). Loimalogia; or, an Historical Account of the Plague in London in 1665. London, 1720; 3rd ed., London, 1721. See, also, #210.

1896. Ranby, John (1703-1773). An Introduction to the History of Physick and Surgery. London, 1752. See, also, #775.

1897. Riollay, Francis (1748-1797). The Doctrine and Practice of Hippocrates in Surgery and Physick. London, 1783. This work exists as an abstract of the Hippocratic canon, in addition to being a complete translation of Hippocrates' aphorisms; see, also, #958.

1898. Rutty, John (1698-1775). A Chronological History of the Weather and Seasons and of the Prevailing Diseases, in Dublin, for Forty Years [1730-1770]. Dublin, 1770. See, also, #226.

1899. Salmon, William (1644-1713). Iatrica: seu Praxis Mendendi. The Practice of Curing Diseases. Being a Medicinal History of near two hundred Famous Observations in the Cure of Diseases, performed by the Author hereof. . . . London, 1681; 2nd ed., London, 1684; 3rd ed., London, 1694. This large work (the third edition extended to 796 pages and included an index, a catalogue of medicaments, and an appendix) bears a dedication to Charles II; see, also, #227.

History (contd.)

1900. Smith, John (1630-1669). King Solomon's Portraiture of Old Age: wherein is contained a Sacred Anatomy both of Soul and Body, a Perfect Account of the Infirmities of Age incident to them both, and in those Mystical and Aenigmatical Symptoms expressed in the six former Verses of the Twelfth Chapter of Ecclesiastes. London, 1666; 2nd ed., London, 1676; 3rd ed., London, 1752. Born in Buckinghamshire, Smith gained admission, as a commoner, to Brasenose College, Oxford (1647); he received the M.D. degree from Oxford; in this curious piece, the writer argues that King Solomon knew about the circulation of the blood and that both the Old Testament monarch and William Harvey stood in perfect agreement relative to that phenomenon.

1901. Templeman, Peter (1711-1769). Curious Remarks and Observations in Physic, Anatomy, Chirurgery, Chemistry, Botany, and Medicine. Extracted from the History and Memoirs of the Royal Academy of Sciences at Paris. 2 vols. London, 1743-1754. The writer studied medicine at Leyden (M.D. 1737); two years later (1739), he came to London to practice medicine, but became interested more in general learning and literature; he associated himself with the British Museum, the Society of Arts, Manufacturers, and Commerce, the Royal Academy of Sciences at Paris, and the Economical Society at Berne.

1902. Walker, Richard (fl.1789-1806). Memoirs of Medicine; including a Sketch of Medical History. London, 1799. 250pp. The writer produced tracts on such curious subjects as the production of artificial cold (1796) and on carrots for curing ulcers and sores (1806).

1903. Wintringham, Clifton the elder (1689-1748). Observations on Dr. [John] Freind's History of Physick. York, 1726. This piece published anonymously; see, also, #1883 and #280.

B. Biography

1904. Adair, James Makittrick (1728-1802). Anecdotes of the Life, Adventures, and Vindication of a Medical Character Morally Defunct. . .by Benjamin Goosequill and Peter Paragraph. London, 1790. 370pp. See, also, #360. This work, although technically biographical, represents one of several of the writer's efforts to eliminate quackery from the medical profession through direct satirical assault upon those whom he believed to be incompetent practitioners.

1905. Aiken, John (1747-1822). Biographical Memoirs of Medicine in Great Britain, from the Revival of Literature to the Time of [William] Harvey. London, 1780. 338pp. The writer studied medicine at Edinburgh and surgery at London, receiving the

History, Biography, Institutions, References   221

          Biography (contd.)
                M.D. degree from Leyden; he practiced at Chester,
                Warrington, Great Yarmouth, and London; in the
                English capital, he turned his attention to
                literature and literary scholarship, particularly
                biography; his sister, Anna Letitia Aiken Barbauld
                (1743-1825), published poetry, hymns, and
                literature for children; his daughter, Lucy Aiken
                (1747-1822), became a noted literary biographer and
                respectable poet.
1906.   ____. A Specimen of the Medical Biography of Great
                Britain. London, 1775. 28pp. This work stands,
                essentially, as a prospectus for #1905.
1907. Alcock, Thomas (1709-1771). Some Memoirs of the Life
                of Dr. Nathan Alcock. London, 1780. 64pp. See,
                also, #1444. Nathan Alcock lectured at Oxford on
                anatomy.
1908. Burton, William (1703?-1750). An Account of the Life
                and Writings of Hermann Boerhaave. London, 1743.
                226pp.; 2n ed., London, 1746. 226pp. The second
                edition includes a dedication to Sir Hans Sloane;
                concerning Boerhaave, see, particularly, #385;
                Burton, an M.D., practiced medicine at Windsor and
                published essays on such subjects as vipers and
                internal cancers.
1909. Duncan, Andrew (1744-1828). An Account of the Life
                and Writings of the Late Alexr. Monro, Senr.
                Edinburgh, 1780. 39pp. Concerning Duncan, see #421;
                for Monro, see #616, #1009.
1910.   ____. An Account of the Life, Writings, and Character
                of the Late Dr. John Hope. Edinburgh, 1789. 31pp.
                Born at Edinburgh, John Hope (1725-1786) studied
                medicine at Edinburgh and Glasgow (M.D. 1750); he
                practiced at Edinburgh and gained admittance to the
                College of Physicians of that city; his interests
                focused upon botany, resulting in his rise to the
                professorship of botany and materia medica at
                Edinburgh; he became the King's botanist for
                Scotland and superintendent of the Royal Garden at
                Edinburgh.
1911. Foot, Jesse (1744-1826). The Life of John Hunter.
                London, 1794. 287pp. See, also, #1104, #5, #199.
1912. Hird, William (fl.1750-1785). An Affectionate Tribute
                to the Memory of the Late Dr. John Fothergill.
                London, 1781. 29pp. See, also, #112, #858.
1913. Hutchinson, Benjamin (fl.1785-1800). Biographia
                Medica: or, Memoirs of Eminent Medical Characters,
                from the Earliest Account to the Present Period,
                with a Catalogue of Their Works. 2 vols. London,
                1789; 2nd ed., London, 1799. The writer belonged
                to the Company of Surgeons at London.
1914. James, Robert (1703-1776). A Medical Dictionary. . .
                3 vols. London, 1743-1745. This encyclopaedic
                work contains significant biographical material;
                see, particularly, #1888 for the complete title.
1915. Leman, Sir Tanfield (fl.1750-1760). Some Memoirs of
                the Life and Writings of the Late Dr. Richard Mead.

Biography (contd.)

London, 1755. 49pp. See, also, #115, #176.
1916. Lettsom, John Coakley (1744-1815). Some Account of the Late Dr. John Fothergill. London, 1783. See, also, #160, #112, #850.
1917. Maty, Matthew (1718-1776). Authentic Memoirs of the Life of Richard Mead. London, 1755. 64pp. Born near Utrecht, the writer studied at Leyden (Ph.D. 1740; M.D. 1740); he came to London in 1741 and established a medical practice in that city; eventually, he rose to become a prominent essayist and biographer, as well as the principal librarian of the British Museum.
1918. Pittis, William (1674-1724). Some Memoirs of the Life of John Radcliffe, M.D. London, 1715. 96pp. The writer graduated from Winchester School and from New College, Oxford; he achieved a reputation as a man of letters: as essayist, poet, historian, and biographer; concerning Radcliffe, see #491.
1919. A Short Account of the Late Dr. John Parsons, Professor of Anatomy in the University of Oxford. Edinburgh, 1786. 24pp.
1920. A Sketch of the Life and Character of the Late Dr. Monsey. London, 1789. 86pp.
1921. Stover, Dietrich Heinrich (1767-1822). The Life of Sir Charles Linnaeus. London, 1794. 435pp. See, also, #502.
1922. Thompson, Gilbert (1728-1803). Memoirs of. . .Dr. John Fothergill. London, 1782. 45pp. Thompson, a Lancashire born Quaker, maintained a school in Lancaster; he then went off to Edinburgh to study medicine, receiving the M.D. there in 1753; he then practiced at London; for Fothergill, see #112, #850.

C. Hospitals, Institutions, and Organizations

1923. An Account of the British Lying-in Hospital for Married Women, in Brownlow Street. London, 1763. 31pp.
1924. An Account of the General Dispensary for the Relief of the Poor, instituted, 1770. London, 1774. 48pp.
1925. An Account of the Hospital for the Maintenance and Education of Exposed and Deserted Young Children. London, 1749. 82pp.
1926. An Account of the Lying-in Charity for Delivering Poor Married Women at their own Habitations. London, 1772. 62pp.
1927. An Account of the Progress made in rebuilding the College of Edinburgh. Edinburgh, 1791. 11pp.
1928. An Account of the Rise and Establishment of the Infirmary, or Hospital for Sick-Poor erected at Edinburgh. Edinburgh, 1730. 32pp.
1929. An Account of the Rise, Progress, and Present State of the Magdalen Charity Hospital. London, 1761.
1930. An Account of the Rise, Progress, and State of the British Lying-in Hospital. London, 1756. 42pp.

History, Biography, Institutions, References   223

            Hospitals, Institutions, and Organizations (contd.)

                 56pp.; four eds. through 1770.
1931. Aiken, John (1747-1822). Thoughts on Hospitals.
      London, 1771. 98pp. See, also, #5, #1905.
1932. Baylies, William (1724-1787). An Historical Account
      of the General Hospital at Bath. London, 1758.
      140pp. See, also, #556, #985.
1933. Bellers, John (1654-1725). An Epistle to Friends on
      the Yearly, Quarterly, and Monthly Meetings,
      concerning the Prisoners and Sick, in the Prisons
      and Hospitals of Great Britain. London, 1724. A
      philanthropist and a member of the Society of
      Friends, the writer lived both in London and in the
      Gloucestershire countryside; he spent most of time
      proposing social reforms, which brought him into
      contact with such various figures of the day as
      William Penn and Sir Hans Sloan; the editor's
      writings generally propose schemes for political
      reform.
1934. Blizard, Sir William (1743-1835). Suggestions for the
      Improvement of Hospitals and Other Charitable
      Institutions. London, 1796. See, also, #35.
1935. Bowen, Thomas (1749-1800). An Historical Account of
      the Origin, Progress, and Present State of Bethlem
      [sic] Hospital. London, 1783. 16pp.; 2nd ed.,
      London, 1784. 1600; a French ed., Paris, 1787.
      56pp. The writer, a Churchman, published a collec-
      tion of his of sermons (1798-1799) and tracts
      urging moral discipline of and religious
      instruction for prisoners (1777-1798).
1936. A Brief Account of the Hospital of St. Elizabeth,
      annexed to the Imperial Monastery of St. Maximum
      the Benedictine. London, 1786. 112pp.
1937. The Celestial Beds: or, A Review of the Voteries of
      the Temple of Health, Adelphi, and the Temple of
      Hymen, Pall Mall. London, 1781. 34pp. Both of
      these "institutions" stood as examples of the less
      legitimate but nonetheless extremely popular
      clinics of the day.
1938. Charleton, Rice (1710-1789). Observations of Cases of
      Patients admitted into the Hospital at Bath. Bath,
      1776. 104pp. See, also, #563.
1939. Cooke, John (1738-1823) and John Maule (fl.1785-1795).
      An Historical Account of the Royal Hospital for
      Seamen at Greenwich. London, 1789. 142pp. Cooke
      appears to have published sermons and accounts of
      others' travels; Sir Christopher Wren and Nicholas
      Hawksmoor built, during 1696-1715, the Greenwich
      Hospital for naval pensioners; the Royal Navy
      College occupied the buildings in 1873.
1940. Dimsdale, Thomas (1712-1800). Observations on the
      Introduction to the Plan for the Dispensary for
      General Inoculation. London, 1778. 136pp. See,
      also, #1035.
1941. Directions and Prayers for the Use of the Patients in
      the Foul Wards of the Hospital in Southwark.
      London, 1734. 24pp.

Hospitals, Institutions, and Organizations (contd.)

1942. Duncan, Andrew (1744-1828). Observations on a Proposal for Establishing at Edinburgh a Public Disepnsary. Edinburgh, 1777. 60pp. See, also, #421.
1943. Eccles, William (fl.1695-1722). An Historical Account of the Rights and Privileges of the Royal College of Physicians and of the Incorporation of Chirurgions in Edinburgh. Edinburgh, 1707. 55pp.
1944. Explanatory Remarks on the Great Utility of Hospitals for the Sick and Poor. Cambridge, 1776. 18pp.
1945. Foster, Edward (d.1780). An Essay on Hospitals. Dublin, 1768. 39pp. See, also, #1741.
1946. Good, John Mason (1764-1827). A Dissertation on the Diseases of Prisons and Poor-Houses. London, 1795. 180pp. See, also, #1885. This tract earned, for the writer, the Lettsome Prize of twenty guineas.
1947. Grimston, Henry (fl.1790-1805). A Short Account of Various Charitable Institutions in Great Britain for the benefit of the Poor and the Infirm. London, 1794. The writer also published an essay on metallic tractors (1804, 1805).
1948. Howard, John (1726?-1790). An Account of the Present State of the Prisons, Houses of Corrections, and Hospitals in London and Westminster. London, 1789. Howard served and contributed as the significant philanthropist and prison reformer of the eighteenth century; he really had no association with the medical profession; in 1777, he visited every prison in Great Britain, publishing the results of his investigations in that same year.
1949. Lee, Samuel ((fl.1750-1775). A Proper Reply to the Serjeant Surgeons Defense of Their Conduct at Chelsea Hospital. London, 1754. 75pp.
1950. Lettsome, John Coakley (1744-1815). Medical Memoirs of the General Dispensary. London, 1774. 362pp. See, also, #160.
1951. Millar, John (1733-1805). Observations on the Practice of the Medical Department of the Westminster General Dispensary. London, 1777. 77pp. See, also, #1162.
1952. The Modern Practice of the London Hospitals, viz., St. Bartholomew's, St. Thomas's, St. George's, and Guy's. London, 1764. 155pp.; 2nd ed., London, 1766. This work includes lists of diets, materia medica, diseases, and treatments of ailments.
1953. A Narrative of Some Proceedings in the Management of Chelsea Hospital. London, 1753. 95pp. Situated on Royal Hospital Road, Chelsea Hospital owes its origins to Charles II, who established the facility for veteran soldiers and appointed Sir Christopher Wren as the architect; Wren constructed the place around three courtyards, and in the center there was placed a statue to Charles II; see The London Encyclopaedia, ed. Ben Weinreb and Christopher Hibbert (Bethesda, Maryland: Adler and Adler), 145-156.

History, Biography, Institutions, References   225

Hospitals, Institutions, and Organizations (contd.)

1954. The Necessity and Usefulness of the Dispensaries lately set up by the College of Physicians in London. London, 1702. 18pp.
1955. Nolan, William (fl.1780-1790). An Essay on Humanity; or, A View of Abuses in Hospitals. London, 1786. 49pp.
1956. Parkinson, James (d.1824). The Hospital Pupil, in Four Letters. London, 1800. The writer began his medical practice prior to 1785, and in that year he attended lectures on surgery delivered by John Hunter; he involved himself in political disputes relative to an attempt to assassinate George III; then, he turned his attention upon chemistry and paleontology; as late as 1811, Parkinson continued to practice medicine at London.
1957. The Practice of the British and French Hospitals. London, 1773. 348pp.; 2nd ed., London, 1775.
1958. The Present State of Dr. Steevens's Hospital, together with a Scheme to enlarge the Fund. Dublin, 1735. A broadside. The hospital had been in existence since 1720, founded by Dr. Richard Steevens and his sister, Griselda; on Thursday, 20 July 1749, John Wesley visited the institution, observing it to have been "far cleaner and sweeter than any I had seen in London. . ." (see The Works of John Wesley. Volume 20. Journal and Diaries, II (1743-1754), ed. W. Reginald Ward and Richard P. Heitzenrater [Nashville, Tennessee: Abingdon Press, 1991] 285).
1959. Reasons for the Establishing and Further Encouragement of St. Luke's Hospital for Lunaticks. London, 1797. 44pp. St. Luke's had functioned, since 1751, as a hospital for the insane.
1960. Rules and Orders for the Government of the Royal Hospitals of Bridewell and Bethlem. London, 1778. 77pp. Prior to 1775, Bridewell stood as the only prison in London to have its own medical staff.
1961. A Short Account of the Institution, Plan, and Present State of the New General Lying-in Hospital. London, 1786. 16pp.

D. Dictionaries, Glossaries, and General References

1962. Barrow, John (fl.1745-1770). Dictionarium Medicum Universale; or, A Dictionary, containing an Explanation of all the Terms used in Physick. London, 1749. See, also, #21.
1963. Bibliotheca Anatomica, Medica. . .containing a Description of the several parts of the body, each done by some eminent Physician or Chiurgeon, wherein all are the Tracts of use that are in the second edition of the Bibliotheca Anatomica of Clericus and Magentus, and many Others. 3 vols. London, 1711-1714.
1964. Blanchard, Stephen (fl.1700-1710). The Physical Dictionary. London, n.d. five eds, through 1708.
1965. Hooper, Robert (1773-1825). A Compendius Medical

Dictionaries, Glossaries, and References (contd.)

Dictionary, containing an Explanation of the Terms in Anatomy, Physiology, and Surgery. London, 1798; six eds. through 1831. Born in London and educated (B.A., M.B.) at Oxford, Hoover received the M.D. degree from St. Andrews in 1805; he practiced medicine and lectured on that subject, specializing in pathology.

1966. James, Robert (1703-1776). A Medical Dictionary. . . 3 vols., London, 1743-1745. See, also, #1888 for the complete title.

1967. Motherby, George (1732-1793). A New Medical Dictionary. London, 1776; 2nd ed., London, 1785; 3rd. ed., London, 1791; 4th ed., 2 vols., London, 1795; another ed., London, 1801; eds. of 1795 and 1801 revised and edited by Dr. George Walls (see #269); born in Yorkshire, Motherby practiced medicine at Highgate, Middlesex.

1968. Prosodia Chirurgica: being a Lexicon Calculated for the use of Young Students in Surgery. London, 1729. 174pp.

1969. Quincy, John (d.1722). Lexicon Physico-Medicum; or, A New Medical Dictionary. London, 1717; 4th ed., London, 1730; 6th ed., London, 1736; 8th ed., London, 1767; a revised ed., London, 1794; a total of eleven eds. through 1811. The writer dedicated this work to John, Duke of Montagu, who had just been admitted (1717) a fellow of the College of Physicians at London; it closely parallels the lexicon of Bartholomew Castellus (Basle, 1628); see, also, #210.

1970. Turton, William (1762-1835). A Medical Glossary. London, 1797; 2nd ed., London, 1802. A native of Olveston, Gloucestershire, Turton practiced medicine at Swansea and devoted his spare hours to the study of natural history; he then moved on to Dublin, Teignmouth, Torquay, and Bideford; he also wrote tracts upon consumption and devoted his efforts to publishing the results of his studies on shells.

XXII

Medical Conditions outside Britain

1971. Anderson, James (d.1826). *A Few Facts and Observations on the Yellow Fever of the West Indies.* Edinburgh, 1798. 47pp.

1972. Baylies, William (1724-1787). *Facts and Observations Relative to the Inoculation of the Small Pox at Berlin.* Edinburgh, 1781. See, also, #556, #985.

1973. Bradley, Richard (1688-1732). *The Plague at Marseilles.* London, 1721. 60pp.; three eds. in 1721. See, also, #37.

1974. Chalmers, Lionel (1715?-1777). *An Account of the Weather and Diseases of South Carolina.* 2 vols. London, 1776. See, also, #896.

1975. Clark, James (d.1819). *A Treatise on the Yellow Fever, as it Appeared in the Island of Dominica.* London, 1797. 168pp. The writer practiced medicine for twenty-five years at Dominica; elected a fellow of the Royal College of Physicians at Edinburgh, he also published widely on fevers associated with the West Indies.

1976. Clark, John (1744-1805). *Observations on the Diseases in Long Voyages to Hot Countries.* London, 1773. 366pp.; 2nd ed., 2 vols., London, 1792. See, also, #900.

1977. Cleghorn, George (1716-1787). *Observations on the Epidemical Diseases in Minorca, from the Year 1744 to 1749.* London, 1751; four eds. through 1779. The writer provides an accurate account of several diseases and conditions that no one had previously observed and recorded; yellow jaundice proves the most graphic; further, the volume contains descriptions of several post-mortems; a native of Edinburgh and an M.D., Cleghorn resided on Minorca for thirteen years as a surgeon for the Thirteenth Regiment; his published works, according to Dr. John Fothergill, proved a model for future writers (see Allibone 1:395).

1978. Coxe, William (1747-1828). *An Account of the Prisons* and Hospitals in Russia, Sweden, and Denmark. London, 1781. 55pp. A native of London, the writer became a fellow of King's College (1768), curate of Denham (1771), rector of Bemerton (1778), canon-residentiary of Salisbury, archdeacon of Wilts, and chaplain of the Tower of London; he traveled widely on the Continent with young members of the nobility, and published a number of narratives relative to those journeys (including this volume).

1979. Gillespie, Leonard (fl.1790-1800). Observations on the Diseases...on the Leeward Island Station. London, 1800. 239pp. The writer held the M.D. degree.

1980. Girdleston, Thomas (1758-1822). An Essay on the Hepatitis and Spasmodic Affections in India. London, 1787. 65pp. See, also, #1516.

1981. Grainger, James (1723?-1767). An Essay on the More Common West Indian Diseases; and the Remedies which that Country Itself Produces. London, 1764. 75pp. See, also, #924.

1982. Harrison, John (fl.1740-1750). A Short Comparative View of the Practice of Surgery in the French Hospitals. London, 1750. 56pp. The writer, an M.D., practiced as a surgeon.

1983. Hendy, James (fl.1774-1790). A Treatise on the Glandular Diseases of Barbadoes. London, 1784. 140pp. The writer held the M.D. degree; see, also #1995.

1984. Hilary, William (d. 1763). Observations on the Changes of the Air and the Concomitant Epidemical Diseases, in the Island of Barbadoes. London, 1759. 360pp.; 2nd ed., London, 1766. 360pp. See, also, #141.

1985. Ingram, Dale (1710-1793). An Historical Account of the Several Plagues that have appeared in the World. London, 1755. 208pp. See, also, #454.

1986. Johnson, Alexander (1716-1799). A Short Account of a Society at Amsterdam...for the Recovery of Drowned Persons. London, 1773. 138pp. The writer held the M.D. degree.

1987. Lind, James (1716-1794). An Essay on Diseases Incidental to Europeans in Hot Climates. London, 1768. 348pp.; 5 eds. through 1792. See, also, #942.

1988. Lind, James (1736-1812). A Treatise on the Putrid and Remitting Marsh Fever, which raged at Bengal. Edinburgh, 1776. 70pp. This Scottish surgeon received the M.D. from Edinburgh in 1768 and served with the East India Company; his interests included astronomy and observations of various fevers; in 1777 he settled at Windsor as a physician to the royal household; his associations included Dr. Charles Burney and the young Percy Bysshe Shelley.

1989. Mathews, Stephen (fl.1780-1785). Observations on Hepatic Diseases Incidental to Europeans in the East-Indies. London, 1783. 214pp.; another ed. in 1785.

1990. Milligen, George (fl.1745-1775). A Short Description

of the Province of South-Carolina, with an Account of the Air, Weather, and Diseases at Charles-town. London, 1770. 96pp.
1991. Monchy, Solomon de (1716-1794). An Essay on the Causes and Cure of the Usual Diseases in Voyages to the West-Indies. London, 1762. 175pp.
1992. A New Discovery of the Nature of the Plague, and the true cause of its Raging in European Cities. London, 1721. 64pp.
1993. Quier, John (b.1740; fl.1770-1780). Letters and Essays on the Small-Pox and Inoculation, the Measles. . .and Intermitting Fevers of the West Indies. London, 1778. The writer also published tracts on small pox and inoculation; these letters had been written to Donald Monro (see #473), who compiled them for publication
1994. Robertson, Robert (1742-1829). Observations on Fevers and Other Diseases which occur on Voyages to Africa and the West Indies. London, 1792. 196pp. See, also, #960.
1995. Rollo, John (d.1809). Remarks on the Diseases lately described by Dr. [James] Hendy. London, 1785. The disease in question proved to have been elephantiasis, then known as "Barbadoes leg"; see, also, #1442; James Hendy, a London physician and M.D., published medical tracts between 1774 and 1790 (see #1983).
1996. ____. A Treatise on Health in the West Indies. London, 1782.
1997. Tennent, John (fl.1700-1742). An Epistle to Dr. Richard Mead concerning the Epidemical Diseases of Virginia. Edinburgh, 1738; 2nd ed., Edinburgh, 1742. 102pp. The writer practiced medicine in Virginia; in this same year, he published (also at Edinburgh) a second epistle to Richard Mead concerning the . . .Bite of a Viper and Its Poison.
1998. Tolver, Alexander (fl.1750-1770). A Treatise on the Present State of Midwifery at Paris. London, 1770. 83pp. See, also, #1677.
1999. Towne, Richard (fl.1725-1750). A Treatise of the Diseases Most Frequent in the West Indies. London, 1726. 192pp; a second ed. at London in 1747.
2000. Trapham, Thomas (fl.1675-1680). An Essay on the State of Health in Jamaica. London, 1679.
2001. Turner, George (fl.1730-1735). A Treatise on the Mineral Waters of Piedmont; from Scippius. London, 1733. The translator held the M.D. degree.
2002. Wade, John Peter (fl.1790-1795; d.1802). An Essay on the Nature of Emetics in Bengal. London, 1792. See, also, #1865.
2003. ____. Select Evidence on Fever and Dysentery in Bengal. London, 1791.
2004. Warren, Henry (fl.1735-1745). A Treatise concerning the Malignant Fever of the Barbadoes. London, 1740. 75pp. The writer held the M.D. degree.
2005. Williams, John (fl.1770-1780). Select Cases in Physick, which have been treated at the Waters of Aix-la-Chapelle. London, 1774. 136pp. See, also,

2006. ____. A Treatise on the Medicinal Virtues of the Mineral Waters of the German Spa. London, 1773.
2007. ____. A Treatise of the Medicinal Virtues of the Waters of Aix-la-Chapelle and Borset. London, 1772. See, also, #658-#659.
2008. Wise, Richard fl.1795-1800). An Hour's Advice to Persons going out to Jamaica, respecting their Health. London, 1798.

XXIII

Professional Concerns

2009. An Account of a Medical Controversy in the City of Cork, in which Five Physicians are Engaged. London, 1749. 60pp.
2010. An Address to the College of Physicians. . . .occasioned by the late Swarms of Scotch and Leyden Physicians. London, 1747. The Royal College of Physicians "jealously guarded" the social prestige of English physicians, admitting only graduates of Oxford, Cambridge, and Trinity College, Dublin, as fellows; it enrolled graduates from other institutions (principally from Scotland, Holland, and Italy, and France) as licentiates; although such universities as Edinburgh and Leyden furnished instruction in medicine that proved superior to that of the English universities, the sons of gentlemen went to Oxford and Cambridge, while students from the middle class attended the foreign institutions (see W.A. Speck, Stability and Strife. England, 1714-1760 [Cambridge, Massachusetts: Harvard University Press, 1977] 50).
2011. Byfield, Timothy (fl.1715-1725). The Devil and the Doctor. London, 1719. 111pp. A poem and a reissue of #2012.
2012. ____. Mandragora; or, The Quacks: A Poem. London, 1717. 111pp. See, also, #2011.
2013. The Case of the Licentiates and the College of Physicians. London, 1796. 11pp.
2014. Celer, Lypsonius (fl.1695-1700). The Late Censors Deservedly Censur'd. London, 1696. The writer, an M.D. who practiced in London, describes the situation of a Dr. Jan Greenfield (or Groenevelt, 1647-1710), who, among other physicians, filed suit against three censors of the College of Physicians, London, because of their supposedly illegal elections to their offices.
2015. The Censor Censur'd; or, the Antidote Examin'd. Wherein the Designs of Dr. [Robert] Pitt and the

Dispensary Physicians are Detected. London, 1704. 109pp. See, also, #488.

2016. Champney, Thomas (fl.1795-1800). A Dissertation on Medical and Chirurgical Reform. London, 1797. This piece exists as one of several pamphlet arguments against the proposals by the Surgeons' Company to change its by-laws and attempt to become a college; Champney identified himself as a London surgeon, apothecary, and midwife; see, also, #53.

2017. _____. A Review of the Healing Art. London, 1797. The writer calls attention to the business aspects of and activities of the Society of Apothecaries, particularly the profits from the sale and supply of drugs to such bodies of the government as the army, navy, and the East India Company.

2018. A Cheap, Sure, and Ready Guide to Health; or, A Cure for a Disease call'd the Doctor. London, 1742. 36pp.

2019. Chevalier, Thomas (d.1824). Observations in Defence of a Bill. . . . London, 1797. The writer, a London surgeon, defends, in this tract, the right of the Surgeons' Company to apply to Parliament for permission to revise its by-laws.

2020. Cunningham, Timothy (d.1789), ed. The Law of Physicians, Surgeons, and Apothecaries: containing all the Statutes, Cases at Large, Arguments, Resolutions, and Judgments concerning Them. London, 1767. 109pp. A London lawyer, Cunningham published tracts on the relationship between laws and the constitution, pleadings, the inns of court and chancery, and the laws of simony; he also compiled a legal dictionary.

2021. Dease, William (1752?-1798). Remarks on Medical Jurisprudence. Dublin, 1793. 32pp. See, also, #737.

2022. Discriminator (pseudonym). The Apothecary's Mirror; or, the Present State of Pharmacy Exploded. London, 1790. 31pp.

2023. Duncan, Andrew (1744-1828). Heads of Lectures on Medical Jurisprudence. Edinburgh, 1796. 87pp. See, also, #421.

2024. Ellis, John (1698-1790). The Surprise; or, the Gentleman Turn'd Apothecary. London, 1739. 139pp. The writer, a literary hack who labored for money rather than for art, spent most of his time translating Latin verse into English and composing poetical epigrams; he translated The Surprise from a Latin version of the original composed in French prose; For Samuel Johnson, Ellis proved an example of the wonders to be found in London: "The most literary conversation that I ever enjoyed, was at the table of Jack Ellis, a money-scrivener behind the Royal Exchange, with whom I at one period used to dine generally once a week" (Boswell, Life of Johnson, ed. R.W. Chapman; a new edition, ed. J.D. Fleeman [London: Oxford University Press, 1970] 732).

2025. An Essay for Reforming the Modern Way of Practicing Medicine in Edinburgh. Edinburgh, 1727. 30pp.
2026. Ferris, Samuel (1760-1831). A General View of the Establishment of Physic as a Science in England. London, 1795. 168pp. The writer argues, in part, against the legality of the College of Physicians in establishing social and educational priorities for the purpose of licensing physicians; an M.D. from Edinburgh, Ferris practiced physic at London.
2027. Gregory, John (1724-1773). Lectures on the Duties and Qualifications of a Physician. Edinburgh, 1772. This work an expanded ed. of #130; the writer defends the right of those candidates for the degrees of doctor of medicine to study and to observe medical practice outside of the secluded environments of medical colleges (at, for instance, hospitals); he argues, further, that time does not permit the medical student to engage in a variety of studies that may be only peripheral to a doctor's theoretical concerns or actual practice.
2028. Gunning, Richard (fl.1785-1805). A Philippic, or Farewell Address to the Company of Surgeons. London, 1790. The most interesting section of this address, delivered by the writer as the Master of the Surgeon's Company, focuses upon the extravagance (both social and financial) of that institution; Gunning also published (1804) a tract on the small pox.
2029. Harvey, Gideon the elder (1640?-1700?). The House Apothecary. London, 1670. The writer, a physician-in ordinary to Charles II. focuses, in this tract, upon upon the excessive charges and large profits of London apothecaries; see, also, #138.
2030. Hody, Edward (1698-1759). An Attempt to Reconcile all Differences between the Present Fellows and Licentiates of the Royal College of Physicians in London. London, 1753. 15pp. See, also, #742.
2031. Lucas, James (fl.1788-1800). A Candid Inquiry into the Education, Qualifications, and Offices of a Surgeon-Apothecary. Bath, 1800. 356pp.
2032. Maddocks, James (fl.1780-1785) and Sir William Blizard (1743-1835). A Treatise of the Expediency and Utility of Teaching. . .Physick and Surgery by Lectures, at the London Hospital. London, 1783. 10pp. See, also, #35.
2033. Marrett, Christopher (1614-1695). A Short View of the Frauds and Abuses committed by the Apothecaries. London, 1669. The writer contends that a man cannot practice medicine without a university education and a knowledge of the classical literatures, the arts, and philosophy; Marrett (naturally enough) held the M.D. degree from Oxford; see, also, #170.
2034. Observations on the Character and Conduct of a Physician. London, 1722. 155pp.
2035. Parker, Samuel (1681-1730). An Essay upon the Duty of Physicians and Patients. London, 1715. 134pp.

Parker, a scholar and bibliophile, had no formal medical associations; he studied for the Church, but refused to take oaths after the revolution of 1688 and, instead, labored for the Bodleian Library, Oxford.

2036. Stanger, Christopher (1754-1834). An Account of the Proceedings of the Licentiates. London, 1798. Stanger describes the various unsuccessful attempts (including his own) to challenge the legality of the by-laws of the College of Physicians; in the courts, judges decided in favor of the College, although they admitted that the by-laws might easily be improved in terms of admitting physicians; see, also, #255.

2037. ____. A Justification of the Right of every well-educated Physician. . . . London, 1798. See, also, #255, #2036.

2038. Wall, Cecil (fl.1700-1705). Why the Apothecary may be supposed to understand the Administration of Medicines. London, 1704. The writer advances the notion that apothecaries' medical education and knowledge generally had risen to the degree that they could practice medicine as well (or perhaps even better) than a number of physicians.

2039. Withers, Thomas (fl.1772-1794). A Treatise on the Errors and Defects of Medical Education. York, 1794. Written as early as 1774, this tract defends the notion of the physician as a "gentleman" and one who must possess sufficient education so as not to discredit the entire medical profession; Withers served as a physician to the York County Hospital; see, also, #282, #1164.

XXIV

Some Contemporary Medical Periodicals

2040. Annals of Medicine. Edinburgh. 1796-1799. 4 vols, ed. by Andrew Duncan (1744-1828). See, also, #421.
2041. The British Physicians. Treating of Your Diet. London, 1716. This journal, obviously, focused upon health and nutrition.
2042. Every Man's Magazine; or, the Monthly Repository of Science. London, September 1771-December 1772.
2043. The Foreign Medical Review. 2 vols. London, 1779-1780.
2044. Hippocrates Ridens; or, Jaco-Serious Reflections on the Imprudence and Mischief of Quacks and Illiterate Pretenders to Physick. London, 1686.
2045. The History of Cradle-Convulsions, vulgarly called Black and White Fits: or, Monthly Observations on the Weekly Bills of Mortality. With References to the Cure of that mad Distemper. London, 1701. Printed for John Nutt. The first issue bears the date of 1 September 1701. Nutt maintained, from 1690 to 1717, shops at Stationers' Hall, Stationers' Court (London), and at the Savoy; his most noteworthy publication proved to have been Jonathan Swift's Tale of a Tub (1704).
2046. The London Medical Journal. 11 vols. London, 1781-1790. This periodical edited by Samuel Foart Simmons (see #351); it continued as Medical Facts and Observations (see #2049).
2047. The London Medical Review and Magazine. 5 vols. London, 1799-1801. This journal came under the editorship of William Blair (1766-1822; see #1082), the eminent surgeon who became involved in the debate over cow-pox inoculation (see #1845).
2048. Man. A Paper for Enobling the Species. London, 1755. Fifty-two numbers betrween 1 January and 24 December 1755. The journal edited by Peter Shaw (1694-1763); see, also, #234.
2049. Medical Facts and Observations. London, 1791-1800. This serial edited by Samuel Foart Simmons (see

#351); it became the successor to the London Medical Journal (see #2046).
2050. The Medical and Chirurgical Review. London, 1799-1908.
2051. The Medical and Physical Journal. London, 1799-1815. This periodical gave way to the London Medical and Physical Journal, 1815-1826.
2052. The Medical Museum. London, 1781.
2053. The Medical Spectator. 3 vols., 48 numbers. London, 1791-1796.
2054. Medicina Curiosa; or, a Variety of New Communications in Physick and Chiurgery. London, 1684. A Total of twelve numbers of this periodal came forth.
2055. The Midwife; or, Old Woman's Magazine. 3 vols. London, 1750-1753.
2056. Memoirs for the Ingenious, containing several Curious Observations in Philosophy, Mathematicks, Physick, Philology, and Other Arts and Sciences. London, 1693. Edited by John de la Crosse and printed for Henry Rhodes and John Harris; twelve numbers, the first dated 1 January 1693; John Harris (d.1698) sold books in Harrow, in Little Briotain (London), between 1685 and 1698; Henry Rhodes (d.1725) operated several book shops in Fleet Street, London, from 1681 to 1709.
2057. The New London Medical Journal. 2 vols. London, 1792-1793.

Index of Subjects

Numbers refer to entries, not pages

Abscess 1354, 1355
Absorbing vessels 309
Agaric 791, 1569
Ague 458, 510, 966, 967, 968
Air 162, 360 377, 438, 484, 545, 860, 1186, 1829, 1837, 1839, 1867, 1984, 1990
Alcohol 905
Alkaline water 578, 615
Almond water 668
Amber 410
Amputation 715, 716, 762, 765
Anatomy 34, 281, 289-358, 744, 785, 800, 1309, 1525, 1545, 1577, 1748, 1770, 1773, 1806, 1819, 1894, 1901, 1963, 1965
Anemia 1795
Angina Pectoris 1526
Animal Calculi 516
Animal motion 103
Animal substances 419, 434
Ankle 1308
Anodyne 397
Anodyne necklace 397
Antibilious alterative pills 526
Antimony 400, 409, 479
Antiscorbutic drops 481
Apoplexy 1330-1332, 1822
Apothecaries 170, 389, 1846, 1885, 2020, 2024, 2029, 2031, 2033, 2038
Argol 523, 573
Arsenic 1366
Arteries 300, 731, 732, 1525
Arthritis 1107, 1296-1297
Artificial teeth 1670
Asthma 1158-1164, 1183
Astrology 33, 229, 231
Asylums 1959
Autumnal disorders 278

Back 1299-1301
Ball metal 384
"Barbadoes leg" 1995
Bark 460, 505
Bath water 217
Bathing 1507
Beech oil 450
Bible 178, 292
Bile 1423, 1427
Biliary concretions 1420
Biliary duct 1419
Bilious diseases 674, 1418, 1422, 1428 1431
Bilious fever 982, 1424, 1426
Black cherry water 668
Bladder 794, 1379, 1380, 1400, 1401, 1406, 1411, 1414
Bleeding 791, 1114, 1562-1571, 1827
Blindness 1630, 1638
Blood 300, 1540-1561
Blood vessels 765, 1543,

1546
Boarding schools 1795
Bones 297, 302, 354, 1302-1317, 1577
Botany 34, 383, 1901
Bougies 504
Bowels 278, 1447-1452
Brain 348, 1219, 1221, 1222, 1605, 1634
Bread 500, 1480, 1481
Bronchocele 798, 1298
Burial 814
Burns 1612, 1613

Cachexias 82
Caesarean section 1698, 1709, 1710
Calculus 893, 1382
Calomel 608, 946, 947
Camphire 608, 946
Cancer 503, 1107, 1206, 1360, 1453-1567
Canine madness 133, 1342
Cataract 1617, 1621, 1637, 1638, 1639, 1641, 1651, 1654, 1655, 1658, 1660
Catarrh 893, 1154-1155, 1226, 1382, 1437
Catheter 1653
Caustic 1354
Cavities 758
Chalybeate water 497, 551, 604
Chemistry 287, 384, 417, 473, 1901
Childbirth 1680-1716
Children 817, 1061, 1062, 1673, 1782-1803
Cinnabar 1336
Circulation 1545, 1550, 1554, 1561, 1571
Clivers 1492
Club foot 1315
Coffee 841, 1483
Cold 1141-1143
Colic 860, 1361, 1444-1446
Common water 665-683, 905
Congenital hernia 827
Consumption 893, 1159, 1165-1184, 1382, 1564
Contagion 686
Cooking 461
Copper 384, 1365
Coroner 813
Cough 854, 1142
Cowhage 1609
Cow pox 1021-1026, 1073, 1074

Croup 1152, 1153
Crystalline lens 1618
Cutaneous eruptions 587

Dentistry 1128, 1676
Dentition 1673
Dephlogisticated nitrous air 736
Diabetes 642, 1516-1519
Dictionaries 1888, 1914, 1962-1970
Diet 1279, 1488, 1489, 1502, 2041
Digitalis 428, 469, 543
Diptheria 1145
Dislocations 771
Dispensaries 1924, 1940, 1942, 1950, 1951
Dissection 725, 808-813, 1575, 1581
Distemper 699, 1319-1323
Dorsal spasm 1301
Dropsy 233, 947, 1213-1223, 1383, 1490
Drowning 703-709, 1185, 1986
Dysentery 1436-1443, 2003
Dyspepsia 587, 1508

Ear 1634, 2664, 1665
Earth 438, 439
Elastic trochar 816
Elbow 1311
Electric fluid bath 378
Elephantiasis 1995
Embalming 814-815
Emetics 424 2002
Epidemic 31, 836-889, 1879, 1997
Epidemic fever 868, 1977
Epidemical madness 700
Epilepsy 1324-1329
Epiphora 1653
Evacuation 365
Exercise 268, 1479
Expectation 138
Eye disease 1622, 1633, 1642, 1644, 1645, 1646, 1649, 1652, 1659
Eye lids 1626, 1644
Eyes 503, 1615-1663

Farmers 1868
Febricula 948
Fetus 1820
Fever 82, 115, 409, 510, 531, 670, 779, 854, 890-976, 1019, 1159, 1382, 1438, 1832, 1876, 2003,

Index of Subjects

2004
Fistula Lachrymalis 1656, 1661
Flux 1448
Food poisoning 1374
Forceps 1693 1707
Fossils 419, 434
Fractures 713, 771, 792, 793

Gallstones 1431
Gangrene 1378, 1866
Glands 691, 1352, 1983
Glaucoma 1637, 1651
Goiter 1298
Gold 489
Golden purging pills 406
Gonorrhoea 1075, 1076, 1081, 1092, 1093, 1096, 1097, 1103, 1115, 111, 1124, 1126, 1131, 1135
Goose grass 1492
Gout 587, 676, 1228-1287, 1288, 1290, 1409, 1502, 1503
Gravel 518, 1379, 1381, 1389, 1396, 1399, 1409
Gums 1667, 1668
Gunshot wounds 803, 804

Haemorrhage 716, 795, 1808, 1820
Haemorrhoids 1357, 1656
Hair 1606-1608
Hanging 1185
Head 710, 1598-1605
Hearing 1627
Heart 300, 1525-1531
Hectic 642
Hectic fever 919, 928, 1181
Hemlock 366, 519
Hepatitis 1980, 1989
Herbals 382, 398, 471, 514
Herbs 33, 514
Hernia 830
Hip 1305
Hosiery 395
Hospital fever 954, 961, 1854
Hospitals 769, 1837, 1854, 1855, 1867, 1923-1961, 1978, 1982
Hydrocele 816, 823, 824, 826, 831, 832, 833, 834, 1213,1215, 1220
Hydrophobia 1319, 1339, 1345, 1346
Hysteria 1324

Impotence 1692
Inanition 905
Indigestion 1506-1508
Infantile fever 1785
Infants 1782-1803
Infection 388, 683, 942, 1377, 1378
Infirmaries 1928
Inflammation 1348, 1349, 1350, 1555
Influenza 1224-1227
Injection 504
Inoculation 163, 984, 985, 987, 996, 999, 1000, 1006, 1009, 1010, 1013, 1016, 1018, 1027-1074, 1972, 1973
Insanity 1319, 1822
Intermittent fever 498, 904, 947, 949, 1993
Internal balsam 511
Intestines 326, 331, 790
Introsusception 1451
Impecacuanha 1158

Jail distemper 1328
Jail fever 930, 954, 961
Jails/prisons 1837, 1946, 1948, 1978
James's powders 446
Jaundice 1432, 1433
Jesuit powder 52
Joints 297, 1302, 1304, 1347, 1469

Kidneys 1379, 1396
Kinkcough 1156
Knee 1306, 1311

Labor 1684, 1686, 1687, 1688, 1690, 1704, 1714, 1758
Lac 410
Lacteal duct 293
Lacteal sac
Lead 437, 1362, 1371
Leeches 1567
Leg 503, 716, 789, 806, 1314, 1351, 1468, 1470, 1471, 1472
Leyden phial 540
Limbs 1586
Lime water 363, 364, 538
Lithotomy 755, 774
Liver 324, 587, 1418-1431
Lock jaw 1333-1334
Looseness 1447, 1449, 1450
Lumbar abscess 710

Lungs 1166, 1179, 1193-1196
Luxations 713

Magnesia Alba 436, 449, 454
Malignant fevers 839, 861, 882, 888, 899, 943
Malt liquor 1514
Mamma 1458
Marsh fever 1988
Materia medica 5, 6, 37, 81, 161, 203, 238, 416, 421, 423, 465, 473, 474, 490, 1119
Measles 888, 1993
Medical biography 1904-1922
Medical colleges 1927
Medical education 283, 2031, 2032, 2039
Medical history 115, 116, 143, 158, 161, 669, 1869-1903
Medical jurisprudence 102, 153, 2020, 2021, 2023, 2036
Medical periodicals 2041-2057
Medical practice 1-287
Medical profession 2009-2039
Medical references 1962-1970
Melancholy 1533
Membrana Tympani 1664, 1665
Mephytic acid 1400
Mercury 385, 387, 390, 401, 445, 453, 462, 470, 489, 509, 522, 529, 991, 1083, 1102, 1112, 1136, 1138
Meteorology 158
Midwifery 1717-1781
Military fever 31, 1844, 1846, 1848
Milk 1477, 1486
Mineral waters 214, 550-664, 1432, 1593, 1884, 2001, 2005, 2006, 2007
Mines 1837
Mithridatum 448
Multiple birth 1695
Muscles 290, 297, 346, 1302, 1574-1590
Muscular motion 1582, 1583, 1585, 1586, 1588
Music 391
Musk 1336
Myrrh 410

Neck 1604
Necrosis 1312
Nerves 55, 1546, 1591-1597

Nervous diseases 674, 937, 1597
Nervous fevers 882, 937
Nervous system 344, 356, 357
Neuroses 82
Newtonian philosophy 221
Nightshade 392, 433
Nitre 402
Nitrous acid 376, 883, 1079, 1080
Nitrous oxide 736
Nitrous vapor
Nursing 1786, 1797, 1799, 1800, 1824
Nutrition 1476-1489

Obstetrics 1681, 1705
Oils 528
Old age 106, 381, 1900
Olecranon 1313
Oleum arthriticum 1273
Oleum terebinthinae 548, 549
Ophthalmia 1128, 1635, 1643, 1653, 1656, 1657, 1663
Opium 368, 412, 441, 531, 542, 547, 905
Optics 1628
Oxygen 367, 451

Pain 759
Palsy 564, 565, 587, 664, 1318, 1330, 1822
Paralysis 539, 578
Passions 59, 100
Patella 1313
Pathology 235, 317, 318, 779, 893
Pectoral drops 373
Perinaeum 1697
Periosteum 1309
Peritonaeum 313
Perkins' metallic tractors 768
Perspiration 710
Peruvian bark 359, 456, 458, 482, 495, 498, 508, 510, 515, 530
Phagedaena 1360
Pharmacopoeia 195, 370, 371, 372, 379, 404, 413, 414, 430, 431, 432, 443, 464, 478, 480, 487, 490, 491, 520, 535, 769
Pharmacy 213, 417, 418
Phlegmatia dolens 1814
Physiology 235, 289-358, 893, 1965
Plague 394, 697, 836-889,

Index of Subjects

1014, 1869, 1872, 1895, 1973, 1985, 1992
Plants 33, 140, 267, 407,
Poison 1360-1376
Poltices 483
Poorhouses 1946, 1947
Pregnancy 1680-1716, 1780, 1805, 1813, 1827
Psrorophthalmy 1657
Pudendagra 1804
Puerperal fever 964, 1682, 1683, 1689, 1696, 1700, 1705, 1713, 1715
Pulse 300, 1536-1539
Pulse watch 107, 1537
Punch 1486
Purging 457
Purulent eye 1657
Pus 1359
Putrefaction 815
Putrid fever 683, 888, 918, 1147, 1499, 1556

Quick-lime 363, 364
Quicksilver 420, 790

Rabies 1335-1346
Regimen 360, 1489
Resin 157
Respiration 1185-1192
Retina 1631
Rheumatism 82, 539, 579, 587, 1233, 1251, 1258, 1259, 1262, 1268, 1285, 1288-1295
Rickets 1316, 1791
Rupture 816-830

Salivation 390, 504, 1679
Scarlet fever 977-979, 1145
Scrofula 503, 674, 1197-1212, 1233, 1234, 1877
Scurvy 233, 509, 893, 1107, 1490-1505
Sea fever 1847, 1976
Sea scurvy 1382, 1497, 1501, 1505
Sea voyages 435
Sea water 688-695
Seamen 1828-1841, 1842-1867
Seton 832
Sexton's powder 1019
Ship fever 961
Silver 489
Silverweed 1492
Skeleton 290
Skin 1609-1614
Slow fever 928

Small pox 211, 888, 893-1020, 1022, 1027, 1030, 1035, 1039, 1049, 1056, 1058, 1059, 1060, 1064, 1068, 1072, 1073, 1074, 1875, 1972, 1993
Snuff 452
Soap 538
Soft palate 1145
Soldiers 1842-1867
Sore eyes 1626-1646
Sore throat 919, 927, 1145-1151
Spasms 1980
Spectacles 1636
Sphacelus 1378
Spine 1299, 1300, 1794
Spirits 1486, 1509-1514
Spleen 1532-1534
Sponge 795
St. Vitus dance 1324
St. Yves's diseases 1647
Stomach 1434, 1435
Stone 506, 518, 538, 1288, 1379-1403
Struma 1210
Styptic balsam 425, 501, 1570
Suffocation 705, 1185
Sugar 1484, 1486
Suicide 1822
Suppuration 1354-1359
Surgery 34, 35, 41, 66, 105, 121, 137, 207, 215, 281, 299, 319, 418, 461, 710-800, 821, 822, 1807, 1838, 1842, 1849, 1859, 1901, 1965, 1968, 1982
Surgical instruments 752
Sweating 1572
Swelling 1347-1350
Swinging 1181
Symphysis pubis 1704
Syphilis 1116

Tape worm 1520-1524
Tar water 696-702
Tartar 523, 573
Tea 1482, 1486, 1487
Teeth 1666-1678
Temperance 268
Tenia 1520, 1524
Tertian intermittent fever 915
Testicles 831-835
Tetanus 532, 802, 1334
Therapeutics 266, 422, 490
Theriaca 448

Throat distemper 31, 1844
Tobacco 1367, 1486
Tourniquet 1568
Tumor 1462, 1473-1475
Typhus 531, 920

Ulcerated sore throat 919,
   1144
Ulcers 789, 1468-1472
Urethra 1404, 1407, 1408,
   1410, 1415
Urinary concretion 1425
Urinary disease 1404-1417
Urine 794, 1412, 1416
Uterus 332, 1748, 1806,
   1808, 1809, 1819, 1820

Vaccination 1034, 1041,1048
Vagina 1812, 1819
Vapor 684-687, 1532, 1533
Variolus infection 1706
Vegetables 396, 419, 434,
   544, 1376
Veins 300, 324
Velnos' vegetable syrup 521
Venereal disease 390, 509,
   1075-1140, 1234,
   1407
Venom 1375
Ventriculus 326

Vesicae lotura 1406
Viscera 292
Vision 1615-1616, 1620,
   1624, 1627, 1662
Vomits 52, 424

Ward's pill and drop 403
Water 438, 550-709, 1828
Watery eye 1653
Weakness 1573
Weather 31, 1898, 1974, 1990
White swelling 1304, 1305,
   1347, 1469
Whooping cough 1156, 1157,
   1162
Willow bark 458, 536
Wine 1486, 1509, 1510, 1511,
   1512, 1515
Womb 1823
Women 664, 1579, 1804-1827
Work-houses 1837
Worm fever 870
Worms 1520-1524
Wounds 673, 729, 744, 758,
   801-807, 1555, 1605, 1857,
   1864

Yellow fever 980-982, 1971,
   1975
Yellow jaundice 233

Index of Names

Arabic numbers refer to <u>entries</u>; Roman numerals refer to pages

Aberdour, Alexander 983, 1017
Abernethy, John 710
Adair, James Makittrick 1, 2, 3, 4, 360, 1904
Adams, George 361, 1615
Adams, Joseph 1360
Adams, William 1379
Addington, Anthony 1828
Addison, Joseph 75
Aiken, John 5, 1905, 1906, 1931
Aiken, Lucy 1905
Aitken, John 288, 711, 712, 713, 714, 1717
Akenside, Mark 1158, 1347, 1436, 1453
Alanson, Edward 715
Albermarle, Earl of 491
Albinus, Bernhard Siegfried 289, 1546
Alcock, Nathan 1907
Alcock, Thomas 1444, 1907
Alderson, John 890
Alexander, Benjamin 290
Alexander, David 1152
Alexander, William 550
Allen, Benjamin 551, 552, 553
Allen, Charles 1666
Allen, John 6
Alleyne, James 362
Alston, Charles 7, 363, 364

Anacreon 1516
Anderson, James 1971
Anderson, John 365, 688
Andree, John (1699?-1785) 366, 554, 1324
Andree, John (fl.1779-1799) 816, 1075, 1418, 1454
Anne, Queen 48, 106, 394, 491, 808, 811, 1630, 1642, 1829, 1848
Anson, George 1498
Anstis, John the elder 1198
Antes, John 1869
Antrobus, Thomas 716
Apperley, Thomas 9
Arbuthnot, John 10, 1829
Archer, Clement 367
Archer, John 11, 1165
Arkwright, Sir Richard 613
Armstrong, Charles 1076
Armstrong, George 1782, 1783
Armstrong, John 12, 13, 14, 1077, 1784
Arnaud, Jasper 15
Arnold, Thomas 1319, 1320
Arnott, James 717
Artephius 228
Arthy, Elliott 1830
Ash, John 555
Astruc, Jean 1765
Atkins, John 718, 1842
Atkins, William 1228
Atterbury, Francis 1829
Aubrey, Thomas 1831

Austin, William   1380
Averell, John   1540
Awsiter, John   368, 1381
Aylett, George   719
Aymes, John   16
Ayscough, James   1616

Bacon, Francis   234
Bacon, Roger   228
Badger, John   1197
Baillie, Joanna   295
Baillie, Matthew   295
Baker, Sir George   17, 860, 984, 1004, 1361, 1437, 1445
Baker, John   836, 837
Baker, Robert   296
Balfour, Francis   891
Balgrave, John   18
Ball, John   19, 369, 350, 892
Banks, Sir Joseph   1048
Banyer, Henry   371
Barbauld, Anna Letitia   5, 1905
Barclay, John   1525
Barker, John   20, 836, 837
Barker, Sir Robert   1052
Barret, Onsow   1229
Barrow, John   21, 1962
Barrow, Sir John   1847
Barry, Sir Edward   1166, 1353
Barry, John Milner   1021
Barwick, Peter   22, 1020
Basse, H.   23
Bate, George   372, 430
Bateman, Charles   373, 374
Bates, Thomas   1832
Bath, Robert   1419
Batting, John   720
Bayford, Thomas   1404
Baylies, William   556, 557, 985, 1037, 1932, 1972
Baynard, Edward   24
Baynton, Thomas   1468
Beale, Bartholomew   25
Beale, Barton   1541
Becket, James   1078
Becket, John Brice   375
Becket, Thomas   721
Becket, William   722, 723, 1198, 1455
Beddoes, Thomas   26, 27, 376, 377, 522, 893, 1079, 1080, 1159, 1167, 1168, 1190, 1382
Bell, Andrew   289

Bell, Benjamin   724, 831, 1081, 1469
Bell, Sir Charles   297, 725
Bell, George   1456
Bell, John (d.1801)   1843
Bell, John (1763-1820)   297, 298, 801, 1302, 1525
Bellers, John   28, 1933
Bennet, Thomas   1230
Bennet, William   1667
Berdmore, Thomas   1668
Berdoe, Marmaduke   378, 1231, 1804
Bergman, Torbern Olaf   502
Berkeley, Bishop George   696, 697, 698
Berkenhout, John   379, 1232, 1335
Berlu, John Jacob   380
Bernard, Charles   1399
Bernard, Christopher   726
Betts, John   29, 1542
Bevis, John   558
Bickerton, George   30
Bidloo, Godfrey   308
Bischoff, Frederick   1617
Bisset, Charles   31, 1844
Black, William   1870
Blackburn, Thomas   32
Blackmore, Sir Richard   839, 986, 1169, 1233, 1383, 1532
Blackrie, Alexander   1384
Blackwell, Elizabeth   382
Bladud, King   626
Blagrave, Joseph   33
Blair, Patrick   34, 383
Blair, William   1082, 1845, 2047
Blake, John   1028
Blakey, William   817, 818
Blanchard, Stephen   1964
Bland, Robert the elder   1680
Bland, Thomas   1325
Blane, Sir Gilbert   1574, 1833
Blicke, Sir Charles   890
Blizard, Sir William   35, 384, 1543, 1934, 2032
Blondel, James   1701, 1702
Blunt, John   1681, 1740
Boag, William   1438
Bodley, James   36
Boerhaave, Hermann   20, 174, 334, 385, 563, 792, 1007, 1009, 1137, 1273, 1327, 1353, 1546, 1660, 1908
Bolaine, Nathaniel   1029

Index of Names 245

Boles, Katherine 819
Bondeloque, Dr. 1746
Booth, Barton 790
Borthwick, George 840, 1618
Boswell, James 271, 340, 1345
Boulcet, Denis Claude 1715
Boulton, Richard 386, 727, 1234
Bowen, Thomas 1935
Bowes, A.R. 1104
Boyle, Robert 234, 444, 559, 575, 1544
Boyle, William 287
Bracken, Henry 1385, 1718
Bradley, Henry 387, 1871
Bradley, Richard 37, 388, 841
Bradney, Joseph 389
Brady, Samuel 1030
Brand, Robert 820
Brand, Thomas 821, 822
Brest, Vincent 390, 1083
Briggs, William 1619, 1620
Brisbane, John 38
Brocklesby, Richard 39, 391
Bromfield, Sir William 392, 728, 987
Brookes, Richard 40, 41, 393, 1321
Broughton, Arthur 1224
Brown, Charles 1199
Brown, John 42, 43, 1873
Brown, Joseph 44, 45, 394, 560, 582, 842, 1545
Brown, Richard 1084
Brown, Sarah 1805
Browne, Andrew 894, 895
Browne, John 729, 730, 1575, 1576
Brownrigg, William 843
Bruce, Alexander 844
Brudenell, Exton 1719
Bryant, Jacob 1872
Bryce, James 981
Brydges, James, Duke of Chandos 238, 1603
Buchan, Alexander Peter 1085
Buchan, William 46, 395, 665, 1086
Burdon, Henry 47
Burges, James 1031
Burke, Edmund 39, 1345
Burkitt, Thomas 1847
Burnet, Sir Thomas 48

Burney, Charles 1988
Burns, John 1348, 1806
Burrows, John 396, 1457
Burton, John 1720, 1721
Burton, William 1908
Bute, third Earl of 340
Butler, Richard 1562
Butler, Thomas 666
Butter, William 731, 732, 1087, 1156, 1386, 1526, 1682, 1785
Buzaglo, Abraham 1235
Byfield, Timothy 2011, 1012
Byrd, William 845

Cadogan, William 1232, 1236, 1238, 1247, 1249, 1277, 1786
Cadwallader, Jonathan 1237
Cam, Joseph 1088, 1089, 1288, 1679
Caroline, Queen 115
Carr, Richard 49
Carrick, Andrew 562
Carter, William 1238
Case, Henry 1490
Castellus, Bartholomew 1969
Cathcart, Lord William Schaw 703
Catherwood, John 1330
Caverhill, John 1239
Celer, Lypsonius 2014
Celsus, Aulus Cornelius 131
Chalmers, Lionel 896, 1974
Chamberlain, John 50
Chamberlaine, William 1609
Chamberlen, Hugh the elder 51, 52, 1722, 1723
Chamberlen, Paul 397
Chambers, John 398
Champney, Thomas 53, 2016, 2017
Chandler, Benjamin 1032, 1331
Chandler, George 1621, 1622
Chandler, John 399, 398, 1141
Chapman, Edmund 1724, 1725
Chapman, Henry 562, 589
Chapman, Samuel 1090
Charles I 54, 372
Charles II 22, 29, 48, 89, 137, 138, 233, 276, 372, 444, 558, 786, 1373, 1402, 1542, 1575, 1899, 1953, 2029
Charles, Richard 400, 1170
Charleton, Rice 563, 564,

565, 566, 1938
Charleton, Walter   54, 300
Charlotte, Queen   17, 148, 587, 1783, 1848
Charsley, William   897
Cheselden, William   301, 302, 303, 538, 735, 752, 775, 781, 1303, 1387, 1390, 1391, 1394
Cheshire, John   1240, 1289
Chesterfield, Lord   1040, 1322
Cheston, Richard Browne   733
Chevalier, Thomas   2019
Cheyne, George   55, 56, 57, 58, 898, 1241, 1322
Childe, Timothy   488
Chisholm, Colin   899
Chishull, Edmund   1892
Chittick, Dr.   1384
Chomel   1151
Churchill, John, Duke of Marlborough   1533, 1872
Claramont, Charles   567
Clare, Peter   401, 529, 1091, 1092, 1354, 1355
Clark, James   1975
Clark, Thaddeus   802, 977
Clark, William   59, 1726
Clarke, John   1683, 1684
Clarke, Matthew   1787
Clarke, William   402
Claromontius, C.   567
Claxton, Marshall   1715
Cleghorn, George   1977
Clement, Samuel   799
Clericus   1963
Clerke, Sir William Henry   61
Clifton, Francis   62, 63
Clinch, William   1874, 1875
Clossy, Samuel   64
Clough, James   1788
Clubbe, John   1093, 1094, 1727
Clutterbuck, Henry   1095, 1362
Clutton, Joseph   403, 901
Coatsworth, William   404
Cockburn, William   65, 902, 1096, 1447, 1448, 1449, 1450, 1834
Coe, Thomas   1420
Coke, John   1363
Colbatch, Sir John   66, 67, 68, 846
Colborne, Robert   405

Cole, Abdiah   69
Cole, William   903, 1326, 1332
Coleman, Edward   1185
Collignon, Charles   70, 304, 305, 306
Colly, Anthony   406
Colman, Benjamin   1058
Coltheart, Patrick   71
Congreve, William   1829
Connor, Bernard   72
Conyers, Richard   1789
Cook, John   307, 410, 1364, 1790
Cooke, James   734
Cooke, John   1939
Cooper, Sir Astley Paston   1664
Cooper, Thomas   1728, 1729
Cope, Henry   73
Copeland, Thomas   1305
Cordwell, John   74
Cornaro, Luigi (Lewis)   75, 244
Cornwell, Bryan   76
Corp, William   1432
Corrie, James   1547
Cotesworth, Caleb   1000
Cotton, Nathaniel   978
Counsell, George   1730, 1731
Couper, Robert   1685
Coward, William   1623
Cowper, Ashley   77
Cowper, William (1666-1709)   301, 308, 1577
Cowper, William (1731-1800)   448
Cox, Daniel   1033, 1535
Coxe, William   1978
Crane, John   568
Crawford, John   1421
Creaser, Thomas   1034
Cribb, William   1097
Crisp, John   1624
Cromwell, Oliver   372
Croone, William   1578
Crosfield, Robert James   1491
Cross, Francis   904
Crosse, William   1625
Crowther, Bryan   1304
Cruikshank, William   309, 1572, 1591
Crumpe, Samuel   412
Cruso, Johann   78
Cullen, William   43, 79, 80, 81, 82, 703, 1179
Culpeper, Nicolas   18, 69, 413

Index of Names

Cumberland, William Augustus, Duke of 954, 1035, 1857
Cunningham, Timothy 2020
Currie, James 905
Curry, James 704
Curry, John 906, 907
Curteis, Thomas 83
Curtis, Richard 1669
Curtis, Sir Roger 1847
Curtis, William 415
Cutler, Sir Joshua 54

Dalby, Joseph 1336
Dale, Samuel 416
Dalton, Robert 84
Daniel, Samuel 1433
Darwin, Charles 1356
Darwin, Erasmus 1168, 1356
Daventer, Henry 1734
Davidson, Samuel 569, 1876
Davidson, William 1193
Davies, Richard 847, 1548
Davis, Richard 1877
Davis, Walter 2044
Davon, M. 1415
Davy, Sir Humphry 736, 856
Dawkes, Thomas 1735
Dawne, Derby 85
Dawson, Thomas 1290, 1626
Deacon, Henry 1098
Dease, William 737, 1099, 1213, 1598, 1736, 2021
De Castro, Tomasso 570
De Chemant, Daniel 1670
Deering, George Charles 989
Defoe, Daniel 420
Degravere, John 86
De Haven, Dr. 174
De la Crosse, John 2056
Denman, Joseph 571
Denman, Thomas 684, 1686, 168, 1688, 1690, 1737, 1808
Dennis, Thomas 87
Derham, Samuel 572
Desault, Pierre Joseph 801
Descherny, David 908, 990, 1242, 1388
Dewell, Thomas 88
Dick, Sir Alexander 1327
Dickinson, Caleb 909
Dickinson, Edmund 89
Dickinson, Robert 1610
Dickson, David 1691
Dickson, Thomas 1563
Dimsdale, Thomas 1035, 1036, 1037, 1038, 1940
Dionis, Pierre 310
Dixon, Roger 90
Dobson, Matthew 1186
Dodd, William 1040
Dolaeus 1279
Dominicet, Robert 91
Dossie, Robert 417, 418
Doude, M.O. 1825
Douglas, Andrew 1809, 1810
Douglas, G. Archibald 1692
Douglas, George 311, 358, 419
Douglas, James 312, 313, 314, 738, 1377, 1390, 1391, 1579
Douglas, John 315, 735, 739, 823, 833, 1101, 1243, 1391, 1725, 1738
Douglas, William (b.1712), 1693
Douglas, William (d.1752), 1739
Dove, William Taube 573
Dover, Thomas 420, 1871, 1878
Dowman, George 1473
Drake, James 316, 910
Drake, Richard 1244, 1245, 1246
Dray, Thomas 92, 1247
Drummond, Alexander M. 911
Dufour, William 1405
Duncan, Andrew 93, 317, 318, 421, 422, 423, 426, 1102, 1909, 1910, 1942, 2023, 2040
Duncan, William 340
Dunn, Edward 740
Dunning, Richard 1041
Durant, Thomas 1201
Dwight, Samuel 424, 912, 1214

Eales, Mary 1476
Earle, Sir James 741, 1215, 1299, 1357, 1392
Eaton, Robert 425
Eccles, William 1943
Edmonstone, William 1202
Edwards, George 94
Edwards, John 1492
Elliott, Sir John 96, 574, 1627
Ellis, John 2024
Ellis, William 1103
Ellison, Thomas 1847
Else, Joseph 824

Emerson, William 1628
Este, Rev. Charles 98
Etherington, Rev. George 913
Eustachius, Bartholomew 1546
Evelyn, John 1332
Ewart, John 1458
Eyre, Henry 576, 577

Falch, Nathaniel 1223, 1835
Falconer, Magnus 319, 1549
Falconer, William 100, 578, 579, 580, 1816, 1249, 1365, 1868
Falkland, third Earl of 611
Farmer, John 742
Farr, Samuel 102, 103, 1564, 1879
Farrer, William 1791
Fascelius 102
Fearon, Henry Bradshaw 1479
Fermor, William 1022
Fern, Thomas 1203
Ferrier, John 428, 1880
Ferris, Samuel 1477, 2026
Fisher, Joseph 104
Fizes, Matthew 1358
Flammel, Nicholas 228
Fleming, James 1694
Fletcher, Charles 1836
Flower, Henry 1250, 1251
Flowerden, Joseph 105
Floyer, Sir John 106, 107, 108, 581, 582, 669, 1160, 1537
Fontana, Felix 1375
Foot, Jesse 1104, 1337, 1338, 1406, 1407, 1408, 1911
Forbes, Murray 1252, 1409
Ford, Edward 1305
Fordyce, George 109, 914, 915, 916, 1506
Fordyce, John 917
Fordyce, Sir William 743, 918, 919, 1105
Fores, S.W. 1740
Forster, William 110, 1478
Foster, Edward 1741, 1945
Fothergill, Anthony 111, 583, 705
Fothergill, John 112, 850, 1144, 1339, 1881, 1912, 1916, 1922, 1977

Fowle, William 991
Fowler, Thomas 114, 1366, 1367, 1565
Fox, Edward 429
Franklin, Benjamin 160, 449, 843
Franklin, Richard 992
Franks, John 920
Fraser, Thomas 1042
Frederick I of Prussia 985, 1440
Free, John 320
Freeman, Samuel 1882
Freind, John 115, 116, 599, 902, 1016, 1030, 1883, 1903
Freke, John 117
Frewen, Thomas 993, 1043, 1069, 1070
Fuller, Francis 1479
Fyfe, Andrew 321, 322, 1306

Galen 20, 1883
Gardiner, John (fl.1700-1705), 1550
Gardiner, John (fl.1771-1804), 1253
Garlick, Thomas 1253a
Garnett, Thomas 119, 584, 585, 586
Garrick, David 140
Garth, Sir Samuel 66
Garthshore, Maxwell 1695
Gataker, Thomas 120, 433, 752, 852, 1629
Gay, John 1829
Geach, Francis 121, 1439
Geber, Dr. 228
Gem, Richard 1393
Geoffrey, Francis 434
Geoffroy, Claude 1393
George I 169, 1630, 1646
George II 234, 775
George III 17, 35, 280, 295, 351, 361, 392, 686, 1440, 1956
George IV 1664
George, Prince of Denmark 491
Ghyles, Thomas 1254
Gibbes, Sir George Smith 587
Gibbs, John 1204
Gibson, Edmund 853
Gibson, John 922, 1422
Gibson, Thomas 323
Giffard, William 1742
Gilchrist, Ebenezer 435, 1323

Index to Names   249

Gillespie, Leonard 1979
Girdleston, Thomas 1516, 1980
Glass, Samuel 436
Glass, Thomas 436, 923, 994, 1884
Glisson, Francis 324, 325, 326
Gloucester, William, Duke of 491, 808
Godbold, Nathaniel 1171
Goddard, Jonathan 122
Godfrey, C.B. 1106
Godfrey, Robert 123
Goldsmith, Oliver 446, 936, 1345
Goldson, William 1812
Gooch, Benjamin 744
Good, John Mason 1885, 1946
Goodall, Charles 1886
Goodwyn, Edmund 1187
Gordon, Alexander 1696
Gordon, Duke of 1685
Gordon, George Alexander 124
Goulard, Thomas 437
Gower, Richard 1792
Graeme, William 125
Graham, James 126, 438, 439, 440, 588
Grainger, James 924, 1981
Grant, Alexander 441
Grant, Roger 1630
Grant, William 854, 925, 926, 927, 1227, 1255
Gravere, Julius de 442
Graves, Robert 443
Greatrakes, Valentine 444
Greenfield, Jan 2014
Greenhill, Thomas 814
Gregory, James 127, 128
Gregory, John 129, 130, 2027
Grey, William de 1256
Grieve, James 131
Griffith, Richard 1566
Grigg, John 1813
Grimston, Henry 1947
Groenevelt, Jan 2014
Grosvenor, Benjamin 132
Guidott, Thomas 589, 590, 591, 592, 611
Gunning, Richard 2028
Guy, Melmoth 1460
Guy, Richard 1461, 1462, 1463
Gwynne, Nell 588

Hales, Rev. Dr. Stephen 698, 701, 1837
Hall, Charles 133
Hall, John 650
Haller, Albrecht von 174, 312, 1440
Hamey, Baldwin the younger 134
Hamilton, Sir David 1848
Hamilton, James 1743. 1744
Hamilton, Robert 1226, 1340, 1849
Hancocke, William 670
Handley, James 745, 855
Hannes, Sir Richard 808
Hanslins, Johann Georg 135
Hardy, James 1271
Harle, Jonathan 1887
Harris, John (bookseller) 2056
Harris, John (physician) 136
Harris, Thomas 445
Harris, Walter 137, 1784, 1793
Harrison, John 1982
Harrison, Thomas 1349
Harvey, Gideon the elder 138, 2029
Harvey, James 139
Harvey, William 22, 300, 333, 1900, 1905
Harvie, John 1697, 1745
Harwood, Sir Busick 327, 328
Harwood, Edward 1318
Hauksbee, Francis 1139
Havers, Clopton 1307
Hawes, William 446
Hawkbridge, John 929
Hawkesworth, John 140
Hawksmoor, Nicholas 1939
Haworth, Samuel 329, 593, 1172
Hay, Alexander 447
Hayes, Thomas 1142
Haygarth, John 995, 996
Hayman, John 1493
Heath, John 1746
Hebrden, William the elder 448
Heister, Lorenz 281
Heming, John 594
Henderson, William 856
Hendley, William 857
Hendy, James 1983, 1995
Henly, Thomas 1747
Hennicken, Gottfried 264
Henning, James 886

Henry, Thomas   449
Hermes   228
Hewson, William   1549, 1551
Hezekiah   1891
Hey, William   1552
Heysham, John   930
Higgs, Joseph   1107
Hill, Aaron   450
Hill, Daniel   451
Hill, James   746
Hill, Sir John   140, 452
Hill, Oliver   1553
Hillary, William   151, 595, 997, 1984
Hippocrates   20, 1873, 1879, 1897
Hird, William   858, 1912
Hoadley, Benjamin the younger   1188
Hobart, Thomas   1326
Hodges, Nathaniel   142, 849
Hody, Edward   1742, 2030
Hoffman, Friedrich   339
Holland, Richard   988, 998
Holliday, John   982
Holwell, John Zephaniah   999
Home, Sir Everard   1359, 1410, 1471, 1554, 1580, 1631, 1665
Home, Francis   143, 144, 145, 596, 1153
Hook, Andrew   146
Hooper, Joseph   147
Hooper, Robert   330, 331, 1965
Hope, John   1910
Hopson, Charles Rivington   1440
Horn, George   1567
Horsburgh, William   597
Houlston, Thomas   1368
Houlston, William   1108
Houlton, Robert   1045
Houstoun, Robert   819, 825, 1394
Howard, John (1726-1790)   1948
Howard, John (d.1811)   453, 832, 1109, 1464
Howgrave, Francis   1046
Huck, Richard   684
Huggenson, John   931
Hughes, Thomas   558
Hull, John   1698, 1709, 1814
Humpage, Benjamin   826
Hungerford, Francis   1566
Hunter, Alexander   598, 1868

Hunter, John (1728-1793)   ix, 5, 199, 766, 801, 1048, 1053, 1095, 1104, 1110, 1359, 1416, 1471, 1551, 1555, 1671, 1672, 1911, 1956
Hunter, John (d.1809)   1850
Hunter, William   ix, 102, 148, 295, 309, 332, 333, 339, 1104, 1110, 1313, 1551, 1683, 1704, 1748, 1768
Hurlock, Joseph   1673
Hussey, Garret   932
Hutchinson, Benjamin   1913
Huxham, John   334, 860, 913, 1145

Ingram, Dale   454, 747, 1257, 1985
Innes, James Dunbar   1111
Innes, John   335, 1581
Ireton, John   336
Irving, Ralph   426, 455, 456, 533
Ixford, Noah   457

Jackson, Alexander   1009, 1308
Jackson, Joseph   150
Jackson, Robert   934, 935
Jackson, Rowland   707
Jackson, Seguin Henry   1611
Jackson, William   1309
James, Lewis   151
James, Robert   446, 537, 936, 1258, 1292, 1341, 1342, 1441, 1888, 1914, 1966
James, Samuel   458
Jay, Sir James   1259
Jay, John   1259
Jeans, Thomas   1260
Jebb, John   1293
Jehoram   1891
Jenner, Edward   ix, 996, 1023, 1026, 1048, 1058, 1073
Jervey, William   1494
Jewel, Edward   1434
Job   1891
Johnson, Alexander   1986
Johnson, James   152
Johnson, Michael   106, 108
Johnson, Robert Wallace   1749
Johnson, Samuel   39, 106, 224, 235, 448, 799, 1010, 1040, 1158, 1345, 1584, 1648, 1888, 2024
Johnston, Alexander   708
Johnstone, James   861, 1592
Jones, John   154

Index of Names

Jones, John Gale 1157
Jones, Philip 1794
Jones, Richard 229
Jones, Robert 155, 937
Jones, Thomas 1815
Jurin, James 803, 1000, 1049
Justamond, John Obadiah 748, 833, 1465

Kalid 228
Keate, Thomas 834
Keill, James 337
Kellie, George 1568
Kelson, Thomas M. 1143
Kemp, William 862
Kennedy, Peter (of Anglesbury) 938
Kennedy, Peter (fl.1710-1738) 459, 863, 1632
Kentish, Edward 1612, 1613
Kentish, Richard 460, 689, 1261
Kephale, Richard 864
Kettilby, Mary 461
Key, George 1112
King, John 599
Kinneir, David 1593
Kirkland, Thomas 749, 939, 940, 950
Kirkpatrick, James (d.1743) 153, 1395
Kirkpatrick, James (d.1770) 815, 1050
Kirwan, Richard 600
Kite, Charles 157, 1189
Knight, Thomas 462, 463, 1556, 1557
Krohn, Henry 1699

Lampard, John 1001
Landford, William 1509
Langrish, Browne 159, 1002, 1582, 1583
Langton, William 1051
Lara, Benjamin 750
Latham, John 1262
Latta, James 751
Lauth, Herr Dr. 891
Lawrence, Thomas 1584
Layard, Daniel Peter 464, 601, 1343
Leake, John 1700, 1750, 1816
Le Dran, Philippe 752
Lee, Samuel 1949
Leeds, Duke of 45
Le Fevre, Dr. 1263

Leigh, Charles 602
Leman, Sir Tenfield 1915
Lempriere, William 1851
Leonardo da Vinci 333
Leslie, Peter Dugud 1227
Lessius, L. 244
Lettsom, John Coakley 160, 809, 941, 1036, 1052, 1451, 1795, 1889, 1916, 1950
Levison, George 1146, 1558
Lewis, Merer 1674
Lewis, Polydore 671
Lewis, William 161, 426, 465, 466
Lind, James (1716-1794) 942, 1495, 1852, 1987
Lind, James (1736-1812) 1988
Linden, Diedrick Wessel 603, 604
Linnaeus, Carl 502, 1921
Lipscomb, George 943, 1161
Lister, Martin 605
Littleton, Adam 134
Litton, Edmund 162
Lobb, Rev. Stephen 163
Louis XV 1765
Lower, Richard 338, 356
Lowndes, Francis 467, 468
Lowther, William 1216
Lubbock, Richard 1496
Lucas, Charles 603, 606, 607, 637, 638, 672
Lucas, James 2031
Luxmore, William 1217
Lynch, Barnard 166
Lynn, Walter 1003, 1004
Lynn, William 1005
Lyons, John 865
Lyser, Michael 810
Lysons, Daniel 608, 946, 947
Lywythlan, Evan David 1053

Macaulay, Thomas Babington 235
MacBeth, William 1510
MacBride, David 167, 1497
Mackenzie, James 1006, 1890
Mackie, John 1333
Maclean, Hector 1853
Maclurin, Robert 35
Macpherson, Robert 709
Madan, Patrick
Maddocks, James 2032
Magenise, Daniel 1350
Magennis, James 469
Magentus 1963
Maillard, Nathaniel 1294

Maitland, Charles 1007
Manning, Henry 168, 753, 1817
Manning, James 1480
Manning, Martin 610
Manningham, Sir Richard 169, 866, 867, 948, 1751
Mansfield, Lord Chief Justice 255
Mantell, Sir Thomas 1796
Maplet, John 611
Markham, Peter 1481
Marrett, Christopher 170, 2033
Marryat, Thomas 171
Marshall, Andrew 1125
Marshall, Rev. Edmund 1263
Marten, Benjamin 1173
Marten, John 172, 1264
Martin, Charles 173, 1265
Martin, John 1129
Martine, George the younger 174
Mary, Queen 491, 811
Mason, Henrich 754, 1527
Mason, Simon 175, 949, 1482
Massey, Edmund 1054
Massey, Isaac 1055
Mather, Cotton 1056
Mather, John 1606
Mathews, Stephen 1989
Maty, Matthew 1917
Mauclerc, John Henry 1633, 1701, 1702
Maule, John 1939
Mauricenus 1722
Mawbray, John 1752, 1818
Maxwell, Archibald 939, 940, 950
May, Nicholas the younger 1057
May, William 868, 1174
Mayow, John 1190
Maywood, Robert 470
McClurg, James 1423
Mead, Richard 115, 176, 177, 178, 179, 180, 210, 490, 842, 849, 869, 873, 954, 1008, 1010, 1370, 1498, 1577, 1888, 1891, 1892, 1915, 1917, 1997
Meadow, Thomas 181
Mears, Martha 1753
Mease, James 1344
Medley, John 613
Meighan, Sir Christopher 614, 673

Memis, John 1754
Menzies, Robert, 1191, 1192
Meyrick, William 471
Middleton, Conyers 1893
Middleton, John 755
Mihlis, Samuel 185, 756
Millar, John 186, 1162, 1951
Milligen, George 1990
Millington, Sir Thomas 810
Millward, John 1847
Milman, Sir Francis 1218, 1499
Misiastrus, Philander 1267
Moeller, J.G. 31
Monchy, Salomon de 1991
Moncreiff, John 615
Monk, Francis 472
Monro, Alexander the elder ix, 616, 1009, 1309, 1909
Monro, Alexander secundus ix, 339, 1581, 1634
Monro, Donald 473, 617, 1854, 1855, 1993
Monro, George 1424
Monro, Hugh 757
Monsey, Dr. 1920
Montagu, John, Duke of 1969
Montagu, Lady Mary Wortley 1058
Montagu, Ralph 1619
Mooney, Matthew 1113, 1268
Moore, James Carrick 474, 758, 759
Moore, Thomas 906
Moore, William 1755
Morand, Sauveur 1393
Morgagni, Giovanni Battista 290
Morgan, Thomas 188, 189
Morland, John 190
Morland, Joseph 1528
Morley, John 1205
Mortimore, Cromwell 191
Moseley, Benjamin 1441, 1483, 1484
Moses 1765, 1890
Moss, William 192, 1797
Motherby, George 1967
Moyle, John 760, 761
Mudge, John 1010, 1155
Murphy, Arthur 1104
Murray, William, first Earl Mansfield 255
Musgrave, Samuel 1594
Musgrave, William 1296, 1297
Mynors, Robert 762, 1599

Neal, Daniel 1058

Index of Names   253

Neal, George   763, 1569
Neale, Henry St. John
    1175, 1595
Neale, Thomas   1114
Nebuchadnezzar   1891
Nelson, Gilbert   1269
Nesbitt, Robert   1310
Nessel, Edmund   618
Nettleton, Thomas   1059
Nevett, Thomas   193, 1176
Nevill, James   1115
Newman, Jeremiah Whitaker
    194
Newton, Sir Isaac   1620,
    1646
Nicholls, William   619
Nichols, Frank   340, 1584
Nicholson, James Francis
    1116
Nihell, James   1538
Nisbet, William   195, 478,
    764, 1117, 1206, 1757,
    1798
Noble, Edward Moore   1635
Nolan, William   1955
Norford, William   1466
Norman, John   1118
Norris, Thomas   479
Northcote, William   342,
    480, 1838, 1894
Norton, John   481
Nott, John   620
Nourse, Edward   343
Nugent, Christopher   1345
Nutt, John   2045

O'Connell, Maurice   196
Ogle, William   1474
O'Halloran, Sylvester   1378,
    1600, 1637
Okes, Thomas   198
Oliver, William (1658-1716)
    621
Oliver, William (1695-1764)
    565, 676
O'Ryan, Michael   482, 1177
Osborne, William   1704,
    1758
Ould, Sir Fielding   1759,
    1774
Owen, William   622

Packe, Christopher   1194
Park, Henry   1311
Parker, Henry   765
Parker, Samuel   2035
Parker, Thomas   951
Parkinson, James   199, 1956

Parry, Caleb Hillier   1048,
    1601
Parsons, James   1411, 1585,
    1705
Parsons, John   1919
Paterson, David   1500
Patterson, William   1219
Paul of Venice   300
Paxton, Peter   200, 201, 202
Payne, Thomas   483
Paytherus, Thomas   1024
Peacock, Henry Barry   1638
Pierce, Zachariah, Bishop of
    Rochester   497
Pearson, George   623, 1025,
    1425, 1518, 1706
Pearson, John   766, 1119,
    1467
Pearson, Richard   203, 484,
    1346, 1426
Peart, Edward   344, 485
Penn, William   1344, 1933
Penrose, Francis   486, 1147
Pepys, Samuel   516
Percival, Thomas   204, 677,
    1061, 1371
Perfect, William   1756
Perkins, Benjamin Douglas
    767, 768
Perkins, Elisha   767
Perkins, William Lee   1148
Perry, Charles   205, 557,
    624, 1396
Perry, Sampson   1397
Pete, Charles   1120
Philander, Eugenius   217, 625
Philips, George   1270
Phillips, Daniel   1011
Phipps, Jonathan W.   1639
Pierce, Robert   626
Pitcairn, Archibald   55, 952,
    1435
Pitcairne, Omelius   1398
Pitt, Robert   206, 488, 2015
Pittis, William   1918
Playfair, James   685
Plot, Robert   627
Pole, Thomas   345, 1761, 1819
Poole, Richard   953
Pope, Alexander   10, 176,
    1829
Pordage, Samuel   276
Portal, Paul   1762
Porterfield, William   1640
Pott, Percival   741, 770,
    771, 827, 828, 1220, 1311,
    1602, 1641
Pouzaire, M.   629

Powell, Richard 1427
Pratt, Edward 217, 628, 772
Prestwich, John 1372
Price, James 489
Price, Philip Parry 208
Priestley, Joseph 449
Priestley, Robert 1428
Pringle, John 872
Pringle, Sir John 872, 954, 1856
Prior, Thomas 698, 699
Profily, John 1121
Prosser, Thomas 209, 1298
Pugh, Benjamin 629, 1763
Pugh, John 346, 1586
Pugh, Robert 630
Purcell, John 1446
Pye, George 873
Pye, Samuel 774

Quier, John 1993
Quin, Charles William 1219, 1221
Quincy, John 210, 211, 212, 213, 490, 874, 1895, 1968
Quinton, John 214, 215, 631, 632, 678, 955

Radcliffe, John 441, 492, 1918
Rainey, John 875
Ramesay, William 1373, 1522
Ranby, John 775, 803, 804, 1857, 1896
Rand, Isaac 493, 494
Randolph, George 633, 634
Rattray, Sylvester 216, 805
Rawlins, Richard 1707
Read, Sir William 1642
Redmond, William 347
Rees, Rev. Abraham 1680
Reeve, Thomas 700, 1149
Reid, Alexander (1586?-1641) 776
Reid, Alexander (fl.1765-1780) 1412
Reid, Andrew 701
Reid, Thomas 690, 1179, 1195
Reide, Thomas Dickson 1858
Relph, John 495
Renny, George 1122
Renwick, William 1859, 1860

Reynolds, Sir Joshua 1010
Reynolds, Thomas 497
Rhodes, Henry 2056
Richardson, Alexander M. 956
Richardson, Samuel 55
Richter, August Gottlieb 249
Riddel, John 957
Ridley, Humphrey 348
Rigby, Edward the elder 498, 1820
Riollay, Francis 958, 1271, 1897
Ripley, George 228
Ritchie, David 1608
Ritson, John 1764
Riverius, Lazarus 217
Roberdes, John 218
Roberts, Daniel 1207
Roberts, John 959
Robertson, Joseph 1374
Robertson, Robert 960, 961, 1994
Robinson, Bryan 499, 1062, 1485
Robinson, Lewis 219
Robinson, Nicholas 220, 221, 500, 1123, 1178, 1272, 1399, 1533
Rodney, George 1574
Roe, Charles 1012
Rogers, John 1273
Rogers, Joseph 876
Rollo, John 1442, 1518, 1519, 1861, 1995, 1996
Rose, Phillip 501, 877
Rosewell, Thomas 878
Rosset, Francis 735
Rotherham, John 426, 502, 679
Rowley, William 222, 223, 349, 503, 504, 962, 1124, 1274, 1351, 1472, 1643, 1644, 1645, 1821, 1822, 1862
Rumball, John 1539
Rush, Benjamin 42
Rushworth, John 505, 577, 778
Ruspini, Bartholomew 1570, 1675
Russell, Alexander 224, 879, 1881
Russell, James 1312
Russell, Patrick 879
Russell, Richard 691, 1352
Russell, William 225
Ruston, Thomas 1063
Rutty, John 226, 506, 507,

606, 635, 636, 637, 638, 1898
Rutty, William   1413
Ruysch, Frederick   1546
Ryan, Michael   508, 1163, 1179
Ryley, Samuel   1765
Rymer, James   692, 779, 1863, 1864

Saffray, Henry   509
Salmon, William   227, 228, 229, 350, 372, 780, 1899
Samber, Robert   880
Samson, William   230
Sanctorius, Sanctorio   174, 212
Sanden, Thomas   1295
Sandford, William   1512
Saul   1891
Saunders, Richard   231
Saunders, Robert   1150
Saunders, William   232, 510, 639, 1400, 1429
Sawrey, Solomon   1125
Scott, John   1275, 1276
Scott, Sir Walter   295
Scott, William   1208
Scribble, Timothy   77
Scrippius   2001
Sedgwick, James   1513, 1514
See, Thomas   511
Selkirk, Alexander   420
Sermon, William   233
Seymour, Thomas   512
Shannon, Robert   513
Sharp, Jane   1766, 1767
Sharp, Samuel   781, 782
Sharp, Thomas   1559, 1560
Sharp, William   1313
Shaw, Peter   234, 640, 641, 2048
Shaw, William   1401
Shebbeare, John   235, 642
Sheldon, John   1314
Sheldrake, Timothy the younger   1300, 1315
Shelley, Percy Bysshe   1988
Sherley, Thomas   1402
Sherwen, John   1414, 1501
Shirley, John   783
Short, Thomas   514, 643, 644, 645, 680, 1486, 1487
Sibly, Ebenezer   236, 1708
Sigault, Jean   1704
Simmons, Samuel Foart   351, 1126, 1180, 1524, 2046, 2049
Simmons, William   1709, 1710, 1711
Simpson, William   881, 963
Sims, James (1741-1820)   237, 882
Sims, James (d.1831)   1741
Simson, Thomas   238, 239, 1603, 1823
Sinclair, Sir John   918
Sintelaer, John   1127
Skeete, Thomas   515
Skinner, Joseph   1375
Slare, Frederick   516
Slaughter, Henricus   964
Sloane, Sir Hans   ix, 28, 62, 382, 424, 790, 1533, 1646, 1908, 1933
Small, Alexander   790
Smellie, William the elder   ix, 51, 240, 1693, 1721, 1722, 1756, 1768, 1769, 1770, 1771, 1772
Smellie, William the younger   240
Smith, Brabazon   241
Smith, Daniel   1277, 1278
Smith, George   784
Smith, Hugh (1736-1789)   242, 646, 1596, 1824
Smith, Hugh (d.1790)   243, 1571
Smith, John (1630-1669)   1900
Smith, John (1648?-?)   681
Smith, Joseph   647
Smith, Timothy   244
Smith, William   245, 246, 247
Smollett, Tobias George   682, 1768
Smyth, James Carmichael   686, 883, 1181, 1328
Smythson, Hugh   248
Soame, John   648
Sobieski, John   72
Solomon   1900
Some, David   1013
Southwell, Thomas   1773
Spaher, Dr.   336
Sparham, Legard   1064
Speed, John   693
Spence, David   1774
Spens, Thomas   249
Spilsbury, Francis B.   250, 1128, 1502, 1503, 1676
Spinke, John   1129, 1130
Spire, John   517
Sprackling, Robert   251
Sprengell, Sir Conrad   252

Squirrel, Robert 253, 1507
Stack, Richard William 254
Stanger, Christopher 255, 2036, 2037
Stark, Dr. Thomas 178
Stark, Rev. Thomas 1416
Ste. Marthe, Scevele de 1800
Stedman, John 352
Steevens, Griselda 1958
Steevens, Richard 1958
Stephens, Joanna 506, 518, 1395
Stephens, John 1182
Stephens, William 1279
Stephenson, David 256
Stern, Philip 1183
Sterne, Laurence 169, 1720
Stevens, J.N. 649, 965, 1604
Stewart, Alexander (fl.1740-1745) 257
Stewart, Alexander (fl.1785-1795) 1608
Stock, Rev. Thomas 1416
Stockton, John 1647
Stone, Sarah 1775
Storck, Anthony 519
Stover, Dietrich Heinrich 1921
Strathmore, Countess of 1104
Strother, Edward 258, 520, 884, 1014
Stuart, Alexander (1673-1742) 1587, 1588
Stuart, Alexander (fl.1702-1740) 785
Stubbs, Henry 650
Stukeley, William 1280, 1534
Sudel, Nicholas 966
Sugrue, Charles 1192
Sury, William 1316
Sutherland, Alexander 259, 603, 607, 651, 652
Sutton, Daniel 1065, 1066
Sutton, Samuel 1839
Sutton, Thomas 1184
Swainson, Isaac 521, 522
Swift, Jonathan 10, 499, 1829, 2045
Sydenham, Thomas 20, 101a, 137, 234, 1278
Symons, John 687

Talbor, Sir Robert 967, 968
Tanner, John 260
Taube, William Dove 523
Tauvry, Daniel 353, 524
Taylor, John the elder 1648, 1649, 1650, 1651, 1652
Temple, Richard 261
Templeman, Peter 1901
Tennent, John 1997
Theobald, John 263, 525
Thicknesse, Philip 1776
Thomas, Robert 264
Thomas, William 1131
Thompson, Gilbert 1922
Thompson, John Weeks 526
Thompson, Thomas 1015, 1281, 1777
Thomson, Frederick 1504
Thomson, George (fl.1648-1679) 885
Thomson, George (fl.1734-1740) 354, 812
Thrale, Hester Lynch 1584
"Three-Fingered Jack" 1484
Threlfal, William 1329
Thurlow, Edward 100
Tickell, William 527
Tissot, Simon Andre (Andrew) 101a, 156, 273
Tofts, Mary 1579
Tolver, Alexander 1677, 1998
Tomkins, Thomas 1415
Tomlinson, Francis 786
Tomlinson, George 1710, 1711
Tonstall, George 694
Torrano, Nicholas 1151, 1778
Touche, Henri Bernard de la 1403
Toulmin, George Haggart 265
Tower, Daniel 1702
Towne, Richard 1999
Townsend, Joseph 266
Trapham, Thomas 2000
Trinder, Rev. William Martin 528, 653, 654
Trismegistus 228
Trotter, Thomas 1505, 1840
Trye, Charles Brandon 1416, 1712
Tryer, Mary 1825
Turnbull, William 529, 829, 1133
Turner, Daniel 787, 788
Turner, George 2001
Turner, Robert 267, 1826
Turton, William 1970
Tweedie, James 268
Tytler, Henry William 1800

Index of Names   257

Umfreville, Edward   813
Underwood, Michael   789,
    1793, 1801, 1802

Valangin, Francis de   1488
Van der Gucht, Gerard   302
Vanhomrigh, Esther   499
Vaughan, John   1824
Vaughan, Walter   355, 530
Vaughan, William   970
Victor, Benjamin   790
Vivignis, Pierre de   1282
Voltaire   262

Wade, John Peter   1865,
    2002, 2003
Wagstaffe, William   1016,
    1030, 1072
Wainewright, Jeremiah   1430
Walker, John   1529
Walker, Joshua   655
Walker, Richard   1902
Walker, Robert   1017
Walker, Sayer   1597
Wall, Cecil   2038
Wall, John   656
Wall, Martin   531
Wall, William   1134
Wallace, Johnson Robert
    1779
Wallis, George   269, 1283,
    1827, 1967
Walpole, Horace   1648
Walsh, Philip Pitt   1713
Walwyn, William   270, 272
Warburton, William   448
Ward, Joshua   403
Ware, James   1653, 1654,
    1655, 1656, 1657, 1658
Warner, Ferdinando   1284
Warner, Joseph   791, 835,
    1659
Warren, George   1135
Warren, Henry   2004
Warren, Martin   971
Wastell, Henry   1136
Wathen, Jonathan   792, 1137,
    1138, 1660 1661
Watkinson, John   1067
Watson, Henry   1313
Watson, Sir William   532,
    1018, 1068, 1334
Watt, James   377
Watts, Giles   1053, 1069,
    1070, 1071, 1714
Webster, Charles   271, 426,
    533, 1435
Weldon, Walter   793, 794

Wellis, Benjamin   1317
Wells, William Charles   1662
Welwyn, William   272
Wemyss, William   1663
Wenzel, M. de   1658
Werenfels, Samuel   1209
Wesley, Charles   1715
Wesley, John   226, 273, 274,
    334, 1715
Whateley, Thomas   806
Wheler, John   1019
White, Charles   795, 796,
    1780, 1866
White, John   972
White, Richard   973
White, Robert   535, 695, 797
White, Thomas   1210
White, William (of Bath)   536
White, William (of York)
    537, 1196, 1931
Whitehead, John   1715
Whyte, William Peter   1285
Whytt, Robert   538, 1222
Wigan, John   116, 974, 1883
Wilkes, Richard   1223
Wilkinson, Charles Hunnings
    539, 540
Wilkinson, John   1841
Willan, Robert (fl.1746-1757)
    1211
Willan, Robert (fl.1757-1812)
    657, 1614
William III   137, 491, 811
Williams, John   658, 659,
    1278, 1286, 2005, 2006,
    2007
Williams Perrott   1072
Williams, William Henry   1867
Willich, A.F.M.   660, 1489
Willis, Francis   275
Willis, Thomas   276, 277,
    356, 357, 541, 886
Wilmer, Bradford   798, 830,
    1376
Wilmot, John, Earl of
    Rochester   276
Wilson, Andrew   278, 683,
    1443, 1452, 1561, 1803
Wilson, Edmund   661
Wilson, Gabriel   278
Wilson, James   1530
Wilson-Philip, Alexander
    Philip   542, 975, 1417,
    1508
Winslow, James Benigus   358
Winter, George   279
Wintringham, Clifton the
    elder   280, 887, 888, 889

1903
Wintringham, Clifton the younger 280
Wintringham, William 280
Wirgman, George 281
Wise, Richard 2008
Wiseman, Richard 799, 807
Withering, William 543, 544, 979, 1159
Withers, Philip 1212
Withers, Thomas 282, 283, 976, 1164, 1573, 2039
Wolveridge, James 1781
Wood, Loftus 545
Wood, Samuel 1287
Wood, William 1531
Woodman, Philip 284
Woodville, William 1026, 1073, 1074
Woodward, John 211, 1020
Woofendale, Robert 1678

Woolcombe, William 1716
Worthington, James 662
Worthington, Rev. Richard 1301
Wren, Sir Christopher 356, 1939, 1953
Wright, John 1515
Wright, Thomas 1589
Wright, William 546
Wurguis 754
Wynel, John 1140
Wynter, John 663, 664

Yarwood, John 285
Young, George 547
Young, James 286, 548, 549, 800, 1605
Ypey, Adolphus 1590
Y-Worth, William 287

Zeiher, Johann Christian 672
Zimmermann, Johann Georg 1440

About the Compiler

SAMUEL J. ROGAL is chair of the Division of Humanities and Fine Arts at Illinois Valley Community College. He is the author/compiler of several books, including most recently *A General Introduction to Hymnody and Congregational Song* (1991), *Calendar of Literary Facts* (1990), and *A Chronological Outline of American Literature* (Greenwood Press, 1987).